THE Women'sHealth

BIG BOOK of

15 MINUTE WORKOUTS

RODALE

© 2011 by Rodale Inc.

All rights reserved. No part of this publication may be reproduced or transmitted in any form or by any means, electronic or mechanical, including photocopying, recording, or any other information storage and retrieval system, without the written permission of the publisher.

Rodale books may be purchased for business or promotional use or for special sales. For information, please write to: Special Markets Department, Rodale Inc., 733 3rd Ave, New York, NY 10017

Women's Health is a registered trademark of Rodale Inc.

Printed in China
Rodale Inc. makes every effort to use acid-free ⊛, recycled paper ❂.

Book design by Elizabeth Neal
With George Karabotsos, design director of *Men's Health* and *Women's Health* Books

Photo editor: Mark Haddad

All photography by Beth Bischoff

Cover Stylist: Kathy Kalafut
Cover Hairstylist: Giovanni Giuntoli at Maxine Tall Management for Redken
Cover Makeup: Lynn LaMorte

Library of Congress Cataloging-in-Publication Data is on file with the publisher.

ISBN- trade 13:978-1-60961-737-0
ISBN- direct 13:978-1-60961-801-8

Trade paperback and direct mail hardcover editions published simultaneously in September 2011.

Distributed to the book trade by Macmillan

10   9   paperback

2   4   6   8   10   9   7   5   3   hardcover

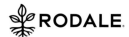

We inspire and enable people to improve their lives and the world around them.
www.rodalebooks.com

Contents

Acknowledgments

It takes a small army to create a big book. And this Big Book was no exception. I can't possibly give sufficient thanks to all those who helped move this project from a simple idea to a big, thick book filled to the brim with really cool, superfast workouts. But I'll try, first by sharing my appreciation for *Women's Health* magazine Editor Michelle Promaulayko and Editorial Director David Zinczenko and the entire *Women's Health* staff for creating such a successful brand that inspires women to live healthier lives. It's my hope that this book helps to forward that mission.

My heartfelt thanks go to editor Jeff Csatari for the opportunity to execute this idea and his calm, unflappable guidance from start to finish.

Stephen Perrine and the entire *Women's Health* Books team, including Ruth Konigsberg for her insightful editing, Debbie McHugh, Ursula Cary, and Erin Williams for catching my mistakes.

Book group Design Director George Karabotsos, and the talented designer on this book, Elizabeth Neal.

Photographer Beth Bischoff for the beautiful chapter openers and workout pictures, assistants Geoffrey Goodbridge and Estaban Aladro, and models Elaine Kwon, Johanna Sambucini, Rebecca Kennedy, Valerie Wong, and Sara Otey for holding those poses so long.

Executive Vice President and Publisher Karen Rinaldi, Chris Krogermeier, Sara Cox, and everyone else at Rodale Books who were so enthusiastic and helpful.

For sharing their invaluable expertise in health, fitness, and nutrition, I thank Sean Armstead; Craig Ballantyne, CSCS; Joan Salge Blake, RD; Traver Boehm; Kurt Brett; Mike Brungardt; Jay Cardiello; Michael A. Clark, DPT; Hannah Davis; Amy Dixon; Gregory Florez; Martin Gibala, PhD; Tony Gentilcore; Bill Hartman, PT, CSCS; Carter Hays; Tom Holland; Katrina Hodgson; William Kraemer, PhD; Christopher Knight, PhD; Jim Liston, CSCS; Ashley Ntansah; Scott Mazzetti, PhD; Mike Mejia, MS, CSCS; Scott H. Mendelson; C.J. Murphy; Stuart Phillips, PhD; Wayne Phillips, PhD; Lauren Piskin; Carrie Rezabek; Craig Rasmussen, CSCS; David Raye; Robert dos Remedios, CSCS; Juan Carlos Santana, CSCS; Jonas Sahratian; Jyotsna Sahni, MD; Michelle M. Seibel, MD; Tina Schmidt-McNulty; Tara Stiles; Patrick Striet, CSCS; Jason Talanian, PhD; Mark Verstegen; Diane Vives; Wayne Westcott, PhD, CSCS; Jordan Yuam, NCEP; Valerie Waters; and Victoria Zdrok, PhD.

And of course, my family. Dave, none of this happens without your undying support; daughter Juniper for hugs and smiles, and Mom and Dad for always lending a helping hand. Thank you.

— Selene Yeager

Introduction:
The 15-Minute Secret

Why a Quarter of an Hour Is All You Need to Lose Weight, Tone Every Inch, and Finally Get the Body You Want.

I

don't have the time. Does that sentence sound familiar? We bet it does. Hands down, it's the number one reason, in survey after survey, that women give for why they can't exercise. And it's true: we are hard-pressed for time. Between work and family commitments and trying to have a social life, there never really seem to be enough hours in the day. But you don't need an hour to start a fitness plan that works. You don't need even half an hour. We're going to let you in on a little secret: All you need to create a slimmer, sexier, healthier body is 15 minutes.

The 15-Minute Secret

That's right, if you use your time wisely, you can get a great, body-transforming workout in just 15 minutes four to six times a week. According to an October 2010 study published in the *European Journal of Applied Physiology,* 15 minutes of resistance training was just as effective as 35 minutes in elevating resting energy expenditure for up to 72 hours after exercising. That means you can burn calories, build muscle, and get the body you want in half the time you thought possible. And you'll actually have a much better chance of slimming down with quick workouts than with lengthy gym sessions. A study in the *International Journal of Sports Medicine* found that women who were trying to lose weight had a much better chance of sticking to an exercise plan if their workouts were chopped down to 15 minutes.

It makes sense. You can always find 15 minutes, right? If you took every single second during which you said or thought "I don't have the time" and added them up, it would equal more than 15 minutes. That's why we've created our revolutionary superfast fitness program composed entirely of 15-minute workouts. These aren't the kind of 15-minute workouts that are half as good as a 30-minute session. They're scientifically designed to be as effective as they are efficient, so you'll achieve the best results in the least amount of time. Every second of exercise will count a little more than it ever has before. Instead of working out longer, you'll be working out smarter and faster.

You'll find workouts to flatten your belly so quickly it's almost instantaneous; workouts that melt fat off your body so fast you'll barely have time to buy a smaller pair of pants before you drop another size; workouts that will turn your jiggly arms and thighs into firm, sleek accessories you'll want to show off every second you can. Each of the workouts in this book has been road tested by our editors and validated by the latest research. Just follow our superfast fitness program and you'll be seeing the fastest results of your life!

To make this book even more useful, the world's top trainers have also provided dozens of cutting-edge 15-minute workouts for just about every form of exercise and just about every situation, such as the yoga metabolism booster in Chapter 15 or workouts for busy travelers designed by Juan Carlos Santana of the Institute of Human Performance in Boca Raton, Florida, that will sculpt lean muscles in no time flat. Some of the advice and exercises in these pages comes from some of the biggest names in performance training, including longtime friend of *Men's Health* Mark Verstegen, the author of the breakthrough book

Core Performance and owner of Athlete's Performance in Phoenix; exercise physiologist Amy Dixon of Equinox in Santa Monica; and Hollywood fitness trainer Valerie Waters in Los Angeles.

That's barely scratching the surface of the sheer volume and variety of workouts we've included. Can't shake nagging headaches? Pain-proof your noggin with the moves provided by Jyotsna Sahni, MD, a sleep specialist in Tucson. We've even created workouts based on your body type, so if you've spent your life trying to whittle down your pear-shaped behind, we've got you covered. And since your body should feel as good as it looks, we've also tapped some experts to bring you a little sexercise (hello, COREgasm!) with a whole chapter on better-sex workouts.

By following our Superfast Fitness Plan, you'll learn how to put all of these workouts together for maximum results. Combine that with our Superfast Weight-Loss System and you'll shed even more pounds, trim even more inches, and get back into your skinny jeans even faster. We'd go on and on about all the tools and resources that are packed into this book, but we don't want to waste your time. Ready to get started? Good. Because who knows when your 15 minutes of fame might arrive.

The 15-Minute Secret

Free Minutes!

15 WAYS TO FIND 15 MINUTES FOR EXERCISE EVERY DAY! (DITCH THE STUFF THAT'S WASTING YOUR PRECIOUS TIME.)

1. FLIP OFF FACEBOOK. We now spend a whopping 7 hours a month on Facebook, according to Neilsen. Let's do the math: Seven hours a month works out to 105 minutes each week or, hmmm, guess what, exactly 15 minutes every single day. You don't have to banish FB from your life entirely, but limit it to two short sessions a day, like once in the morning over coffee and later in the evening. Then log out and stay off.

2. SAY "NO!" Women have a very hard time with this one. But we think you'll really like it once you try it. Next time someone (not your big boss) asks you to do something you really don't want or need to do, say, "I'm sorry. No. I just can't," and feel the freedom— and all that free time— wash over you.

3. PLAN YOUR PEAKS. We all have certain times of the day when we are most focused and productive. Schedule your biggest task for that time (for many people it's in the morning, say 9:00 a.m.). You'll get it done more quickly and efficiently than if you wait to tackle it during a natural low point (like midafternoon).

4. DO ONE THING AT A TIME. We pride ourselves on being supreme multitaskers, but trying to do too many things at once means getting nothing done. Sit down with your to-do list. Pick an item, and do it and only it. You'll be shocked by how quickly each task gets done when you give it your full energy and attention.

5. RECORD YOUR SHOWS. A typical hour-long TV show contains just 40 to 42 minutes of real content—the rest is commercials. Watch two shows and that's 40 to 45 minutes you could have spent doing something else. It's well worth investing in a digital TV recorder so you can watch just what you want when you want, and free up hours (and, by the end of the year, days) to pursue more healthful activities, like 15-minute workouts.

6. DON'T BE A NEATNIK. Is it really all that important that your apartment is spotless? Stop wasting precious time straightening your sheets just so and polishing picture frames, and aim for adequate instead.

7. BE DECISIVE! You can easily waste hours choosing what color to paint your walls or which brand of sneakers to buy (it's called analysis paralysis). At some point, you need to stop waffling and move forward. Set a time limit, say 45 minutes, for comparison shopping, weighing pros and cons, etc., then make a decision and go forth.

8. BUY TIME. Yes, you actually can buy more hours in the day by paying for services that suck up tons of time. Before you pooh-pooh the idea of hiring a laundry or cleaning service, sit down and do a little math. What is an hour of your time worth? How do you spend your disposable income? When you consider that you might be blowing a few hundred bucks on shoes and bags you don't really need while you slave away all your spare time scrubbing the tub, it's time to reconsider your expenditures. Hire a cleaning service to do the heavy-duty stuff twice a month, look into premade meal plans, and buy yourself hours every week.

9. INK IT ON YOUR CALENDAR. Amazing how you find time for everything on your calendar, right? That's because it's there in black and white, demanding your attention (and time). Block out your workouts as you would work appointments and you won't miss a one.

10. USE AN EGG TIMER. Certain activities are black holes for time. All the little things you plan to do for just a few minutes—surfing the Web, playing games on your phone, "window shopping" all the new apps for your iPhone or iPad—can suck away hours if you're not careful. Keep an egg timer on your desk. When you sit down, set it for 15 or 20 minutes. Then shut down when the bell rings.

11. TOUCH IT ONCE. When a paper comes across your desk (or in the mail), deal with it immediately. Piling up stacks of paper not only creates distracting clutter, you also waste time revisiting each issue again (and again) or, worse, losing something important. (Try it with email too!)

12. MAKE A CALL. IM-ing and emailing can be great time-savers. But sometimes it takes 15 messages to accomplish what you could do in a 40-second phone call. As soon as it starts getting complicated, pick up the phone.

13. PUT THINGS IN THEIR PLACES. I used to waste minutes (hours...days) looking for my keys. At any given time they could have been anywhere, and I mean anywhere—coat pockets, drawers, messenger bags, the clothes dryer, my car, or my personal favorite, hanging from the door lock. Finally, I bought a 75-cent hook, hung it by the phone as my designated key spot, and have not lost my keys since. Try this trick with anything you lose regularly. It works.

14. SET OUT YOUR STUFF. This one is repeated more often than *It's a Wonderful Life* at Christmastime, but it works. Setting out your exercise clothes at night makes it far more likely that you will get up and get moving for a morning workout, instead of hitting snooze (or worse, skipping the whole affair entirely) because it's too daunting to get up and start rummaging around for your workout gear.

15. GET UP 15 MINUTES EARLIER. Ridiculously simple, right? Yep, and it works. Vow to get up and work out at 5 a.m. every day and you'll never do it. But even the most nocturnal of night owls can set their alarms (and roll out of the sack) a mere 15 minutes earlier in the morning. Even if you don't use that extra time for your workout, it gets you out the door and to your office earlier than usual, so you get more done earlier in the day. So you're more likely to feel entitled to take that 15 minutes for yourself later in the day.

Chapter 1:
The Genius of the 15-Minute Training Plan

When It Comes to Exercise,
It Really Is About Quality, Not Quantity.

The Superfast Workouts Help You Become
Leaner, Sexier, and Healthier in Half the Time!
And That's Just Plain Smart.

In our *Biggest Loser* culture we have a tendency to believe that if a little exercise firms and burns, *a lot* of exercise will transform us into Victoria's Secret models. Even though I'm a trainer and triathlete and I should know better, I've been guilty of buying in to this notion myself. A few years back, I laced up my running shoes and started hitting the street for an hour a day, believing that if only I sweated more, my skinny jeans, which were on the verge of becoming my asphyxiation jeans, would never get too snug. But to my dismay, I didn't really get any leaner. I lost a little bulk, sure. But I also got softer, especially in my belly. Then a running coach gave me some advice that stuck (because it worked!): If you want to scorch calories and burn fat, go harder, not longer. I picked up the pace and haven't looked back since.

The Genius of the 15-Minute Training Plan

The more-is-more mind-set is more than a waste of time; it also derails people from their fitness goals. If we think we have to do a ton to get results, we sometimes don't exercise at all. It's a mentality that sets us up for failure before we even start. As it turns out, it is far more important to know what kind of exercise to do rather than how long to do it for. Because much of what we think is going to make us thin or keep us fit actually does neither. Case in point, a study published in the *International Journal of Sports Nutrition and Exercise Metabolism* in which researchers asked a group of women to do 45 minutes of steady, moderate cardio exercise (like a brisk elliptical workout) 5 days a week for 12 weeks. The result? At the end of the study, the women experienced no change in their body composition compared with women who didn't exercise or diet.

Depressing huh? Not at all. The good news is that you have permission to stop wasting your time. You can finally free yourself from marathon gym sessions. Instead scientists are now saying you can shed fat, firm trouble spots, boost your heart health, and fend off a host of ills, mental and physical, not by doing more, but by doing less. You can do this in as little as 15 minutes if you do the right exercises. But you need the inside knowledge.

Short Workouts, Sweet Rewards

That's exactly what you get with the *Women's Health Big Book of 15-Minute Workouts*: a scientifically proven, insider shortcut to losing weight permanently. We've pooled all our expertise and pored over the latest research to create the Superfast Fitness Plan. At the heart of it is resistance training. Hands down, resistance training is the quickest way to burn fat and build a lean, beautiful body. When you create resistance—whether with weights or your own body—you cause microscopic tears in your muscle fibers, which sounds like a bad thing, but is actually the first step to slimming down and getting strong. This fiber breakdown speeds up a process called muscle protein synthesis that uses amino acids to repair and reinforce those fibers—and voilà, you've built some new muscle.

Muscle works magic in many ways. First, all that lifting and rebuilding burns calories not just while you're exercising, but long after you're done. Secondly, muscle is metabolically more active than fat, meaning it burns more calories just to sustain itself. Finally, being stronger makes you more active. Research finds that people are more spontaneously active when they start lifting weights because they're stronger and even hard physical tasks suddenly feel easier. Worried that building muscle will make you bulky? Don't be. A pound of muscle takes up 20 percent less space than a pound of fat. So you'll actually be smaller, but stronger. Didn't we tell you less is more?

The best part: You can get all these body-shaping benefits in no time—just 15 minutes is all it takes. How? We've condensed the workout by removing all the sitting around and resting between moves for a supereffective program. It's not only time efficient, it also increases your energy expenditure both during and afterward. Researchers from Southern Illinois University recently found that one set of 10 reps of 10 exercises (which took 15 minutes to complete, by the way) raised resting energy expenditure (the calories you burn when you're just sitting around) as much as three sets, which took the volunteers 35 minutes to do.

Finally, to turbocharge your results, we've added cardio to the mix. Not the 45-minutes-to-an-hour-a-day variety that may barely budge the scale, but the superfast-fat-burning variety, known in scientific circles as high-intensity interval training (or HIIT) that, like resistance training, builds muscle and burns fat fast. While the government keeps upping the ante on its cardio exercise recommendation—up a half hour from 60 minutes a day to 90 minutes a day for weight loss—a large and growing body of research is saying the opposite thing: that HIIT is drastically superior to regular cardio workouts in improving cardiovascular functioning, increasing insulin sensitivity, and, of course, burning calories. What determines whether or not you shed fat is not the duration of your workouts, but the intensity. In other words, it'll take many hours to walk away that extra weight. But you can sprint it off in no time.

HIIT builds up lactic acid in your muscles because you're working harder and faster than your body has a chance to clear it, which triggers a release of human growth hormone, a powerful natural elixir that promotes fat loss and may crank your metabolism to Maserati speed. And it works fast. Just 30 seconds of sprinting on a stationary bike is enough to send your levels of human growth hormone—that chemical that boosts lean muscle and burns fat— soaring by 530 percent. Another study, published in the *Journal of Applied Physiology,* reported that just 2 weeks of alternate-day interval training boosted eight active women's fat-burning ability by 36 percent. Importantly, your metabolism stays elevated for far longer—up to 24 hours, burning up to 120 additional calories (twice as many as low-intensity exercise)—after a high-intensity workout, so you see results fast.

All that fat burning translates into a leaner you in half the workout time. In a study of 18 women, Australian researchers found that those who performed superfast fat burning workouts that included 8-second sprints followed by 12 seconds of recovery 3 days a week lost about 5½ pounds during the

The Genius of the 15-Minute Training Plan

study period while a similar group who pedaled twice as long at an average pace actually gained a pound of fat over the same period. Even better, the weight you lose is pure fat. In one study from Laval University, researchers found that even when HIIT exercisers burned half as many calories during their actual workout sessions, they still lost nine times more fat after 15 weeks of working out than their traditional long-cardio-bout peers did after 20 weeks.

The benefits don't stop at weight loss. HIIT workouts also help you get fitter faster (so you have more energy for everything you love to do). In a striking head-to-head showdown, Canadian researchers found that a group of exercisers who cranked out short stationary bike workouts that included a series of 30-second sprints 3 days a week improved their fitness by about 30 percent—nearly identical to the improvements made by a similar group of exercisers who pedaled for $1\frac{1}{2}$ to 2 hours at a lesser intensity. Interval training is also the ticket for better health. Researchers in Norway reported that interval training was far more effective for reducing blood pressure, controlling blood sugar, and improving cholesterol than traditional one-speed workouts.

When you stop and think about how your body works, all of this seemingly counterintuitive science suddenly makes a lot of sense. Our bodies are built to adapt to the work we demand of them. When you get up and go out the door for

33

Percent more calories you burn after doing back-to-back sets of two different exercises (supersets) compared with sets that let you rest between moves, according to the *Journal of Strength and Conditioning Research.*

a leisurely jog, you're asking your slow-twitch (endurance) muscle fibers to wake up and get to work, but all those fast-twitch (speed and power) muscle fibers go largely untapped. Over time, many of the neurons that once served fast-twitch fibers will get rewired to serve their slower counterparts. Others will die off. Turning up the intensity of your workouts not only gives you firmer, more shapely muscles by tapping in to all those unused fibers (think Dara Torres), but also fast-tracks your fitness gains, says HIIT training researcher Martin Gibala, PhD, professor of kinesiology at McMaster University. "High-intensity exercise kind of shocks your system. Your body thinks, 'She's making me do some really hard work,' so it increases your total exercise capacity—your ability to use oxygen and burn fat—in a fraction of the time than if you'd exercised less intensely," he says. In fact, according to neuromuscular researcher Christopher Knight, PhD, of the University of Delaware, there's an almost immediate effect when you tap into your fast-twitch fibers with strength training and/or high-speed intervals. "We've found that you can increase your fast-twitch firing rates after just 1 week of training," he says.

That's the genius of the Superfast Workout Plan. You combine 15-minute resistance-training workouts with 15-minute HIIT workouts to lose the most weight. Scientists already know that combining cardio and resistance training works faster and better than either alone. When Pennsylvania State University researchers put three groups of overweight people on a diet and then had them do cardio, resistance training and cardio, or no exercise at all, they found that though each group lost roughly 21 pounds, the lifters dropped 6 more pounds, or 40 percent more, of fat (which, remember, takes up more room than muscle and doesn't look nearly as nice). That's right, nearly every ounce they lost was in the form of fat, while the other two groups dropped precious metabolism-revving muscle as well. Now you get to reap all these rewards in a fraction of the time you ever thought possible.

But the 15-minute secret doesn't just give you the shortest, most effective workout on the planet. You'll also:

1. Trade Fat for Muscle

Whether you want to be bikini ready or are just looking to boost a sagging bottom, 15 minutes is all it takes. Premiere strength-training researcher

Wayne Westcott, PhD, CSCS, instructor in the exercise science department at Quincy College in Massachusetts, confirms that when you choose your exercises wisely, a handful of moves— just four in some cases—is all you need to change your body composition. "Navy research shows you can get tremendous overall improvement—losing 4 pounds of fat and adding 2 pounds of muscle in 8 weeks—by doing just four exercises that work every major muscle," he says. The four moves are the squat, chest press, row, and abs curl. Do them during several rounds of a 15-minute workout for total body transformation.

2. Burn More Calories

Even better, the calorie-burning benefits of even the shortest strength-training bout keep coming long after you've left the gym. In a study from Southern Illinois University, researchers found that when volunteers did just one set of nine exercises, or about 11 minutes of strength training, 3 days a week, they increased their resting metabolic rate (the calories burned when just hanging out) and fat burning enough to keep unwanted weight at bay. And then even more great things will happen.

3. Stay Young

Unless you do something to stop it, your body loses about half a pound of muscle a year after age 20, says Tina Schmidt-McNulty, exercise specialist at Purdue University Calumet. That may sound nearly insignificant,

The Genius of the 15-Minute Training Plan

but when you consider that muscle is your body's biggest calorie burner—burning five times as many calories per pound as fat—it's like "taking your foot off the gas pedal of your metabolism right as you enter adulthood," explains McNulty. That metabolism meltdown can lead to a creeping weight gain of 1 to 2 pounds per year. Little wonder then that the average American woman loses a metabolism-stalling 15 pounds of muscle and adds 45 pounds of fat between the ages of 20 and 50.

4. Fit Into Your Clothes
Even if the scale doesn't take a wild downhill ride, that lean muscle tissue minus the fat will keep you in those skinny jeans forever. How's that? Because 1 pound of fat takes up 20 percent more space on your body than 1 pound of muscle. Resistance training—just 15 minutes a shot—is all it takes to keep your youthful muscle (and figure) for life.

5. Sleep Better
High-intensity exercise helps you sleep like a baby, which in turn helps you keep pounds at bay. Australian researchers recently reported that men and women who did total-body resistance training for 8 weeks enjoyed a 23 percent improvement in their sleep quality. Even better, they were able to fall asleep faster and slept longer than before they started working out. That's important because poor sleep wrecks your waistline. In fact, Stanford University scientists have found that body weight rises proportionally as hours of sleep drop below 7½ a night, likely because sleep deprivation triggers the hunger hormone ghrelin and the fat-storage hormone cortisol.

6. Get Stronger
Resistance training is second to none for building bones. Unfortunately, women build their peak bone mass in their teens and early twenties and then start a skeletal slide around 35, when bone thins at a rate of about 1 percent a year; it's two to three times that following menopause. A study of 124 men and women published in the journal *Osteoporosis* recently reported that high-intensity exercise like that found in our superfast workouts increased bone density in high-risk spots like the spine, hips, and legs in just 40 weeks. By contrast, those doing low-intensity exercise actually lost bone mineral density over the same time.

7. Become More Flexible
Flexibility is the first thing to go, as your muscles shorten over time. Left unchecked, you can lose a full 50 percent of your flexibility over adulthood, which means waving a long-distance good-bye to your toes...from your knees. Using those muscles through a full range of motion, like you will in these 15-minute workouts, will keep all your limbs limber. In a study published in the *International Journal of Sports Medicine*, scientists reported that men and women doing just three full-body

workouts a week for 16 weeks increased their range of motion in their hips and shoulders and also improved their sit and reach test scores by 11 percent. You'll find specific stretching and strengthening workouts for even greater flexible benefits in our workouts.

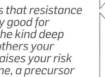

TIP: *Research shows that resistance training is particularly good for burning visceral fat, the kind deep in your belly that smothers your internal organs and raises your risk of metabolic syndrome, a precursor to type 2 diabetes.*

8. Prevent Heart Attacks

Regular resistance training strengthens your most important muscle—the heart—and improves the health of your entire cardiovascular system. In a study published in the *Journal of Applied Physiology,* scientists reported that volunteers who strength trained just 3 days a week for 8 weeks lowered their systolic blood pressures (the top number) by an average of 9 points and their diastolic blood pressures (the bottom number) by an average of 8 points. That's enough to slash your risk of stroke by 40 percent and bring down your risk of heart attack by 15 percent.

9. Avoid Diabetes

Muscle is simply good medicine. A 2003 study from the University of Sydney, Australia reported that resistance training could improve insulin sensitivity, which means fewer blood sugar spikes and crashes as well as fewer of those binge-eating episodes low blood sugar can trigger. Research also shows that resistance training is particularly good for burning visceral fat, the kind deep in your belly that smothers your internal organs and raises your risk of

metabolic syndrome. Even if you have diabetes, it's not too late to benefit. Austrian scientists found that men and women with type 2 diabetes who started strength training were able to significantly lower their blood sugar levels and improve their conditions.

10. Prevent Cancer

Resistance training fends off cancer-causing free radicals, according to a study from the University of Florida. Researchers there found that people who did resistance-training workouts 3 days a week for 6 months had significantly less oxidative cell damage than their non-lifting peers. High-intensity exercise, like the kind found in our HIIT workouts, also has been shown to protect against breast cancer.

11. Get Smarter

No dumb jocks, here. Canadian researchers found that a year of just once-weekly strength training boosted brain power among women volunteers by nearly 13 percent. Other research has reported that strength training improves short- and long-term memory, verbal reasoning, and attention span. Now that's a mind–muscle connection!

The Genius of the 15-Minute Training Plan

12. Stress Out Less

Survival of the fittest is especially true when it comes to handling stress. Scientists at A & M University discovered that the fittest people have significantly lower levels of stress hormones than their couch potato counterparts. Scientists at the Medical College of Georgia have also found that blood pressure levels return to normal faster after a stressful situation in people with more lean muscle tissue compared to those with less.

13. Be Happier

Pushups may work as well as Paxil for improving your mood. Researchers from the University of Sydney recently reported that people who did strength training on a regular basis were far less likely to suffer symptoms of major depression. Short bouts of cardio may be equally powerful. Scientists from Bowling Green State University reported that as little as 10 minutes of cycling improved mood in 21 men and women, compared with a similar group who did nothing during that time.

14. You'll Have More Time

In the pages that follow, you're going to find all the information you need to follow the Superfast 15-Minute Plan. And then you're going to have hours (heck, days!) for everything else!

How to Start

So if 15-minute workouts are so great, why aren't more people using them?

Because you have to know how to put them all together to make them work for you. That's why we set our minds to creating the most comprehensive guide possible to unleash the magic of the 15-minute secret. And even we were amazed at how the Superfast Fitness Plan can be adapted to every kind of exercise to meet every conceivable goal.

This plan is the most versatile you'll find. You don't need to be bench-pressing barbells or even stepping foot in a gym (unless you want). You'll find dozens or workouts you can do right in your living room. You can swim, bike, jump rope, elliptical train, and even power walk for your superfast fat-burning workouts. You'll even find workouts to help you perform better on the tennis court or in road races, if that happens to be your weekend passion. You'll also find an entire chapter of workouts based on the most popular workout equipment (and even some household items), including the ever-popular kettlebell, stability ball, Bosu, and even paper plates!

Following the schedule that we provide on page 21, you'll be choosing three strength-training workouts and one HIIT workout each week. You'll find at least two versions of most strength training workouts because it's important to switch up your exercises as often as possible to keep your results coming. "Your body adapts to meet the specific challenges you place on it," says strength-training researcher Wayne Phillips, PhD, founding partner in the STRIVE Wellness Corporation. "If you constantly challenge it in different ways, it will continue adapting and you'll be less likely to hit a plateau. You're also less likely to get bored with your work-outs." That's why we've included multiple workouts to surprise your muscles with new and different challenges.

Which workouts should you choose? If you're looking for a major makeover, you'll probably want to start with the total-body workouts, which you do 3 times a week for 3 or 4 weeks. If you're looking to work on a specific part of your body, there's a wide array to choose from and you can mix them up during the week, alternating between, say, the Michelle-Obama-Arms Workout and the Thinner Inner Thighs Workout. The Superfast Fat Burn (HIIT) workout you choose depends on what you like to do (i.e., elliptical train, bicycle, etc.). Just look through Chapter 8 so you can plan which ones you want to do ahead of time. For your down days, when you're under the weather or recovering from a medical condition, we even have workouts that will address your woes, mental and physical.

There you have it. It takes no time. You can do it anywhere with your favorite equipment or none at all. No more excuses standing between you and your best body ever. Flip the page and let's get started.

■

Chapter 2:
All of Your
15-Minute-Workout
Questions Answered

Everything You Need to Know to Get
the Most Out of the Superfast Workouts in This Book.

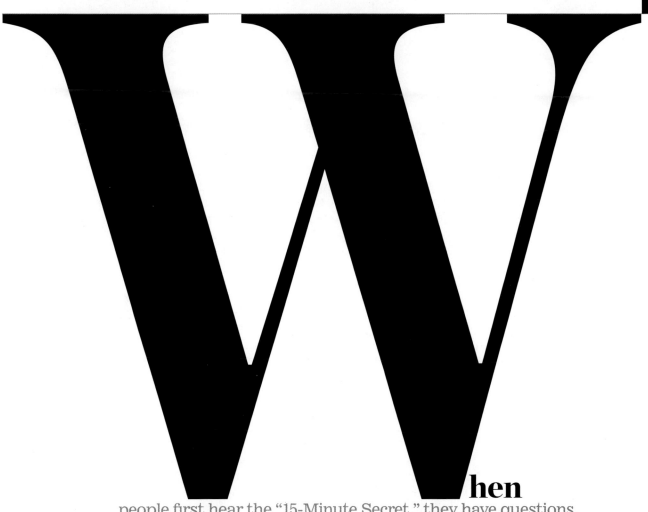

When people first hear the "15-Minute Secret," they have questions. Lots of questions. How does it work? When do I see results? What equipment do I need? That's why we've already put together a list of FAQs that will help you reap maximum rewards from your short workouts. We want you to be armed with all the answers you need to feel confident in the gym, at home, and when your friends say, "Fifteen minutes? No way!" You can just smile, finish your workout, and enjoy all that free time you have left in your day.

Your 15-Minute-Workout Questions Answered

Fifteen minutes is half the standard recommendation of 30 minutes a day. How can it work?
Great question. Because it's actually not half the standard recommendation. In fact, these 15 minutes exceed the standard exercise recommendation. It's true. What most people don't realize is that the 30 minutes a day the Centers for Disease Control and Prevention (CDC) recommends of is for moderate exercise, like brisk walking or washing your car. If you do moderate exercise only, you need to do 150 minutes a week, or about 30 minutes a day, to get benefits. But if you work out more vigorously, using the 15-minute secret, those official exercise recommendations are slashed in half to 75 minutes a week, or about 10 to 15 minutes a day. And in the end, those faster workouts work better. Remember: In a study by Australian researchers, exercisers who did 20-minute workouts that included high-intensity sprints 3 days a week shed fat pounds while their peers who did 40 minutes of cardio actually gained weight.

Do I need to use a stopwatch?
No. To make the program easy, we've designed every workout to take 15 minutes or less. Now, if you take longer rest periods, your workout may extend a few minutes longer, but our goal in this book is to give you the most effective and efficient workout possible in just 15 minutes. On days when you might have more time, go ahead and add more circuits or double up on the workouts. That's cool, too. But you don't have to do that, and, in fact, trying to overreach might derail your progress altogether. A study in the *International Journal of Sports Medicine* found that women had a much better chance of sticking with an exercise routine if it was limited to just 15 minutes.

What should I eat before a workout?
You don't need to have any special foods before your superfast workouts. In fact, because the workouts can be intense, especially the Superfast Fat Burning HIIT routines, it's best not to have a belly full of food. If it's been more than 3 hours since you've eaten, you might want to have a small snack, like half a banana or a handful of trail mix, just to raise your blood sugar and give you an energy boost 30 to 45 minutes before you plan on exercising.

How quickly will I see results?
Depending on which workouts you do, anywhere from 2 to 4 weeks. (If you combine two of the workouts into one 30-minute power session, you'll be losing weight and sculpting even faster.) Since women tend to carry less weight in their

upper bodies, if you do our workouts for arms, shoulders, and back, you'll start to see new definition in as little as 2 weeks.

How much weight should I lift?

The short answer: More than you think. Study after study shows that women tend to err on the side of using weights that are way too light when they resistance train, especially newbies. In a study where novice weight lifters were allowed to select the weight of their choice for their exercise sessions, not a single volunteer chose one that was heavy enough to stimulate muscle growth. Stuart Phillips, PhD, of McMaster University in Hamilton, Ontario, put it to me more bluntly: "A woman doing traditional squats with 10-pound dumbbells is likely activating zero fast-twitch muscle fibers." That's bad news because these are the fibers that go first, says William Kraemer, PhD, professor of kinesiology, physiology, and neurobiology at the University of Connecticut in Storrs. "With age, you naturally lose this type of lean muscle tissue," he says. "That loss doesn't slow down if all you do is cardio and lift 5-pound dumbbells. Those fibers only respond to heavier loads."

The good news is that by lifting heavy loads—such as 15-, 20-, even 25-pound weights depending on the exercise— occasionally (it doesn't need to be, nor should it be, every time; your muscles need recovery), you can fire up those fast-twitch fibers and maintain (or regain) strength and shapely muscle tone. Before you shake your head and dismiss this as too hard, think about the last time you went grocery shopping or to the airport. I'm going to bet that your grocery bags were about 10 pounds each (at least)—and that overstuffed suitcase? Thirty pounds, easy. We women are far stronger than we give ourselves credit for being.

Here's how to figure out a proper weight, using the bent-over row with dumbbells as an example: Grab, say, 20-pound dumbbells and do a set of 10 repetitions of the bent row. The weight is appropriate if you can do 8 or 9 reps with perfect form but you start to struggle or pull more slowly on the 9th or 10th rep. If you struggle earlier in the set or lose form by twisting your torso or trying to use momentum (i.e., cheating), the weight is too heavy. Try 15-pound weights.

How many times do I do each exercise?

You'll find a range of set and rep recommendations in the Superfast Workouts. As a rule of thumb, you'll be doing as many sets as you need to to complete about 25 to 30 repetitions for a muscle group. There's an inverse relationship between sets and reps. If you're doing a high number of reps, like 15, you'll only do two sets. If you're lifting heavier weights for fewer, like 8 to 10 reps, you'll do 3 sets. The goal is to challenge your muscles for an appropriate amount of time no matter how many reps you're performing. Simply follow the instructions for each workout.

Your 15-Minute-Workout Questions Answered

Do I stop each between each exercise?

In general, no. Most of the Superfast Workouts are done circuit style, which means you do a series of exercises in succession without resting between sets, before starting from the top and completing the circuit again. There's an important strategy behind this: Because you never let your heart rate come down between moves, you get a calorie-burning cardio workout as well as a muscle-firming strength challenge. Circuits are an extremely efficient way to exercise, which is why they make up the bulk of the workouts in this book. But don't worry, your body will also be getting rest, it's just active rest. These workouts are ordered so the exercises alternate between upper- and lower-body exercises. So, for example, you would do a squat followed by a chest press followed by a hip bridge followed by a dumbbell row and so forth, with little or no rest between them. That way your upper body gets a break while your lower body works.

You'll also be doing supersets, which are similar to circuits except you flip-flop between pairs of exercises before moving on to the next pair. By working different muscle groups back-to-back with no rest between, you not only save precious time (that you would otherwise be using for recovery), but also, some experts believe, you increase the rate at which your body breaks down and rebuilds muscle protein, which in turn boosts your metabolism for hours afterward.

Can I do all my Superfast Workouts on consecutive days or should I spread them out?

Spread them out. You'll be doing three resistance-training workouts per week. Those should be on alternate days, with a day of recovery between them. On "off" days you can choose specialty workouts like one of the healing workouts, such as headache relief or a foam roller stretch/massage workout. One day a week will be reserved for the HIIT workout of your choosing and 1 day is for complete rest.

Researchers at the University of Texas Medical Branch in Galveston have generated a tall body of research that confirms that this strategy of every-other-day-lifting works wonders for your metabolism. In short, they found that muscle protein synthesis, which is what happens as your muscles are being repaired (this also raises your metabolism), is elevated for 48 hours after a resistance-training bout. So if you hit the kettlebells Tuesday at 10 a.m., your body remains in muscle toning and firming mode until 2 days later, when muscle synthesis returns to normal. So Thursday at 10 a.m. it's time to fire it up again with another workout.

What about cardio? Shouldn't I be doing that four times a week to lose weight?

HIIT workouts are actually much better than traditional cardio for losing weight. But the truth is, even on your superfast resistance-training days, you'll be raising your heart rate and getting your blood flowing, which counts as cardio. We now know that weight training and the sprint-type training characteristic of HIIT strengthens your heart and lungs, lowers blood pressure, controls cholesterol, and shapes up your cardio-vascular system as well, if not better than, classic aerobic exercise. So nearly any workout you choose in this book will count as cardio.

And don't worry, you'll still be burning plenty of fat, even though you're working well above the "fat burning" zone. Vigorous exercise may burn more stored carbs while you're doing it, but it burns far more fat in the long run. Hard efforts trigger the release of hormones such as epinephrine that stimulate fat release from your fat cells. "Your body also responds to hard efforts by building more mitochondria and producing more fat-burning enzymes, so you become better at burning fat, not just glycogen [stored carbs] during exercise," says HIIT researcher Martin Gibala, PhD, professor of kinesiology at McMaster University, whose research found that exercisers who did sprint work improved their VO$_2$ max levels (how much oxygen the body is capable of using—a key element in fat burning) by 30 percent, identical to a group who slogged along for more than 90 minutes in the fat-burning zone. Even better, your metabolism stays set to high for up to five times longer after a hard workout than an easy one, so you're torching fat long after you're done.

Do I need to lift superslow?

Nope. In fact, you'll make greater gains if you speed things up a bit and lift a little faster. "By picking up the pace, you recruit more of your unused fast-twitch muscle fibers, which take a lot of energy to move," explains resistance-training researcher Scott Mazzetti, PhD, of Salisbury University in Salisbury, Maryland. Mazzetti and his coworkers found that when volunteers performed springy, split-second reps during their strength-training sessions, they recruited more muscle and increased their calorie burn by about 28 percent— that adds up to 72 extra calories, or the amount you'd burn walking a mile, over the course of a full-body workout. Ramping up your repetition rate also revs up your metabolism for hours after you're done. The same study reported that fast pace reps boost afterburn, the calories you burn for about an hour after you're finished, by 5 percent.

Should I join a gym?

You can. But you don't need to. You can do many of the 15-minute workouts in your living room with minimal (some-times no) equipment. And for a couple hundred bucks, you can put together the perfect home gym. But there's no question that belonging to a good gym opens up a world of workout possibilities that would likely not exist at home. There also are some people (I am one) who simply work out harder and longer and give just a bit more in a gym envi-ronment. Many women are also inspired

Your 15-Minute-Workout Questions Answered

by being surrounded by kindred spirits. A recent Stanford University study of nearly 3,000 women found that women (who are social by nature) are more motivated to exercise when they see others doing the same.

My advice: Start immediately. Do the workouts you can with what you've got and see how it goes. If you're happy, but don't feel like you have quite enough equipment to get the job done, check out "What gear do I need" on pages 18 and 19 and gear up if you need to. If it really isn't working for you, it's time to check out the local fitness clubs. Treat this "purchase" as you would shopping for a car. Do some research. Look around. Ask friends for their opinions. And most importantly, give the place a test drive. Any club worth your cash will give you a trial membership so you can come and use the facilities for a few days before making up your mind. Be sure to check it out during the times you'll most likely be using it, especially if that's during peak hours, like before and after work. The same gym that is pleasantly buzzing at 9 a.m. may be a madhouse at 6 p.m. Here are a few other factors to consider before signing on the dotted line at a health club or gym.

• **Convenience.** First and foremost, is the place convenient for you to get to? It doesn't matter if you find the Shangri-la of fitness clubs. If it's out of the way, you will not go. Period. Think about it: If it takes you 20 minutes to drive to the club and 20 to get home, plus time to change in the locker room, your 15-minute Superfast Workout has suddenly transformed into a superslow waste of time. Your health club or gym needs to be along your normal daily path and open during hours that you can easily accommodate. If not, take a pass and keep looking.

• **Does it feel good?** The right club should feel good immediately. First impressions count. If you walk in and think, "Wow," that's a good start. If you're trying to talk yourself into it, leave.

• **The staff.** Committing to a gym is like buying a car, but you shouldn't feel like you're at a used-car dealership when you walk in the door. The staff and trainers should be sharp, credentialed, helpful, and engaging. But ultimately the place should sell itself. You shouldn't be pressured with a hard sell.

• **Affordability.** Obviously, you shouldn't blow your budget on a gym, but don't shortchange yourself, either. Joining a cheap, so-so gym you never go to ultimately wastes more money than spending a few extra bucks a month on one you really love. Your health, strength, and fitness are sound investments.

If I work out after lunch, should I eat a recovery meal afterward?

You don't have to scarf something immediately, as you would if you had skipped the preworkout lunch. The idea that you need to eat a fast-acting recovery meal or shake as soon as possible after training is rooted in research on endurance athletes who were doing

$2\frac{1}{2}$-hour workouts. Your 15-minute Superfast Workout—even if it's really intense—won't deplete your glycogen stores. Besides, you ate lunch, so your body isn't running on empty.

How do the body-specific workouts work? I always heard you couldn't lose weight in one place.

That's a great question. You know, because 10,000 other trainers and I have told you a million times, that you can't get rid of belly fat by doing dozens and dozens of crunches. That's still true. You cannot spot reduce. But what you can do is spot tone, which many of the Superfast Workouts will do. When your muscles are untrained, they will be soft and, in the case of those affected by gravity, like your triceps and tush, saggy. If you have excess fat on the backs of your arms or on your behind, you will not make it go away by doing kickbacks and squats. But you will tighten, tone, and firm those muscles, which will improve the appearance of those areas. Because you're burning calories during your workouts, you're also shedding fat, which means you'll be able to see those newly toned muscles shine through sooner.

How do I know if I'm working my muscles hard enough?

If you have the breath to ask, you may not be. Seriously, for strength workouts, use the guidelines under "How much weight should I lift?" The final repetition or two should be very tough. You should need to work hard to complete it with proper form and not be able to easily do more. For your HIIT workouts, simply use the talk test, which measures how many words you can spit out while you're cranking out your efforts. Researchers have found to be very accurate way to judge exercise intensity without a heart rate monitor or other equipment. Those same researchers recommend using the Pledge of Allegiance as your guide. It works like this:

- **Low-intensity activity (warmup):** You should be able to say the entire pledge—all 31 words—comfortably, breathing at the usual pauses.
- **Moderate aerobic activity:** While working at this level you should be able to easily recite four to six words of the pledge at a time. You shouldn't have to strain to get the words out of your mouth. You'll be working at this intensity during most of the resistance-training circuits.
- **High-intensity activity (intervals):** This is an all-out effort (where you should be during the hardest parts of your HIIT workouts). When cranking it at this intensity, you should be able to speak only a word or two between breaths. (You'll know you're fully recovered from these efforts when you can say the whole pledge comfortably.)

Do I need a spotter?

Not often. Most of the workouts in this book involve bodyweight exercises or lightweight dumbbells that won't get you into trouble. However, anytime you are using heavier weights or lifting a barbell over your head or chest (think bench press), it's a good safety measure to ask a friend for a spot. Accidents happen every year, and you don't want to add to the statistics.

What gear do I need?

You don't need anything more than your own body to get rolling on some of the 15-minute workouts. But a little equipment can open a lot of body-sculpting doors, especially if you don't belong to a fitness club. Here's a rundown of the gear required to do many of the Superfast Workouts in this book.

DUMBBELLS: Hand weights are must-haves. With a few sets of dumbbells, you can work every body part; they don't take up much space, and they're relatively cheap (about a dollar a pound, but shop around). For the best results, invest in three sets: light (5 to 8 pounds), medium (10 to 12), and heavy (15 plus). Another good option is an "all in one" adjustable set like PowerBlocks or the Speed Pac from Reebok. In the case of the Speed Pac, each of the dumbbells adjusts from 2.5 pounds using the handle only to 12.5 pounds using all the weights. Each weight plate allows you to increase the weight by 2.5 pounds—a feature many women appreciate because it allows you to increase your weight in smaller increments rather than making a 5-pound jump as you might have to do with traditional dumbbell sets. The all-in-one package also takes up less space, if storage is a concern. One other

benefit of dumbbells: They are safer to use than barbells, especially if you don't have a spotter.

BENCH: Technically, you don't need a bench. You can use a stability ball, chair, or even the floor for many traditional bench moves. But a bench does make it easier to lift a heavier weight with proper form, so an exercise bench is worth the investment if you're going to be working out at home. Look for one that is adjustable, so you can perform exercises on both an incline and a decline. You can find adjustable benches at most sporting goods stores.

BARBELL AND WEIGHT PLATES: Go to the gym and use the standard 7-foot Olympic barbell. They weigh in at about 45 pounds and are great for squats, lunges, deadlifts, and a variety of lower-body exercises. You can buy smaller, lighter barbells for home use if you find you like them.

KETTLEBELL: These little weighted balls with handles originated in Russia decades ago, but have recently been getting a lot of love here in the States. Because the kettlebell's weight is off center (hanging beyond your hand), it makes traditional dumbbell moves more difficult because your body's stabilizing muscles must work overtime to control your movement. The handle also allows you to perform a variety of explosive and swinging movements. These exercises build strength and endurance in your back, legs, shoulders, and core. You'll find two kettlebell workouts starting on page 214. Like dumbbells, kettlebells come in a range of weights. Or you can invest in an adjustable set like the 20-pound Weider PowerBell for about $100. It comes with a 5-pound handle and adjustable 2.5-pound plates, which allows you to have seven different weights in one bell.

MEDICINE BALL: I love medicine balls. With them, you can tone your abs and strengthen your core without doing a single crunch. They're also second to none for sports-specific training. You'll find a wide array of medicine balls in all sizes, weights, and materials at PerformBetter.com. For the biggest bang for your buck, look for one that is rubberized and bounces so you can toss it against the wall or floor. Check out pages 230 and 236 for a full medicine ball workouts.

STABILITY BALL: Also known as a Swiss ball and a physioball, this large inflated exercise ball is the perfect addition to any home gym. As the name implies, stability balls are ideal for balance training and they make great core-toning tools. In a study of 41 exercisers, researchers at Occidental College in Los Angeles found that muscle activity spiked in the upper abs, lower abs, and obliques by 31 percent, 38 percent, and 24 percent, respectively, when crunches were performed on the ball instead of flat on the floor. You also can use one

instead of a bench for chest presses and seated exercises. These days, you can buy stability balls in nearly every big-box store such as Target and Wal-Mart and even in some supermarkets. PerformBetter.com offers heavy-duty balls if you're looking for extra durability.

EXERCISE BAND: If you travel a lot, pick up a few exercise bands. They're feather light, dirt cheap (less than 20 bucks), and put a complete gym in your tote bag. In fact, few workout tools beat the efficiency of the multitasking resistance band. You can step on the middle and grab the ends for arm curls, hold the ends at your shoulders for squats, and choke up on the band and perform some upright rows without even changing position. You also can tie the ends together and use it as a large band to perform assorted hip, leg, and glute moves. Exercise bands come in a variety of thicknesses for more or less resistance. A good brand is Thera-Band, which offers latex-free bands. Or try Superbands, extra-strong, long resistance bands that are designed for heavy-duty use. You can also by a band utility strap that allows you to easily affix the band to doorjambs and poles.

FOAM ROLLER: You can't beat these pressed foam cylinders for a self-massage that will keep you in the game. Roll your achy body parts along one and say, "Ah." (You'll find a 15-minute foam roller workout on page 370. Either 6 by 18 inches or 6 by 36 inches is fine. Find them at sporting goods stores or order online for $10 to $25.

VALSLIDES: These foam-topped slippery plastic disks turn any carpeted, hardwood, or linoleum floor into an ice rink. Use them to add challenge and intensity to lunges (especially side lunges) and for working your core. You'll find a workout on sliding moves on page 250. If you don't have special sliders, you also can use paper plates. They're not quite as slick, but they'll get the job done.

JUMP ROPE: Really, any jump rope will do. But for the best jumping experience, go with a beaded jump rope, which stacks short pieces of plastic tubing over a thin rope. The beading adds heft to the rope, so the rope maintains a wide U-shape to jump through and makes it easier to maintain momentum.

BOSU BALANCE TRAINER: Half stability ball, half wobble board, the Bosu trainer, which looks like half of a stability ball on a platform, helps build strength and coordination. With the ball side up you can do crunches, squats, even plyometric hops. Then flip it over and do pushups, or try standing on it for advanced balance work.

STEP OR BOX: A step, like the Reebok aerobic step, gives you a sturdy platform for stepups, elevated pushups, and plyometric jumping moves. For a higher, more intense platform, you also can invest in an adjustable squat box (elitefts.com). It provides a stable, no-slip surface to lift from, and you can quickly raise and lower the height of this box for stepups, split squats, and any number of upper- and lower-body moves and jumps.

How To Use This Book

Your easy guide to a leaner, fitter, sexier you—in half the time!

Pick three superfast resistance-training workouts a week: Choose from any of the workouts to do, say, on Monday, Wednesday, and Friday. You can do one particular workout all 3 days (although you should start to mix them up after 3 weeks so it doesn't get too easy for your body) or you can do three different 15-minute workouts in 1 week. You can pick from workouts that target specific areas of your body or workouts for the whole enchilada, workouts that prepare you for a particular sport or workouts that get rid of PMS. Note, if you have time-specific goals (such as an upcoming class reunion), you should do one of our total-body workouts on all 3 days to get the fastest result. But once you've achieved that goal (and high school is once again ancient history), you can switch over to another workout. This book is your personalized plan that you can keep on personalizing over time to meet your ever-changing fitness needs.

Pick two specialty workouts: Two days a week, you have the option of choosing a specialty, non-resistance-training 15-minute workout like the one for PMS or a stretching workout. Or you can just do some light cardio like a quick jog or bike ride if you wish.

Pick one HIIT workout: Once a week, say on a Saturday, you will commit to doing a HIIT workout, your secret weapon to burning fat and losing weight.

Take off 1 day a week: That's it! Now you'll have tons of time to do everything else you love!

Sample Week on the 15-Minute Exercise Plan

Monday	Tuesday	Wednesday	Thursday	Friday	Saturday	Sunday
Fit-Into-Your-Skinny-Jeans Workout	Brisk walk (optional light cardio, specialty workout, or rest)	Age Eraser Workout	Yoga stretches in the evening (optional light cardio, specialty workout, or rest)	Tighter Tush Workout	Elliptical HIIT Workout	Use all the time you saved for something completely indulgent!

Chapter 3: The Superfast Weight-Loss System

Eating Healthy Doesn't Have to Complicate Your Life.

In This Chapter, You'll Find Quick and Simple
Diet Advice That Works Fast.

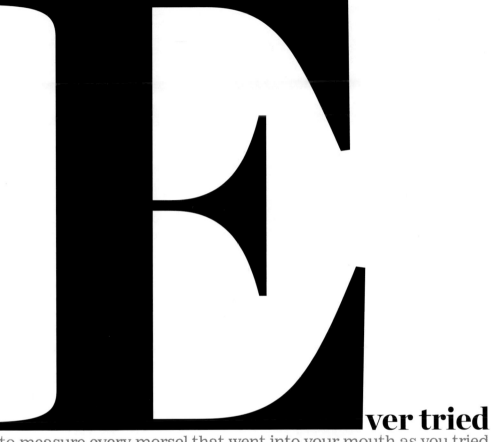

Ever tried

to measure every morsel that went into your mouth as you tried to finally shed those stubborn saddlebags, only to see your cup size shrink while your thighs stayed just as wide? Then you know that the true ticket to a hot body isn't just lowering the numbers on the scale, but rather improving your body composition—building shapely, lean, metabolism-revving muscle while shedding unwanted fat. That's why we developed the Superfast Weight-Loss System, a simple and easy plan that is grounded in lean, healthy protein—which your body uses to form muscle—as well as special fat-burning foods to complement the superfast exercise plan and fast-forward your weight loss.

The Superfast Weight-Loss System

Trim Carbs, Pump Protein, Drop Pounds

The Superfast Weight-Loss System is based on groundbreaking research from a team of diet and exercise scientists at the University of Connecticut. They found that by tweaking your diet to match your workouts, you can maintain shapely lean muscle mass while shedding fat fast. In fact, in one of their studies of overweight men and women, those who followed a reduced-carb diet like the one presented here and lifted weights three times a week shed 22 pounds, nearly 2 pounds a week. Here's the best part: Nearly all of it (97 percent) came from fat.

For a more powerful impact, we've pumped up the protein, as well. Study after study shows that for building and maintaining lean muscle while burning off flab, you can't beat the power of protein. In a study published in *Nutrition and Metabolism*, dieters who increased their protein intake to 30 percent of their diet ate nearly 450 fewer calories a day and lost about 11 pounds during the 12-week study. What's more, high-protein diets seem to let you keep on losing weight longer than their high carbohydrate counterparts. When London researchers compared the effects of a high-protein versus a high-carb diet on 48 overweight men and women who had lost weight on a liquid diet, they found that the high-protein

eaters kept shedding pounds, losing another 5 pounds during a 12-week follow-up, compared with the high-carb eaters, who actually gained weight.

The superfast exercise and diet plan is quite simply the fastest, most efficient way to lose weight. In a study of 48 women, University of Illinois researchers found that those who combined a resistance-training plan with a high-protein diet lost 22 pounds (and only 1 pound of muscle) during the 11-week study whereas a group eating the same number of calories in a high-carb diet lost only 15 pounds and 2 pounds of muscle. And those Connecticut researchers also reported that those eating fewer carbs didn't just lose more weight, they also enjoyed significant reductions in total cholesterol and triglycerides. Their levels of insulin plummeted 32 percent and C-reactive protein—a marker of inflammation—fell 21 percent. They got healthier—inside and out.

Just as the superfast workouts were designed to be done in 15 minutes, so too is the Superfast Weight-Loss System. And by that, we don't just mean nearly instant results, but also that it takes no extra time and barely any effort to follow. You'll find a special section on 15-minute recipes and a 15-minute kitchen makeover, as well as a list of 15 top fat-burning foods. Consider this your 4-week fast lane to the body of your dreams.

Everything You Need to Know to Start Eating Healthier and Losing Pounds

With the Superfast Weight-Loss System, you eat more, not less, but what you eat will trigger your body to burn fat stores. At the same time you'll pump up your protein and savor a fair share of delicious natural fats, which research shows helps people better control blood sugar, hunger, and cravings. The end result: You'll lose weight faster than you ever have before, kibosh your cravings, and never feel deprived!

What to Eat

This plan is incredibly simple. Eat any combination of the foods from three categories: high-quality proteins, low-starch vegetables, and natural fats. (See chart on page 29.) Snack on nuts and seeds or low-calorie fruits. Eat until you feel satisfied—who has time to count calories?—and you'll automatically lose fat. Fast workouts, fast weight loss, fast results. That's what this book is all about: speed.

The Guidelines

Put high-quality protein on your plate at every single meal. Protein helps you incinerate pounds on nearly every weight-loss front. For one, just eating it burns energy! About 25 percent of the protein calories in your food are burned off in digestion, absorption, and chemical changes in your body, so protein has less of a caloric impact than most foods. And as we've learned, it's also nature's appetite suppressant because it takes longer to digest. Protein also preserves

The Superfast Weight-Loss System

your hard-earned, metabolism revving muscle tissue while you're losing fat. A recent study in *Medicine and Science in Sports & Exercise* found that a weight-loss diet with 35 percent of its calories from protein preserved muscle mass in athletes, while a diet with just 15 percent protein led to an average loss of 3½ pounds of muscle in just 2 weeks.

It's particularly important to start the day with a protein-packed meal. A Purdue University study found that eating lean protein (such as Canadian bacon, egg whites, or low-fat yogurt) at breakfast keeps you satisfied longer than it would if you consumed it at other times of the day. "Try to get at least 1 ounce (30 grams) of protein at breakfast," recommends Joan Salge Blake, RD, a clinical associate professor of nutrition at Boston University. Remember, eating protein stimulates muscle growth. In fact, every time you eat at least 10 to 15 grams of protein, you trigger a burst of protein synthesis, which means your body is repairing and building muscle (it also means a greater calorie burn because of all of this metabolic activity). And when you eat at least 30 grams, that period of synthesis lasts about 3 hours—and that means even more muscle growth all day long.

Embrace a little fat. You'll recall what happened when we all tried to trim every ounce of fat from our diets? We all got fatter. We now know that dietary fat plays a critical role in calorie control and fat metabolism. Oleic acid, an unsaturated fat found in olive oil, nuts, and avocados, helps quash hunger, according to a study in the journal *Cell Metabolism*. During digestion, it's converted into a compound that indirectly triggers hunger-curbing signals to your brain. (Bonus benefit: Oleic acid has been shown to lower bad cholesterol without affecting the good HDL.) Omega-3 fatty acids found in naturally fatty foods like salmon and other cold-water fish and avocados also helps reduce body fat, lower triglycerides, and raise healthy HDL cholesterol. Just keep portions in check by eating fat in balance with the other elements of the superfast weight-loss system. As long as pounds are peeling off your frame, your fat intake is fine.

Set limits on starch. Since 1980, our food intake has grown by up to 500 calories a day, nearly 80 percent of which can be attributed to carbohydrates; in that time, the prevalence of obesity has increased by 80 percent. The lesson: Cap your consumption of the most carbohydrate-dense foods, such as breads, pasta, rice, beans, candy, baked goods, and potatoes. Think of starch as sugar in disguise. (One of my favorite descriptions of spaghetti: Sugar on a string.) In fact, starch is nothing more than neatly packaged bundles of glucose, the basic building block of sugar, stuck together by chemical bonds. These bonds start to dissolve the moment they make contact with the saliva in your mouth, immediately freeing the glucose to surge into your bloodstream. As a result, starch has an even greater impact on blood sugar than sucrose. It also encourages your body to store fat. When you do eat starch, have it in the form of whole grains or a small sweet potato, which at least contain some fiber to slow the down the surge. Or even better, try quinoa, a protein-packed grain with more fiber and fewer carbs than most. Limit yourself to two servings of starch a day. Here's a tip for those special occasions at your favorite Italian restaurant when you must have spaghetti and meatballs: doggie-bag one-half to three-quarters of your pasta entrée before you dig in. The portion the chef piles on your plate is likely three or more actual servings' worth.

Pile on the produce. These filling, good-for-you foods are your ticket to sticking with it. And they cannot be overdone. When researchers at the State University of New York Downstate Medical Center in New York City surveyed more than 2,000 low-carb dieters, they discovered that, on average, those who were most successful downed at least four servings of low-starch vegetables every day. That's likely because these foods are brimming with filling fiber and water that leave you full and satisfied on very few calories. Keep your fruit intake a bit more in check. While low-calorie fruits like berries and melons are encouraged in the superfast diet, bananas and other commonly consumed fruits like pineapple, oranges, grapes, and pears are high in sugar and/or starchy carbs.

Snack on nuts, seeds, and/or low-calorie fruits. Add nuts to your daily diet, but don't shovel fistfuls mindlessly—a serving of nuts should total 1 ounce, which is about 35 peanuts, 24 almonds, or 18 cashews. Limit yourself to two servings a day. A serving of low-calorie fruit is $1/2$ cup. You can also help yourself to a protein shake when midafternoon hunger hits (or any time of day!).

THE 15 BEST FAT-BURNING FOODS

These are foods that start winnowing your waistline the moment they leave your fork and enter your mouth. They build muscle, promoting fat burning, or simply use energy (i.e., burn calories) just to digest them! Stock up today.

Almonds and other nuts (with skins intact)
Build muscle, reduce cravings

Dairy products (fat-free or low-fat milk, yogurt, cheese)
Build strong bones, fire up weight loss

Eggs
Build muscle, burn fat

Turkey and other lean meats
Build muscle, strengthen immune system

Berries
Improve satiety, prevent cravings

Enova oil (soy and canola oil)
Promotes fullness, not easily stored as fat

Continued on page 28

The Superfast Weight-Loss System

Peanut butter
Boosts testosterone (a good thing even in women), builds muscle, burns fat

Fatty fish (such as salmon, tuna, mackerel)
Trigger fullness, fire up fat burning

Grapefruit
Lowers insulin, regulates blood sugar and metabolism; be sure to eat the fleshy white membranes

Green tea
Fires up fat burning

Chili peppers
Spikes metabolism

Spinach and green vegetables
Fight free radicals and improve recovery for better muscle building

Whole grains (quinoa, brown rice, whole grain cereal)
Small doses prevent body from storing fat

Beans and legumes
Build muscle, help burn fat, regulate digestion

Whey
Builds muscle, burns fat

Meal-by-Meal Guidelines

Remember, this is supposed to be quick and easy, so don't complicate it. Build your meals around protein and veggies and you're good to go (and lose!). Here's an at-a-glance look at what 24 hours of 15-minute weight-loss eating might look like.

MORNING: Crack those eggs. No matter how you scramble or serve them, they're a perfect part of the morning meal. Add some cheese, toss in some sliced peppers and tomatoes, and add a serving of meat such as lean sausage or Canadian bacon, and start your day.

MIDMORNING: A handful of nuts, low-fat yogurt, a protein shake, or some string cheese and grapes will keep you moving through any morning lull.

NOONISH: Lunch should be a big meaty salad. Mix up tons of greens and veggies with tuna, chicken, beef, or the meat of your choice. For a change, you might want a burger with no bun, some egg salad or tuna wrapped in Romaine leaves, or simply the leftovers from last night's dinner.

MIDAFTERNOON: Pump up the protein to shake the sleepy 3 p.m. dip. A smoothie or some nut butter on celery will do the trick.

EVENING: Dinner is easy. Just pair your favorite meat with a heaping serving of recommended vegetables and you're on the program. Don't limit yourself to chicken and broccoli (though that's a stellar combination) every night or you'll get bored fast. Try roasting cauliflower and brussels sprouts in some olive oil and garlic for a savory side. Grill asparagus and a skirt steak. Use your imagination and watch the pounds peel away.

For more ideas, check out Chapter 16 for "15 Delicious Muscle-Building, Fat-Fighting Meals You Can Make in 15 Minutes or Less" (page 378).

What to Drink

Fill your cup with beverages that have 5 calories or fewer per serving. Water is a no-brainer, but a bit boring. Stock up on herbal teas, pick up some Crystal Light, go ahead and enjoy your coffee (just skip the sugar). Diet soda is okay on occasion, but opt for healthier beverages when possible.

As for alcohol, close the bar after one or two drinks per day, whether it's wine, beer, or hard alcohol. And watch the mixers. Juice, soda, and sugary blended drink mixes amp up the sugar and calories fast. Skip them.

HIGH-QUALITY PROTEINS	LOW-STARCH VEGETABLES*		NATURAL FATS
Beef	Artichokes	Leafy greens	Avocados
Cheese	Asparagus	Mushrooms	Butter
Eggs	Bok choy	Onions	Coconut
Fish	Broccoli	Peppers	Cream
Pork	Brussels sprouts	Radishes	Nuts and seeds
Poultry	Carrots	Spinach	Olives, olive oil, and canola oil
Whey and casein protein powder	Cauliflower	Tomatoes	
Soy	Celery	Turnips	Full-fat salad dressings
	Cucumbers	Zucchini	

Any vegetables besides potatoes, peas, and corn are fair game.

How to Make It Work

If this way of eating is completely new, you might encounter a few bumps at first. Here's a troubleshooting guide for common glitches.

Mood swings. When you change the way you eat, your body sometimes protests by making you grumpy or tired. This should only last a couple of days. If it lingers a week, be sure you're taking in enough fluids to stay hydrated. And by all means, eat enough fat. This diet is designed to make you a better fat burner, so you absolutely need to eat this important source of fuel.

Tummy troubles. Introduce the high-fiber veggies a bit at a time, so your body can make the enzymes you need to digest them. If you suspect you're not getting enough fiber because you're eating fewer grains, try taking some Metamucil or Benefiber once a day.

Stuck scale. If the weight isn't coming off, do a quick calorie check. Multiply your target body weight by 10 to 12. That's how many calories you should aim for each day. Count them out for a few days so you know what that amount of food looks like. Many of us don't have a sense of proper portions.

AVOID THE SUGAR SPIKERS

Foods high in starch and sugar spike your blood sugar too quickly and cause a crash, slowing down your superfast route to a new body. Some common culprits to avoid (or in the case of fruit, simply limit):

Bananas

Biscuits

Candy

Chips

Cookies

Doughnuts

Grapes

Ice cream

Pasta (refined)

Rice (white)

Soda

Sweet tea

White bread

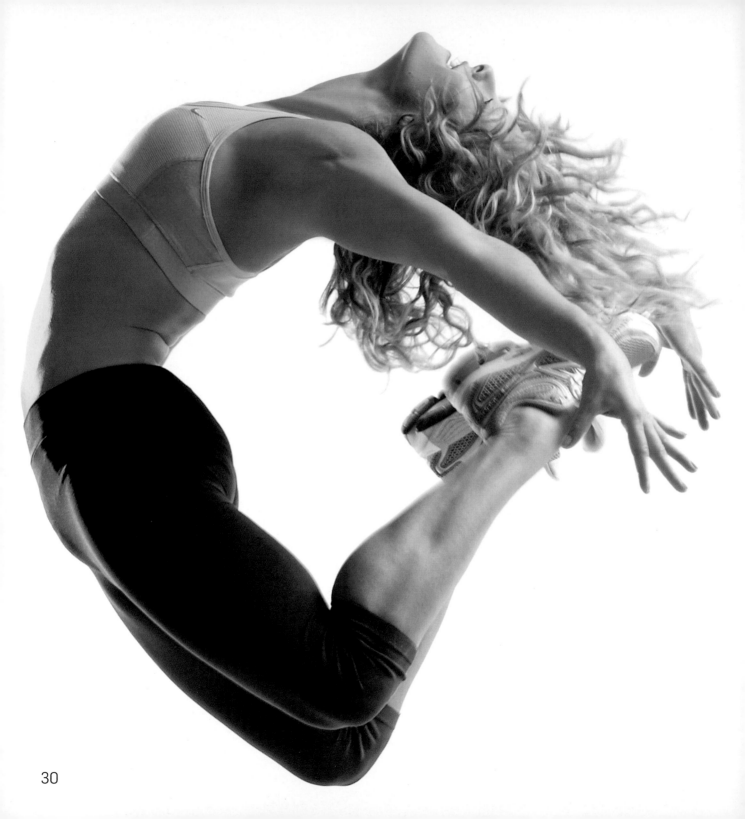

Chapter 4:
15-Minute Total-Body Workouts

The Fastest Way To Burn Calories, Lose Weight,
And Tone Muscles Everywhere is Right Here.

Superfast Total-Body Workouts

In this chapter you'll find power-packed workouts specially designed to help you fry flab and sculpt lean, shapely muscle from head to toe—fast. These total-body workouts do that using an exciting mix of high-energy, challenging exercises that fire up every muscle fiber. The more varied your movements, the more motor units you recruit, which activate and build more muscle fibers. As a bonus (because your body also includes your brain), we've added mind–body workouts, like the 15-minute mood-lifting routine, too. They're a perfect complement to resistance training and can be done on your 2 open workout days to let you feel as good as you look.

Start with the basics...

Brand new to strength training? The workouts in this chapter are excellent, but might be a bit outside your comfort zone straight out of the gate. So, cut your teeth (and jump-start body sculpting) with a simple routine of four basic moves. The Basic Superfast Total-Body Workout (page 34) is designed to get you up to speed, fast. Focus on form and use light weights (5 to 8 pounds) until you feel confident that you're performing the movements smoothly and

steadily. Then try the more advanced routines. For the best results, do all of the workouts in the goal area of your choice each week. For example, if you want to shape up for your high school reunion, do both of those workouts and one special area workout (like a lower-body workout) each week. Do the prescribed number of sets and reps for each exercise, opting for a weight at which you can barely squeeze out the last rep of your final set with spot-on form.

Find It Quick: Your 15-Minute Total-Body Circuit Plan

HOW TO DO A CIRCUIT

Circuits are fast and efficient workouts that combine the heart rate–elevating benefit of aerobics and the muscle building of resistance training. In a circuit, you do one set of each exercise, resting only briefly—10 to 30 seconds if at all—between exercises before moving to the next. Only after completing the list of exercises do you go back and repeat them. Rest for 1 to 3 minutes between circuits.

Basic Superfast Total-Body Workout

Four moves. That's all it takes to fire up your fat burning and build lean, metabolism-charging muscle. As mentioned in Chapter 1, you can lose 4 pounds of fat and add 2 pounds of muscle in just 8 weeks by doing a basic routine that hits all your major muscle groups. If you're new to resistance training, master these before moving on.

START HERE:

Do these moves one after another with no rest in between. Then repeat the circuit for a total of three times, with 1 minute of rest between circuits.

Squat

WORKS your entire lower body.

A

- Stand with your feet hip-width apart, holding dumbbells at your sides.

B

- Squat down like you're sitting in a chair until your thighs are nearly parallel to floor (don't let knees jut past your toes).
- Slowly return to the starting positon.

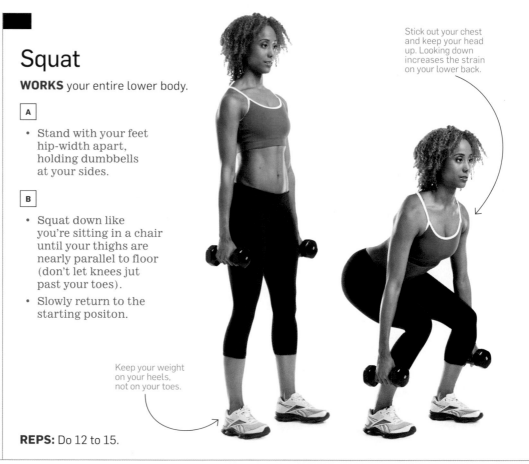

Stick out your chest and keep your head up. Looking down increases the strain on your lower back.

Keep your weight on your heels, not on your toes.

REPS: Do 12 to 15.

Chest Press

WORKS the pectoralis major, the largest muscle in the chest.

A

- Lie back on an exercise bench while holding dumbbells at arm's length over your chest.
- Your palms should be facing out, but turned slightly inward.

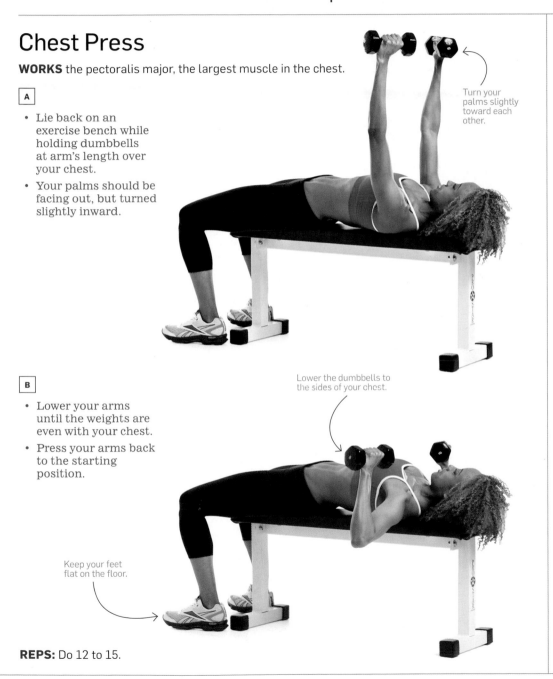

Turn your palms slightly toward each other.

Lower the dumbbells to the sides of your chest.

B

- Lower your arms until the weights are even with your chest.
- Press your arms back to the starting position.

Keep your feet flat on the floor.

REPS: Do 12 to 15.

KNOW SQUAT

A typical beginner squat mistake is bending forward, which puts too much stress on your joints and sends your weight onto your toes. To fix it: As you squat, imagine that you're sitting down into a chair. Push your hips back first instead of beginning by bending your knees, says Dan John, a strength coach in Burlingame, California. Be sure to sit back into your heels. To make that easier, pretend that you're standing on a paper towel, says Charlie Weingroff, lead physical therapist for the U.S. Marine Corps Special Operations Command at Camp Lejeune, North Carolina. "Then imagine trying to rip the towel apart by pressing your feet onto the floor and outward." This activates your glutes, which also helps you move on to heavier weights.

BONUS TIP: You can do squats without dumbbells. Follow the same form using only your bodyweight.

Basic Superfast Total-Body Workout

Bent-Over Row

WORKS your upper back, rear deltoids, and rotator cuffs.

Your lower back should be naturally arched.

Squeeze your shoulder blades toward each other.

Keep your torso still as you raise the weights.

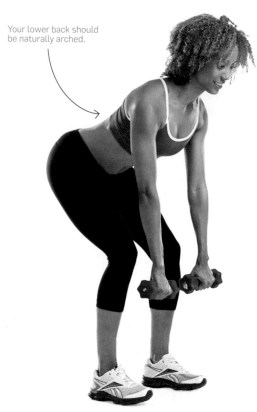

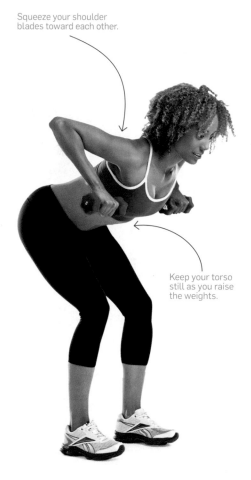

A

- Stand, grasping dumbbells at your sides.
- Bend forward from your hips until your back is nearly parallel to the floor, with your arms hanging down, palms facing backward.

REPS: Do 12 to 15.

B

- Squeeze your shoulder blades together and pull the dumbbells to your chest.
- Then lower the weights back to the starting position.

Bicycle

WORKS your rectus abdominis and obliques.

A

- Lie on your back, knees bent to 90 degrees and legs lifted so your calves are parallel to the floor.

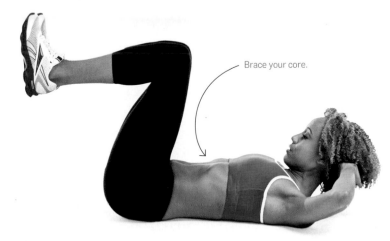

Brace your core.

B

- With your hands behind your head, lift your right shoulder off the floor and curl toward your left knee as you extend your right leg.
- Then curl toward your right knee as you bend it and extend your left leg.

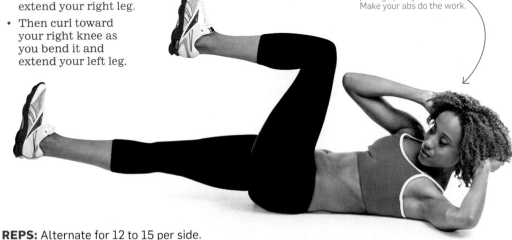

Don't stress your neck by pulling up on your head. Make your abs do the work.

REPS: Alternate for 12 to 15 per side.

RESET YOUR CLOCK

Want to work out in the morning, but can't seem to rouse yourself? Try this trick to flip your circadian switch: For 4 weeks force yourself to get up 15 minutes earlier than normal and do any type of physical activity (walking, for instance). "Make it so easy that you don't even have to change into your workout clothes," says John Raglin, PhD, an exercise researcher and professor at Indiana University Bloomington. As you near the end of the 4 weeks, you'll have a new habit and will then be able to progress to greater amounts of exercise.

High School Reunion Workout 1

Need to drop down a pants size or two in a month? These routines work their magic by challenging multiple body parts as well as balance and core stability with each move, so every major and minor muscle has to fire up to keep you moving with good form. The challenging, multimuscle moves also raise your heart rate so you burn more calories, and hone your balance to prevent injury.

START HERE:

Do these moves one after another with no rest in between. Rest for 60 seconds at the end. Then repeat the circuit once more.

Test-the-Water Squat and Biceps Curl

WORKS your biceps and entire lower body.

- This is a time-efficient combination lift. Grab a pair of 8- to 10-pound dumbbells and stand on a 1- to 2-foot-high step or bench with your feet together and your arms at your sides with your palms facing forward.
- Lift your left foot off the bench .

B

- Squat down a few inches, curling the dumbbells up to your shoulders as you squat. That's 1 rep.
- Next, lift your right foot off the bench, curling the dumbbells as you squat.

REPS: Do 12 to 15, then repeat the exercise, this time squating with your right leg.

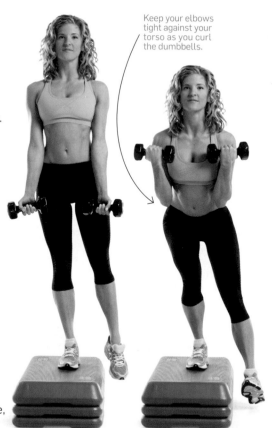

Keep your elbows tight against your torso as you curl the dumbbells.

Take a Walk

WORKS your triceps and core.

10

Optimum number of minutes for a nap. A brief snooze immediately wards off fatigue and boosts brainpower for at least 2½ hours, according to an Australian study.

Engage your core muscles.

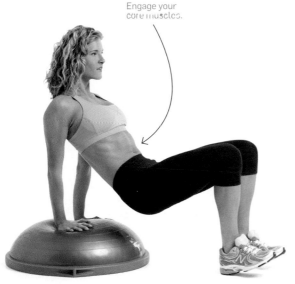

A

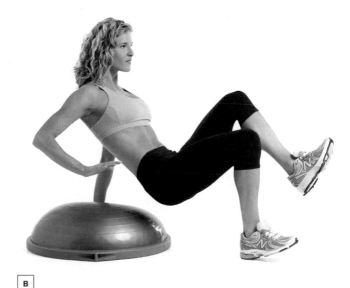

B

- Place a Bosu on the floor and sit on the dome's center. Place your palms on the dome alongside your hips with your fingertips facing forward, and position your heels on the floor about 2 feet from the base of the Bosu.
- Straighten your arms and lift your hips off the ball.

REPS: Do 15 to 20.

- Simultaneously lift both your right hand and your left foot a few inches.
- Hold for 1 second, then lower and repeat with the other hand and foot. That's 1 rep.

High School Reunion Workout 1

Rotational Lunge and Shoulder Press

WORKS your shoulders and entire lower body.

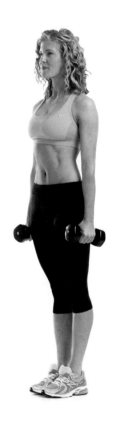

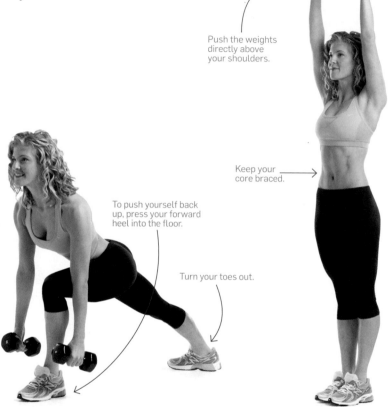

Push the weights directly above your shoulders.

Keep your core braced.

To push yourself back up, press your forward heel into the floor.

Turn your toes out.

A

- This is another combination lift. Grab a pair of 8- to 12-pound dumbbells and stand with your feet together and your arms at your sides.

B

- Take a giant step back with your right leg, landing with your toes turned out.
- Sink into a lunge until your left thigh is parallel to the floor, then lower the dumbbells and your torso until the weights are on each side of your left ankle.

C

- Straighten your left leg without locking your knee and stand up, straightening your torso and bringing your right leg forward so your legs are together.
- At the same time, press the dumbbells overhead with your palms facing each other. That's 1 rep.

REPS: Do 8 to 10, then repeat the exercise while lunging back with your left leg.

Warrior 3 Triceps Extension

WORKS your triceps, core, back, glutes, and hamstrings.

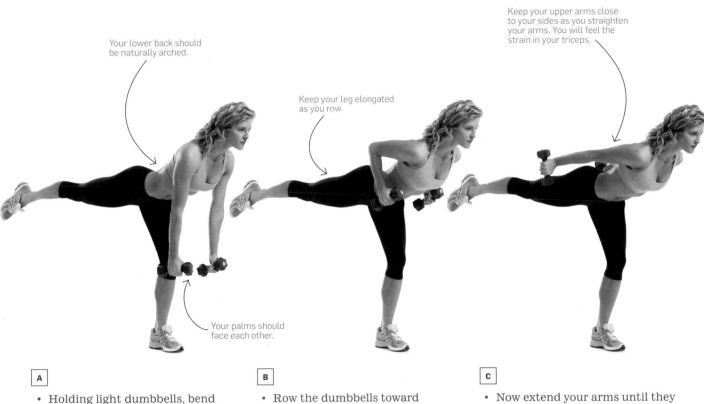

Your lower back should be naturally arched.

Your palms should face each other.

Keep your leg elongated as you row.

Keep your upper arms close to your sides as you straighten your arms. You will feel the strain in your triceps.

A

- Holding light dumbbells, bend forward. Raise your right leg behind you until your leg and torso form the top of a T and your arms hang straight down.

REPS: Do 12 to 15.

B

- Row the dumbbells toward your ribs until your elbows pass your torso.

C

- Now extend your arms until they are straight, pressing the weights backward.
- Return to a standing position, both feet on the floor. Repeat the exercise, this time raising your left leg behind you. That's 1 rep.

High School Reunion Workout 1

Plank with Front Raise

WORKS your shoulders and core.

A

- Grab a pair of lightweight dumbbells and assume a plank position with your hands on the weights directly below your shoulders and your palms facing each other.

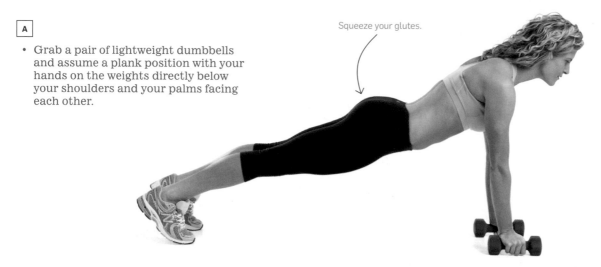

Squeeze your glutes.

B

- Brace your abs and, keeping your left arm straight, raise it in front of you to shoulder height.
- Return the weight to the floor, then repeat, raising your right arm straight in front of you while balancing on your left. That's 1 rep.

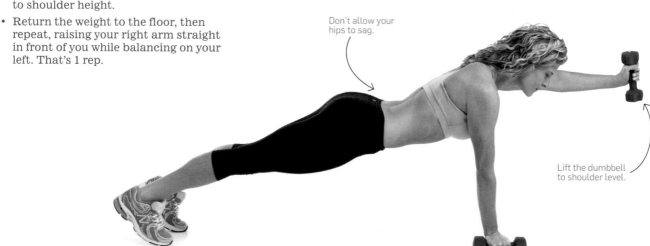

Don't allow your hips to sag.

Lift the dumbbell to shoulder level.

REPS: Do 12 to 15.

Sumo Squat Side Knee Raise and Side Crunch

WORKS your arms, core, and lower body.

⇓

> **TIP:** *Start with an 8-pound ball. Don't increase the weight until you've mastered the move with perfect form.*

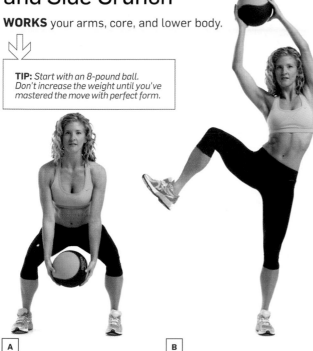

A
- Standing with your legs wider than shoulder-width apart, hold a medicine ball in front of your body.
- Squat until your thighs are almost parallel to the floor.

B
- Press back up, keeping your right knee bent. Lift the leg while rotating your hip so your inner thigh faces forward. Balance on your left leg as you lift your right leg out and up until your knee is past your hip.
- At the same time, circle the ball counterclockwise until it's above your right shoulder and crunch your upper body to the right.

REPS: Do 12 to 15, then repeat on the other side.

Lying 1-2 Punch

WORKS your core, chest, and arms.

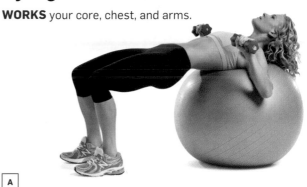

A
- Grab a dumbbell in each hand and rest your midback on a stability ball.
- Hold the dumbbells at your shoulders as if you're ready to do a chest press.

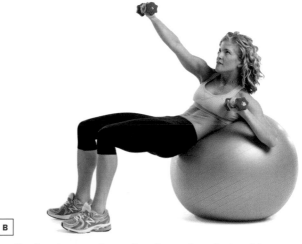

B
- Contract your abs and curl your head, shoulders, and torso off the ball. Extend your right arm across your body while twisting slightly to the left.
- Immediately lower the weight to your shoulder and repeat with the left arm while twisting slightly to the right. That's 1 rep.

REPS: Do 8 to 10.

High School Reunion Workout 2

A terrific followup to reunion workout 1, this routine focuses on the large muscles of the chest, back, and legs. Remember: Good form and quickness will help you burn more calories.

START HERE:

Do these moves one after another with no rest in between. Rest for 60 seconds at the end of the circuit. Then repeat the circuit once more.

Legs Up Pushup

WORKS your chest, arms, shoulders, and core.

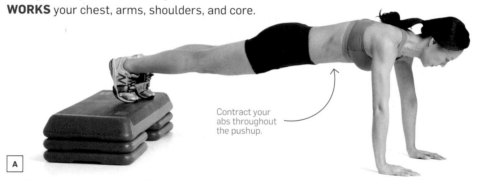

Contract your abs throughout the pushup.

A

- Assume a pushup position with your feet on a low step or sturdy stack of books propped against a wall and your hands on the floor directly below your shoulders.

WHAT IT DOES:
Researchers say this move focuses on muscles that stabilize your shoulders.

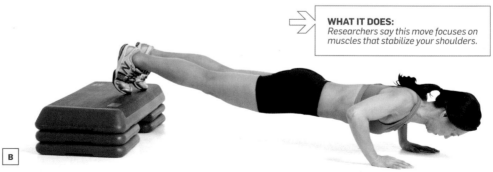

B

- Bend your elbows and lower your chest until your upper arms are parallel to the floor.
- Press back to the starting position.

REPS: Do 12 to 15.

Single-Leg Toe Touch Squat

WORKS your glutes, quads, hamstrings, and calves.

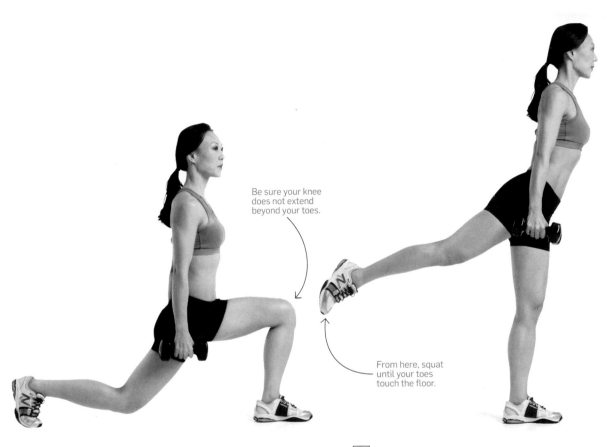

Be sure your knee does not extend beyond your toes.

From here, squat until your toes touch the floor.

A

- Grab a dumbbell in each hand and keep your arms at your sides.
- Stand in a lunge position with your left foot forward and both knees bent so your right knee grazes the floor.

B

- Stand by straightening your left leg; extend and lift your right foot off the floor behind you, pointing your toes.
- Bend your left leg into a squat while keeping your right leg extended and allowing only your toes to touch the floor. Repeat.

REPS: Do 12 to 15 with your left leg, then repeat with your right leg for just as many.

High School Reunion Workout 2

Scoop and Press

WORKS your arms, shoulders, glutes, quads, and hamstrings.

A dumbbell biceps curl with palms facing in instead of up is known as a hammer curl.

Keep your palms facing each other as you press.

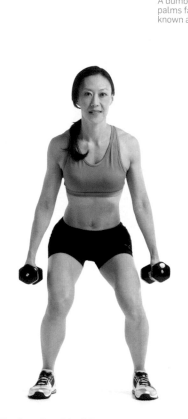

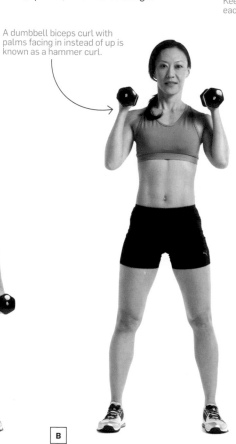

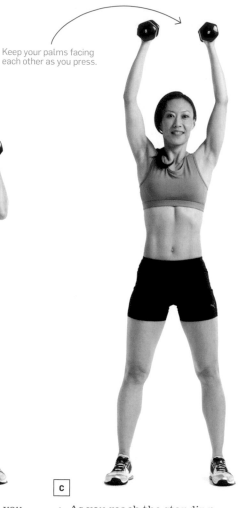

A

- Grab a dumbbell in each hand and stand with your feet hip- to shoulder-width apart.
- Your palms should face your thighs. Now bend your knees and drop your butt back as though you're sitting in a chair.

B

- Push back to stand up while you bend your elbows and curl the dumbbells, keeping your palms facing in, to your shoulders.

C

- As you reach the standing position, immediately press the weights overhead.
- Lower the dumbbells to your shoulders and then to your sides. That's 1 rep.

REPS: Do 12 to 15.

Pedal Crunch

WORKS your core.

90

Percentage of back problems that can be solved with exercise, physical therapy, and lifestyle fixes instead of with surgery, according to the American Association of Neurological Surgeons.

MAKE IT HARDER:
To turn this move into a more challenging Cycling Russian Twist, hold your arms straight out in front of you with your palms together and reach to the outside of the knee that's bent.

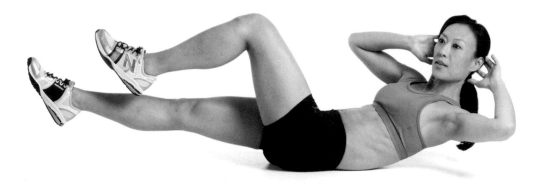

A

- Lie faceup on the floor with your feet raised, knees bent, and calves parallel to the floor.
- Place your hands loosely behind your head.
- Pull your navel to your spine and contract your abs to bring your head and shoulders off the floor.
- Twist your right shoulder toward your left knee as you straighten your right leg (extend your right arm to the outside of the knee for a bonus challenge).
- Return to the starting position and twist your left shoulder toward your right knee while straightening your left leg. That's 1 rep.

REPS: Do 12 to 15.

High School Reunion Workout 2

Curtsy Salute

WORKS your shoulders, glutes, quads, and hamstrings.

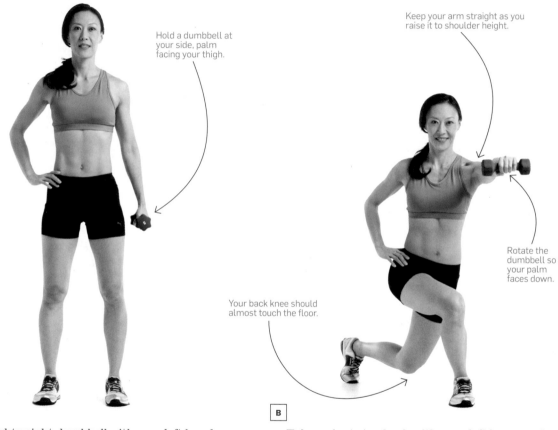

Hold a dumbbell at your side, palm facing your thigh.

Keep your arm straight as you raise it to shoulder height.

Rotate the dumbbell so your palm faces down.

Your back knee should almost touch the floor.

A

- Grab a lightweight dumbbell with your left hand and stand with your feet hip-distance apart.
- Place your right hand on your hip.

B

- Take a giant step back with your left leg, crossing it behind your right as in a curtsy.
- Bend your knees and lower your hips until your right thigh is parallel to the floor.
- At the same time, raise your left arm straight out in front of you to shoulder height. Return to the starting position.

REPS: Complete 12 to 15, then repeat the exercise with the dumbbell in your right hand and stepping back and across with your right leg for another 12 to 15 reps.

Wide Row

WORKS your biceps, shoulders, and upper back.

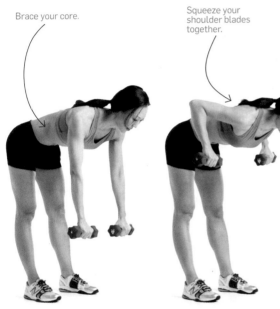

Brace your core.

Squeeze your shoulder blades together.

A

- Grab a 3- to 8-pound dumbbell in each hand. Stand straight and keep your arms at your sides, palms facing backward.

- Bend forward at the hips, allowing your arms to hang straight.

B

- Squeeze your shoulder blades together and pull the dumbbells to the sides of your ribs, then lower them to the starting position.

REPS: Do 12 to 15.

Butterfly Plié

WORKS your biceps, glutes, quads, and hamstrings.

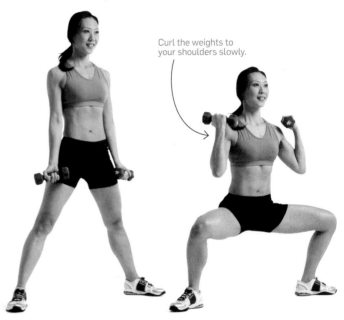

Curl the weights to your shoulders slowly.

A

- Grab a dumbbell in each hand and let your arms hang naturally at your sides, palms facing forward.

- Stand in a wide straddle stance with your toes pointed outward.

B

- Squat until your thighs are parallel to the floor. Your knees should not travel past your toes, and your butt should not dip lower than your knees.

- As you squat, bend your elbows and curl the weights toward your shoulders. Return to the starting position.

REPS: Do 12 to 15.

Bikini Body Workout 1

This program firms up those notorious flabby spots that spill out around your bikini by pairing two powerful moves in every exercise. Doing two at the same time—each targeting an unrelated muscle group—allows you to train harder without exhausting a single group too quickly, says trainer Katrina Hodgson, cofounder of Tone It Up studio in Los Angeles, who helped design this workout.

START HERE: ▇

Do these moves one after another with no rest in between. Rest for 60 seconds after completing a full circuit, then repeat the circuit once more.

Reverse Lunge with Rotation and Biceps Curl

WORKS your biceps, core, obliques, quads, hamstrings, and glutes.

A

- Hold dumbbells at your sides and stand with your feet hip-width apart.

B

- Step back with your left foot and bend both knees to lower your body until your right knee is bent to about 90 degrees.

- At the same time, rotate your upper body toward your right leg and curl the dumbbells to your chest.

- Reverse the movement by lowering the weights and rotating your chest to face forward, then return to the standing position. That's 1 rep.

- Now step back with your right foot and rotate to the left while curling.

REPS: Alternate sides for 10 to 15 per side.

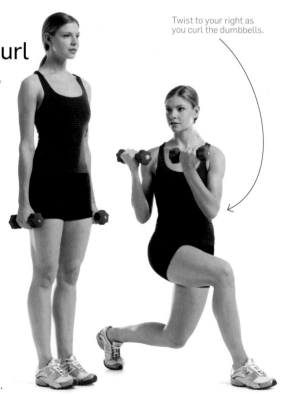

Twist to your right as you curl the dumbbells.

Deadlift to High Pull

WORKS your shoulders, upper back, hamstrings, and glutes.

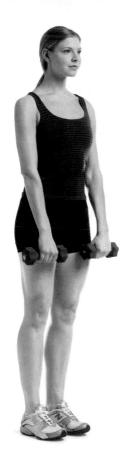

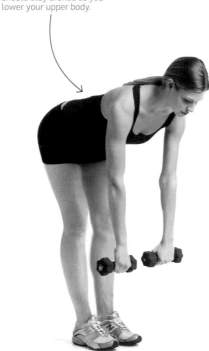

Don't round your back; it should stay arched as you lower your upper body.

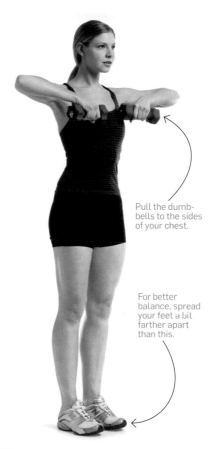

Pull the dumbbells to the sides of your chest.

For better balance, spread your feet a bit farther apart than this.

A

- Stand with your feet hip-width apart, and your knees slightly bent and hold dumbbells in front of you, with your palms facing your thighs.

REPS: Do 15.

B

- Keeping your back slightly arched and your core engaged, hinge forward at the hips and slowly lower your torso until it's almost parallel to the floor. Allow your arms to hang straight.

C

- Pause, then squeeze your glutes and push your hips forward to return to standing while pulling the dumbbells to your chest by bending your elbows out to the sides and raising your forearms.
- Return to the starting position. That's 1 rep.

Bikini Body Workout 1

Plank Hold and Single-Arm Row

WORKS your upper back, lats, shoulders, core, and glutes.

A

- Assume a pushup position with your hands gripping a pair of dumbbells; your hands should be slightly wider than shoulder-width apart and your feet slightly wider than hip-width apart.

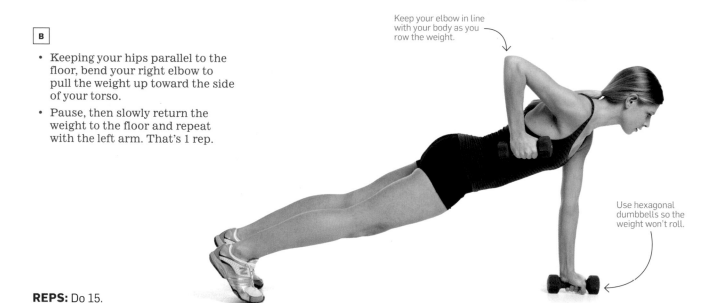

Engage your core and glutes throughout the exercise.

Your hands should be directly under your shoulders.

Keep your elbow in line with your body as you row the weight.

B

- Keeping your hips parallel to the floor, bend your right elbow to pull the weight up toward the side of your torso.
- Pause, then slowly return the weight to the floor and repeat with the left arm. That's 1 rep.

Use hexagonal dumbbells so the weight won't roll.

REPS: Do 15.

Squat with Leg Abduction and Lateral Raise

WORKS your upper back, lats, shoulders, core, and glutes.

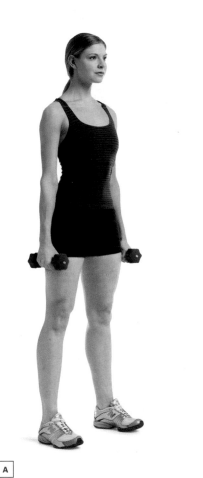

Sit your hips back to squat.

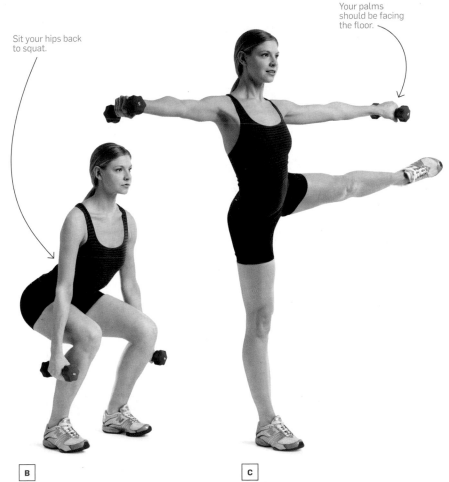

Your palms should be facing the floor.

A

- Hold a pair of dumbbells at your sides and stand with your feet shoulder-width apart.

B

- Brace your core and lower your body into a squat.

C

- As you return to standing, lift your left leg out to the side while raising your arms until they're in line with your shoulders.

REPS: Do 16 to 20, alternating lifting the right and left legs.

Bikini Body Workout 1

Hamstring Curl with Chest Press

WORKS your chest, core, glutes, and hamstrings.

A

- Hold a lightweight dumbbell in each hand and lie faceup on the floor with your calves resting on a stability ball.

- Straighten your arms and hold the dumbbells perpendicular to the floor above your chest, palms facing your knees, and raise your hips to form a straight line from shoulders to feet.

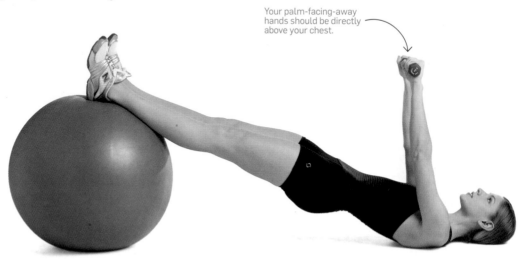

Your palm-facing-away hands should be directly above your chest.

B

- Bend your knees to roll the ball toward your butt while lowering the dumbbells to your chest.

- Reverse the movement to return to the starting position. That's 1 rep. (If you lose balance during the return, do it in two movements: First, straighten your legs, then press the weights.)

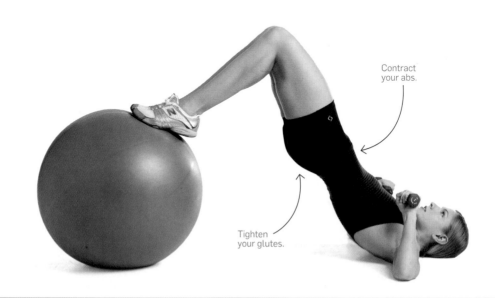

Contract your abs.

Tighten your glutes.

REPS: Do 15.

54

V Sit with Incline Press

WORKS your biceps, triceps, shoulders, upper back, core, and quads.

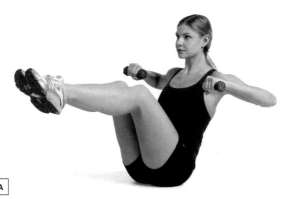

A

- Hold a pair of light dumbbells in front of your shoulders and lean back so your torso is at a 45-degree angle. Raise your lower legs until they are parallel with the floor, keeping your knees bent.

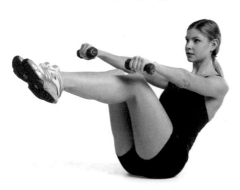

B

- Balancing in this V position, engage your core and press the dumbbells up and away from your body until your arms are straight.
- Return to the starting position. That's 1 rep.

REPS: Do 12 to 15.

Side Plank with Rear Fly

WORKS your shoulders, upper back, obliques, and core.

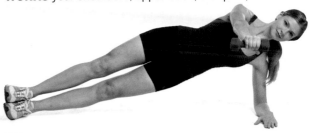

A

- Grab a dumbbell with your right hand and lie on your left side, then prop yourself up on your left forearm and raise your hips so your body forms a straight line.
- Extend the weight in front of you at shoulder level.

Resist the urge to drop or rotate your hips.

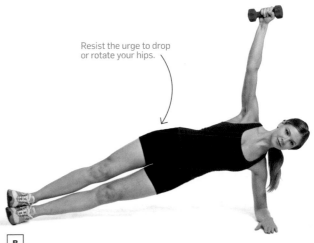

B

- Slowly raise the weight toward the ceiling, keeping your arm straight and pulling your shoulder blades together.
- Return to the starting position. That's 1 rep. Do a full set, then switch to a right side plank and lift the weight with your left arm.

REPS: Do 12 to 15 per side.

Bikini Body Workout 2

If the thought of slipping into a string bikini has you running for cover, do this workout and you'll be ready for the beach in just 4 weeks. Another combo workout, it boosts total-body tone and fixes muscular imbalances that can cause injury.

START HERE:

Do these moves one after another with no rest in between. After completing one circuit, rest for 60 seconds. Then repeat the circuit once more.

Dumbbell Thruster

WORKS your lower body and shoulders.

- Grab a pair of dumbbells and hold them, arms bent, in front of your shoulders with your palms facing each other.
- Position your feet shoulder-width apart, then quickly lower your hips until your thighs are almost parallel to the floor.

B

- Explode back up and push the dumbbells above your head until your arms are straight.
- Hold for 1 second, then lower the dumbbells as you squat back down.

REPS: Do 10 to 15.

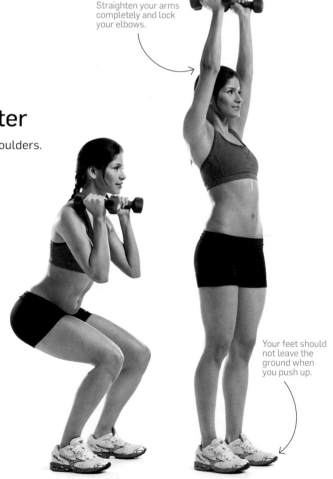

Straighten your arms completely and lock your elbows.

Your feet should not leave the ground when you push up.

Dumbbell Pushup and Row

WORKS your chest and upper back.

A

- Assume a pushup position with your arms straight, your feet slightly wider than shoulder-width, and your hands resting on a pair of dumbbells directly below your shoulders.

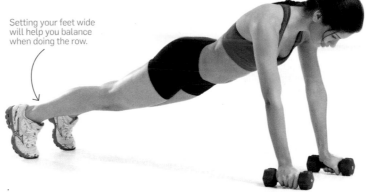

Setting your feet wide will help you balance when doing the row.

B

- Lower your body to the floor, pause, then push yourself back up.

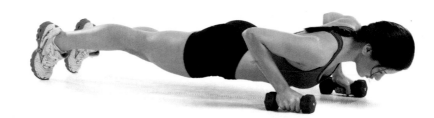

C

- Then, from the up position, lift your right elbow toward the ceiling until your elbow passes your torso.
- Lower the weight, do another pushup, then row the left dumbbell. That's 1 rep.

REPS: Do 10 to 15.

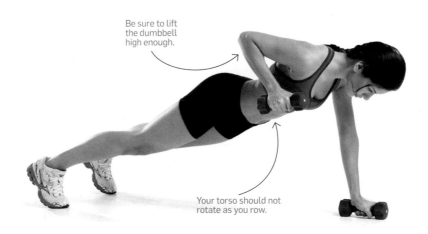

Be sure to lift the dumbbell high enough.

Your torso should not rotate as you row.

Bikini Body Workout 2

Dumbbell Reverse Lunge and Curl

WORKS your quadriceps, calves, and biceps.

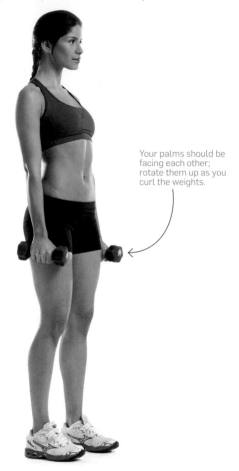

Your palms should be facing each other; rotate them up as you curl the weights.

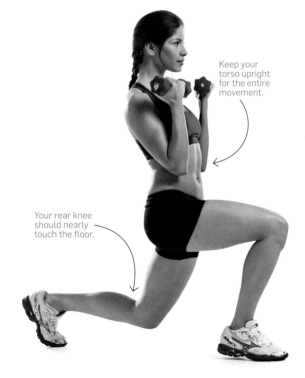

Keep your torso upright for the entire movement.

Your rear knee should nearly touch the floor.

A

- Grab a pair of dumbbells and hold them at your sides with palms facing your thighs.

REPS: Do 10 to 15.

B

- Step back about 3 feet with your left leg, simultaneously curling the dumbbells toward your shoulders as you lower your hips until your right knee is bent to 90 degrees and your left knee is just above the floor.

- Push back up and lower the dumbbells. Repeat, this time stepping back with your right leg. That's 1 rep.

Triceps Dip and Reach

WORKS your triceps and hip extensors.

FIGHT FLABBY ARMS
Most people ignore their triceps, the backsides of their upper arms. By building these muscles with dips, you'll firm and tone your arms faster than by focusing only on your biceps with curls.

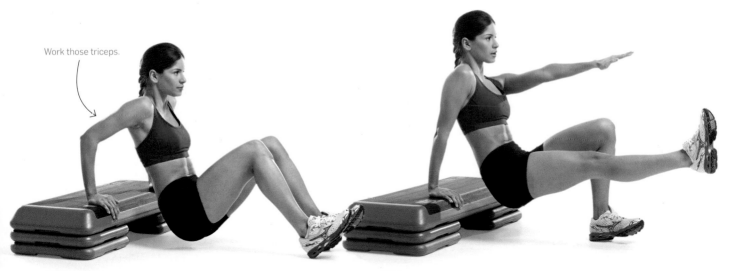

Work those triceps.

A

- Sit on the floor with your knees slightly bent and your back against a 12-inch-high step.
- Grab the edge of the step with your hands slightly more than hip-width apart.
- Push your heels into the floor as you straighten your arms. Perform a dip.

REPS: Do 10 to 15.

B

- After straightening your arms, reach your left arm straight out in front of your body at shoulder height while lifting your right leg.
- Hold for 2 seconds, then repeat, starting with a dip, then lifting the other arm and leg. That's 1 rep.

Bikini Body Workout 2

Sumo Squat

WORKS your glutes, hamstrings, and quadriceps.

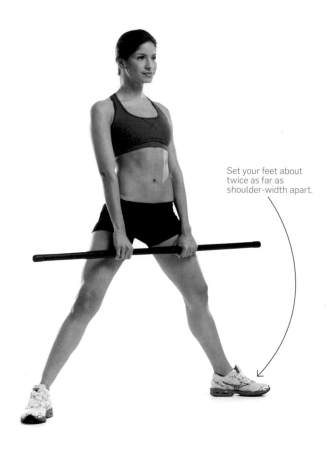

Set your feet about twice as far as shoulder-width apart.

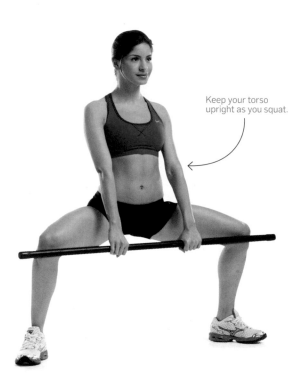

Keep your torso upright as you squat.

A

- Grab a barbell or weighted fitness bar with an overhand grip, hands shoulder-width apart.
- Position your feet wider than shoulder-width, toes pointed out to the sides, and let the bar hang a few inches in front of your thighs.

REPS: Do 10 to 15.

B

- Squat down until your thighs are parallel to the floor.
- Immediately stand back up. That's 1 rep.

Barbell Lunge and Press

WORKS your core, glutes, hamstrings, quads, shoulders, and triceps.

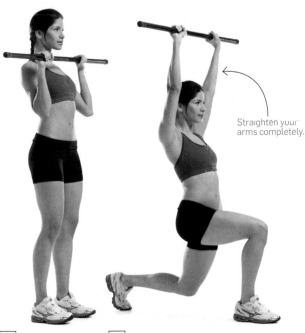

Straighten your arms completely.

A

B

- Grab a fitness bar with an overhand grip, hands shoulder-width apart.
- Keeping the bar close to your body, lift it until it's just above your collarbone.

- Lunge forward with your right foot and lower your hips until your right knee is bent to 90 degrees and your back knee is just a few inches from the floor, simultaneously pressing the bar straight overhead.
- Return to the starting position as you lower the bar. Repeat with the opposite leg. That's 1 rep.

REPS: Do 10 to 15.

Balancing Pushup and Barbell Rollout

WORKS your chest, core, shoulders, and triceps.

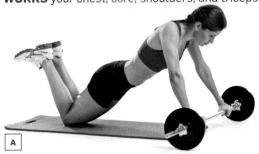

A

- Attach a 5-pound weight plate to each end of a barbell and place it on the floor. Kneel about arm's length from the bar.
- With your hands shoulder-width apart and arms straight, lean forward and grab the bar.

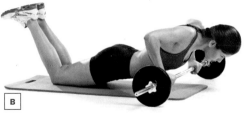

B

- Roll the bar underneath your shoulders and perform a modified pushup with your knees on the floor.

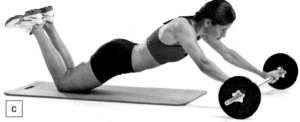

C

- Then roll the bar as far forward as you can without arching your back.
- Use your core to roll the bar back to the start position. That's 1 rep.

REPS: Do 10 to 15.

Get My Body Back Workout 1

If your once-hard body has grown soft and maybe a little saggy, these workouts will get you back to your old self fast. Routines like this one, designed by Gregory Florez of the American Council on Exercise, take classic moves like rows and squats and add unexpected twists to fire up all those stabilizing muscles in your core and extremities that become weak from disuse.

START HERE: ▬

Do these moves one after another with no rest between them. After completing 1 circuit, rest for 60 seconds, then repeat the circuit once more.

Stability Ball Back Extension

WORKS your lower back, hips, and thighs.

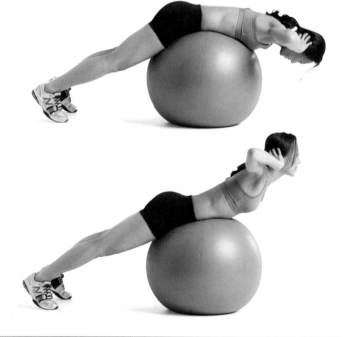

- Lie facedown on a large stability ball so it supports your pelvis.
- Keep the balls of your feet on the floor. Lightly touch your fingertips to the back of your head. (If this makes the exercise too hard, then simply hold your arms at your sides.)

- Next, tighten your glutes and gently lift your chest.
- Hold for 3 seconds, then lower to the starting position.

REPS: Do 10 to 12.

Split Jump with Bar

WORKS your lower body; builds explosive power.

TIP: *Start slowly, jump in control, and don't sink all the way into a lunge.*

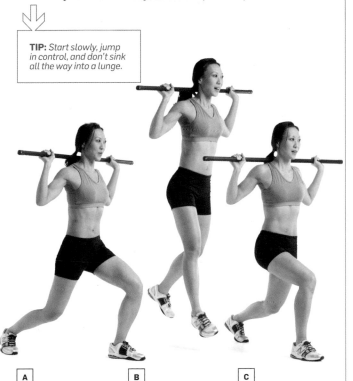

A
- Stand holding a fitness bar gently at the back of your neck, feet shoulder-width apart with the left foot 3 feet in front of the right. Bend your knees slightly.

B
- Drop your hips and then jump up, switching leg positions in the air so your right foot lands about 3 feet in front of the left.

C
- Bend your knees, then immediately jump up and switch legs again.

REPS: Alternate for 15 per side.

Stability Ball Chest Press

WORKS your chest, triceps, and core.

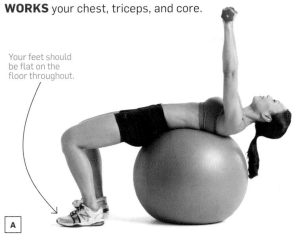

Your feet should be flat on the floor throughout.

A
- Grab a pair of dumbbells and lie on a stability ball (positioning it underneath your upper back). Raise your hips so your body forms a straight line from knees to shoulders.
- Hold the dumbbells with straight arms above your shoulders, palms facing forward.

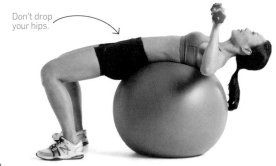

Don't drop your hips.

B
- Lower the dumbbells to the sides of your chest while using your abs to keep your body still.
- Pause, then press the weights back to the starting position.

REPS: Do 10 to 12.

Get My Body Back Workout 1

Weighted Bicycle Crunch

WORKS your core, especially the obliques.

Holding a medicine ball against your chest adds weight resistance to the crunch.

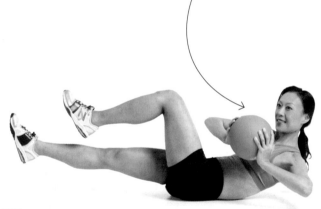

A

- Lie on your back with your knees bent. Hold a medicine ball directly on your chest.
- Curl your upper body as you lift your left leg.
- At the top of the crunch, rotate your torso so that your right elbow meets your left knee.
- Extend your right leg at the same time, as if you're pedaling.
- Return to the starting position and repeat on the other side. That's 1 rep.

REPS: Do 12.

Bosu Balance and Sit

WORKS your lower body; strengthens your ankle muscles.

CAUTION: *This is a challenging exercise and can cause injury if you lose balance. You may wish to master it without dumbbells first.*

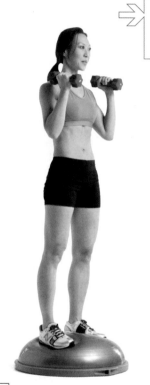

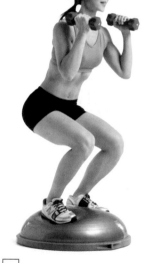

A

- Holding lightweight dumbbells at your shoulders, palms facing in, stand on a Bosu with your knees slightly bent.

B

- Keeping your back straight, bend your hips and knees and squat back until your thighs are nearly parallel to the floor.
- Pause. Then return to start and repeat.

REPS: Do 10 to 12.

Side Stepup with Triceps Kickback

WORKS your quadriceps, calves, and triceps.

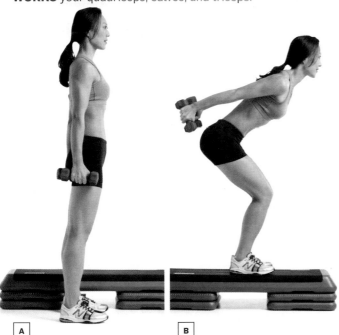

A

B

- Stand sideways next to a step, holding dumbbells with your arms in a relaxed position and your elbows slightly behind your body.

- Step laterally one foot at a time onto the step.
- Tighten your abs and lean forward slightly. Press the dumbbells behind you and straighten your arms.
- One stepup and kickback counts as 1 rep. Step down to the right and repeat.

REPS: Do 15, then repeat the exercise (15 reps) while standing to the left of the step and stepping to the right onto the platform.

Traveling Lunge with Biceps Curl and Shoulder Press

WORKS your quadriceps, calves, biceps, and shoulders.

Palms should face in at the top of the curl.

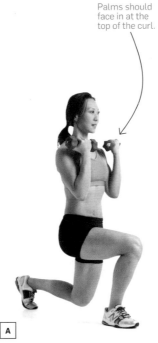

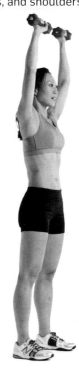

A

B

- Holding dumbbells at your sides, step forward with your right leg into a lunge.
- Make sure that your upper right leg is parallel to the floor, keeping your knee behind your toes.
- Curl the dumbbells to your chest as you sink down.

- As you rise, rotate your wrists so that your palms face forward and press the dumbbells overhead when you are in the standing position.
- Lower the dumbbells. Then repeat, stepping your left leg forward. That's 1 rep.

REPS: Do 15.

Get My Body Back Workout 2

Mix up your workouts with challenging new exercises like these to keep your muscles guessing. The routine below is especially good for firming up the butt and strengthening the core muscles that support your spine and improve your posture.

START HERE:

Do these moves one after another with no rest in between. Rest for 60 seconds. Then repeat the circuit once more.

Boat with a Twist

WORKS your core.

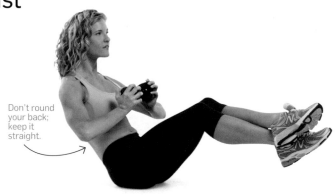

Don't round your back; keep it straight.

A

- Sit with your knees bent and hold a dumbbell by the ends in front of your chest, elbows pointed out.
- Lift your feet, cross your ankles, and lean back 45 degrees, keeping your back straight.

B

- Rotate to the right and lower the weight toward the floor.
- Immediately repeat to the left. That's 1 rep.

REPS: Do 10 to 12.

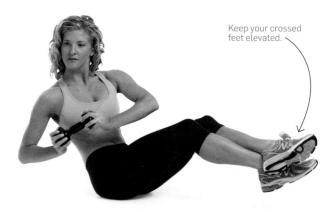

Keep your crossed feet elevated.

T Row

WORKS your back shoulders, arms, and core.

A

- Grab a dumbbell in each hand and let your arms hang at your sides, palms facing in. Stand with your feet hip-width apart.

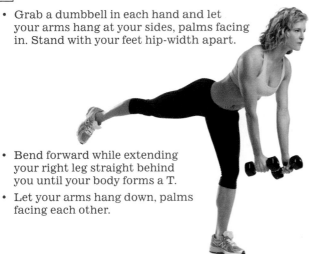

- Bend forward while extending your right leg straight behind you until your body forms a T.
- Let your arms hang down, palms facing each other.

B

- Squeeze your shoulder blades together and bring your elbows toward the ceiling.
- Return to the starting position. Do all the reps on one side, then switch legs.

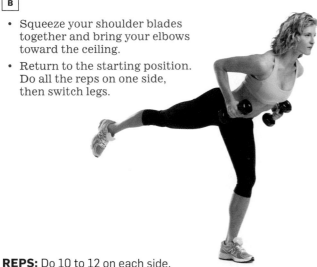

REPS: Do 10 to 12 on each side.

Hamstring Curl and Triceps Kickback

WORKS your hamstrings, glutes, and triceps.

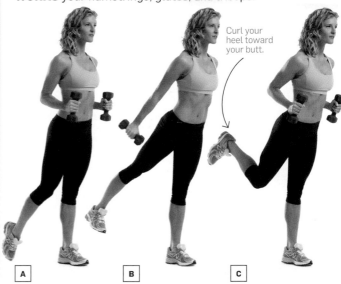

Curl your heel toward your butt.

A

- Stand and hold dumb-bells at your sides, palms facing in.
- Extend your right leg behind you, keeping your toes on the floor.
- Bend your elbows 90 degrees so that the weights are at either side of your torso.

B

- Lean your upper body slightly forward and extend your arms straight back.

C

- Bring the weights back to the starting position, while curling your right heel toward your glutes.
- Lower your leg to the starting position. That's 1 rep.

REPS: Do 5 to 6, then switch legs and repeat.

Get My Body Back Workout 2

Side Stepup and Kick

WORKS your glutes, hips, quads, and hamstrings.

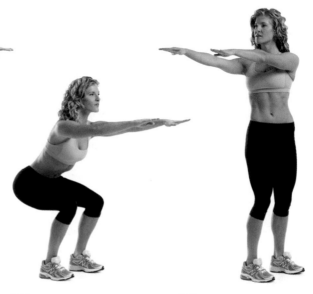

A

- Stand with your right side next to a step and hold a dumbbell in your right hand, elbow bent, weight at your shoulder, palm facing in.
- Plant your right foot on top of the step and raise your left arm straight out to the side at shoulder height, palm facing the floor, for balance.

B

- Straighten your right knee as you raise your left leg straight out in front of you to hip height, toes pointed.
- Return to the starting position.

REPS: Do 10 to 12 then repeat to the other side.

Swivel Squat

WORKS your glutes, hamstrings, quads, and core.

A

- Stand with your feet hip-width apart and raise your arms out in front of you, parallel to the floor. (To make this move more difficult, you can hold a light-weight dumbbell in your hands.)
- Sit your hips back into a squat until your thighs are parallel to the floor. Pause.

B

- Press your heels into the floor to stand while simultaneously rotating your torso and arms as far to the right as is comfortable without moving your feet.
- Rotate back to center as you dip into another squat.
- This time rotate to the left as you straighten your legs to stand. That's 1 rep.

REPS: Do 10 to 12.

Butterfly Squat and Curl

WORKS your biceps, glutes, hamstrings, and quads.

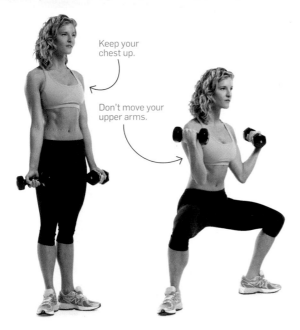

Keep your chest up.

Don't move your upper arms.

A

- Stand with your heels together, toes turned outward to least 45 degrees.
- Hold a dumbbell in each hand by your thighs, palms facing forward.

B

- Take a giant step to the left and squat down, keeping your knees aligned with your toes.
- Simultaneously, bend your elbows, rotating your arms out to the sides as you do, and curl the weights up to the sides of your shoulders.
- Return to the starting position and repeat, this time stepping to the right side. That's 1 rep.

REPS: Do 10 to 12.

Front Loaded Split Squat

WORKS your glutes, hamstrings, and quads.

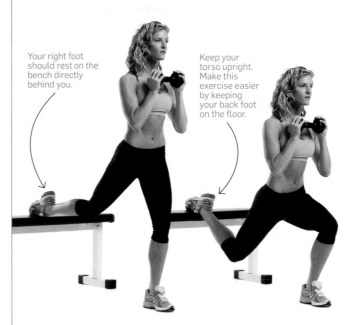

Your right foot should rest on the bench directly behind you.

Keep your torso upright. Make this exercise easier by keeping your back foot on the floor.

A

- Stand with your back facing a bench that's 2 to 3 feet behind you and hold a dumbbell by the ends in front of your chest, your elbows bent.
- Swing your right leg back and place the top of your foot on the bench.

B

- Keeping your abs tight and your back straight and tall, bend your left leg and lower your hips toward the floor until your front thigh is nearly parallel to the floor.
- Press back to the starting position.

REPS: Do 10 to 12, then repeat the exercise with your right leg forward.

Stress-Busting Workout 1

Send stress packing with these four explosive moves created by Kim Blake, a trainer at Nike World Headquarters Sports Center in Portland, Oregon. You'll push your bodyweight off the floor and then absorb it when you land.

START HERE:

Do these moves one after another, resting for 15 seconds between exercises. When you've finished all four, rest for a minute, then repeat the circuit two more times.

Runner's Lunge to Knee Skip

WORKS your quadriceps and calves; builds explosive power.

A

- Start in a pushup position, then bend your right knee and place your right foot between your hands.

B

- Push through your right foot, raise your torso, and drive your left knee and right arm into the air, hopping off the floor.
- Return to the starting position, then place your left foot between your hands and hop with your right leg. That's 1 rep.

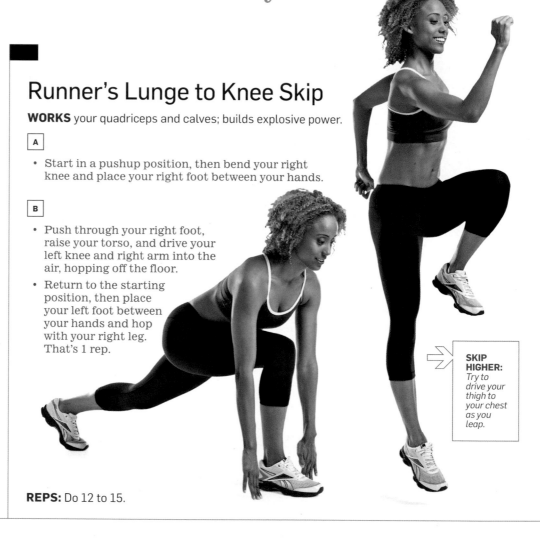

SKIP HIGHER: *Try to drive your thigh to your chest as you leap.*

REPS: Do 12 to 15.

Plié Jumping Jacks

WORKS your upper and lower body and heart.

A

- Stand with your hands at your sides and your feet hip-width apart.
- Now bend your knees and jump into the air, bringing your arms overhead and spreading your feet wide, knees and toes turned out.

B

- Land lightly and lower yourself into a squat.
- Quickly jump back to the starting position. That's 1 rep.

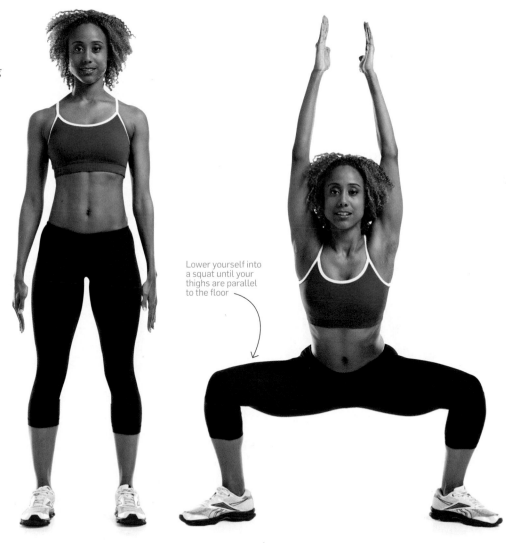

Lower yourself into a squat until your thighs are parallel to the floor

REPS: Do 12 to 15.

Stress-Busting Workout 1

Quarter-Turn Squat Jump

WORKS your quads, calves, glutes, and lower back.

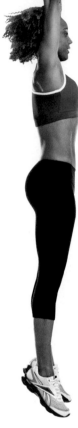

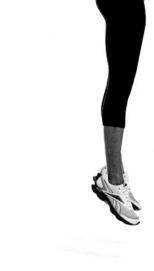

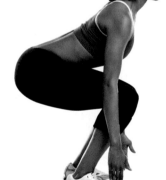

 TIP: *This also is a good warmup exercise to improve mobility and prep muscles for any activity.*

A

- With your feet shoulder-width apart, lower into a squat, and bring your arms toward the floor. Then jump up, swinging your arms overhead and rotating yourself 90 degrees to the left while in the air.

REPS: Do 12 to 16.

B

- Land softly and lower into a squat, then jump up and rotate to the right. That's 1 rep.

Donkey Kick

WORKS your shoulders, glutes, and hamstrings.

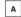

- Start in a pushup position, legs extended directly behind you and hands under your shoulders.

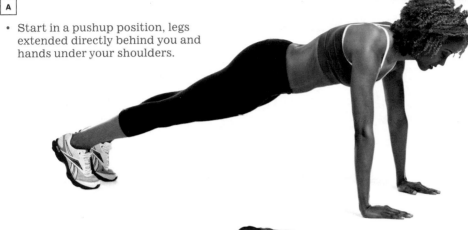

B

- With your legs together, brace your core and glutes, then kick both legs into the air, bending your knees to bring your feet toward your butt.

- As your lower body descends, straighten your legs and try to land softly on the balls of your feet. That's 1 rep.

REPS: Do 12 to 16.

Stress-Busting Workout 2

Martial-arts-style maneuvers are much more than self-defense. Launching fierce jabs and kicks is a great stress blaster. As a sweet side benefit, this workout boosts your metabolism and sculpts your arms, shoulders, abs, thighs, and butt into a stunning (and serene) physique. Enjoy all these killer body benefits—and Zenlike mental state— with this series of fighter-inspired moves.

START HERE:

Perform as many reps as you can in 60 seconds (or as indicated), then move to the next exercise. Continue until you've completed all seven moves. Rest for 60 seconds, then repeat the entire circuit.

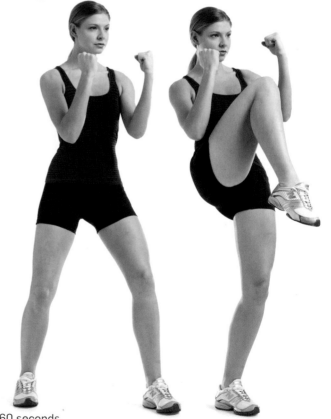

Knee Thrust

WORKS your hip flexors and other core muscles.

- Stand with your feet in a left-foot lead stance (left foot at the front left corner of an imaginary square, right foot at the back right corner), knees slightly bent, fists in front of your chin, palms facing in.

- Quickly raise your right knee toward your chest, drive it back down, and without changing your left-foot lead stance, do the same with your left leg.

REPS: Do as many as you can in 60 seconds.

Squat Thrust with Knee Thrust

WORKS your quads, glutes, and hip flexors.

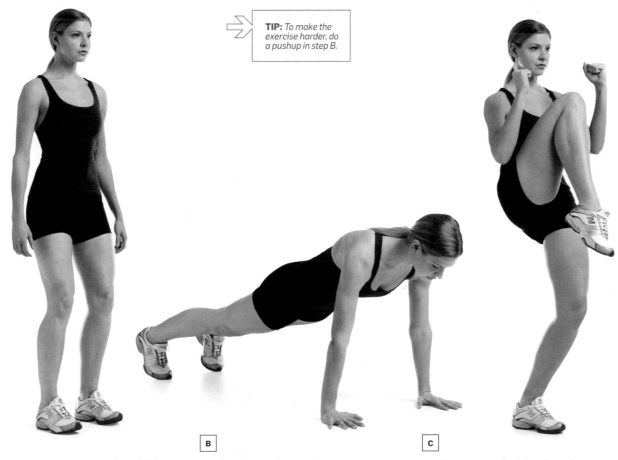

TIP: *To make the exercise harder, do a pushup in step B.*

A

- Stand with your feet hip-width apart, your arms at your sides.

REPS: Do as many as you can in 60 seconds.

B

- Bend your knees, lower your hands to the floor, and jump both feet back so you're in a pushup position.

C

- Jump your feet back up to your hands, quickly stand up, then bend your right knee and pull it up toward your chest.
- Return to the starting position, then do another squat thrust and a knee thrust with the left leg. Keep alternating this way.

Stress-Busting Workout 2

Speed Jump Rope

WORKS your calves, quads, and heart.

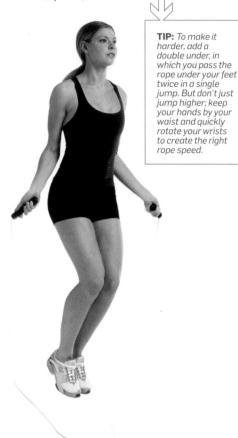

TIP: To make it harder, add a double under, in which you pass the rope under your feet twice in a single jump. But don't just jump higher; keep your hands by your waist and quickly rotate your wrists to create the right rope speed.

A

- Hold the ends of a jump rope with your feet hip-width apart and your knees slightly bent.
- Push off the floor with the balls of your feet and point your toes downward while making small circles with your wrists.
- Land softly on your toes, immediately pushing off again. Focus on jumping over the rope as quickly as possible.

REPS: Jump for 60 seconds.

Situp with Punch

WORKS your rectus abdominis and obliques.

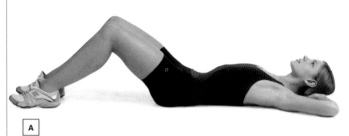

A

- Lie on your back with your knees bent and feet flat on the floor.

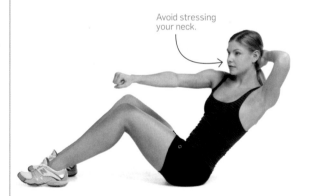

Avoid stressing your neck.

B

- Brace your abs, sit up, and punch across your body six times with one arm.
- Return to the starting position; repeat with the opposite arm.

REPS: Do as many as you can in 60 seconds.

Front Kick

WORKS your hip flexors and quads.

TIP: *Slow it down! Your underused hip flexor muscles will have to work that much harder to control the movement.*

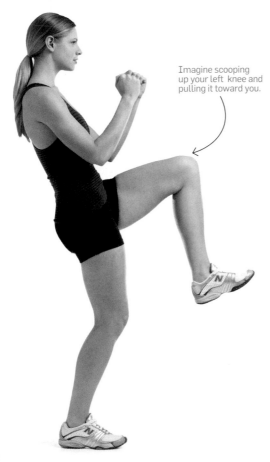

Imagine scooping up your left knee and pulling it toward you.

A

- Stand with your feet in a left-foot lead stance, fists at chin height.
- Raise your left knee toward your chest.

REPS: Do as many as you can in 60 seconds.

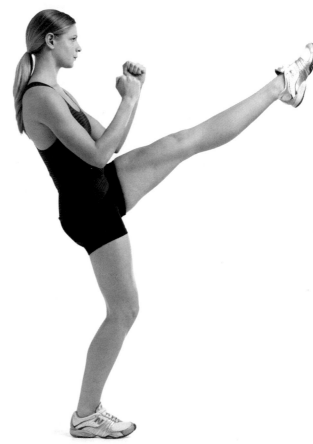

B

- Then kick straight out as if you're slamming a door closed with your heel.
- Quickly bring your leg back, placing it staggered behind your right. Repeat with your right leg, then continue alternating.

Stress-Busting Workout 2

Spiderman Pushup

WORKS your chest and obliques; enhances your hips' mobility.

Keep your back flat
and brace your core.

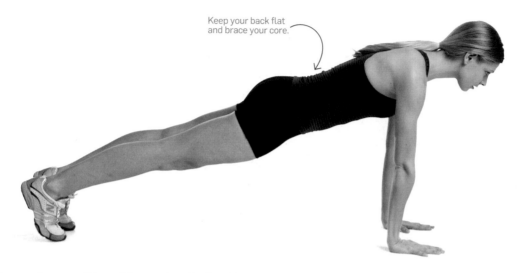

A

- Start in a pushup position with your hands directly under your shoulders.

Try to touch your
knee to your elbow.

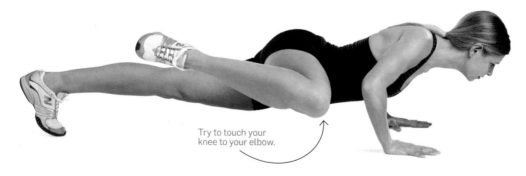

B

- As you lower your chest to the floor, turn your right knee outward and bring it toward your elbow.
- Slowly return to the starting position and repeat with the left leg. If the regular pushup position is too difficult, try doing Spiderman Pushups from your knees instead.

REPS: Do as many as you can, alternating legs, in 60 seconds.

Side Kick

WORKS your back, quads, shoulders, and hip flexors and abductors.

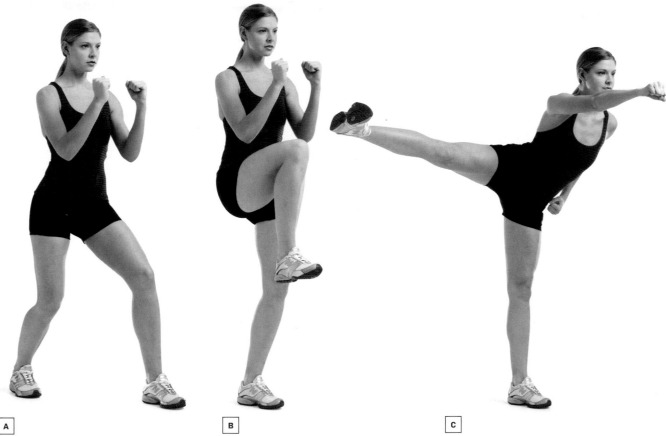

A
- Stand in a left-foot lead stance with your knees slightly bent and your fists up.

B
- Raise your right knee and pull your thigh toward your chest.

C
- Rotate your hips and right foot and kick your right leg to the side, pushing through the heel, while punching with your right arm.
- Quickly bring your right leg down, placing it staggered in front of your left.
- Repeat the kick with your left leg, punching with your left arm. Continue alternating sides.

REPS: Do as many as you can in 60 seconds, alternating sides.

Mood-Lifting Workout

Sometimes what your body needs most is to feel calm and content. Recent research shows that yoga poses can reduce fatigue and adjust the level of the stress hormone cortisol—too little of which can zap your energy. This sequence of poses engages your core muscles and energizes your system from the inside out. These poses challenge your balance, which sharpens your focus. They require deep, even breathing, which increases your oxygen intake to help you feel more alert and alive. Stretching also relieves those tightened muscles and leaves you feeling limber, relaxed, and happier when you're done.

1-Minute Warmup

Scrap your preexercise stretching routine for this dynamic yoga flow. "Warmups should involve flowing, gentle movements to get blood pumping," says Sara Ivanhoe, instructor at YogaWorks in Santa Monica, California. This Chair Pose Vinyasa Warmup sequence works the whole body. Hold each part of the move for one deep breath.

DO IT: Stand with your feet hip-width apart and lace your fingers behind the small of your back, keeping your arms straight. Drop your head back as if you're doing a mini-backbend. Next, exhale and bend forward as far as you can while stretching your still-laced fingers toward the ceiling. Release your hands, swinging them down in front of you. Bend your knees about 45 degrees and lift your chest, raising your arms above your head so they're in line with your ears, palms facing each other. Repeat the sequence 10 times.

START HERE:

Do each of these moves in order, holding the poses for 10 deep breaths (about 60 seconds). Repeat the sequence on the other side of your body, and continue alternating until you've done the pose twice on each side.

Modified Down-Dog Split

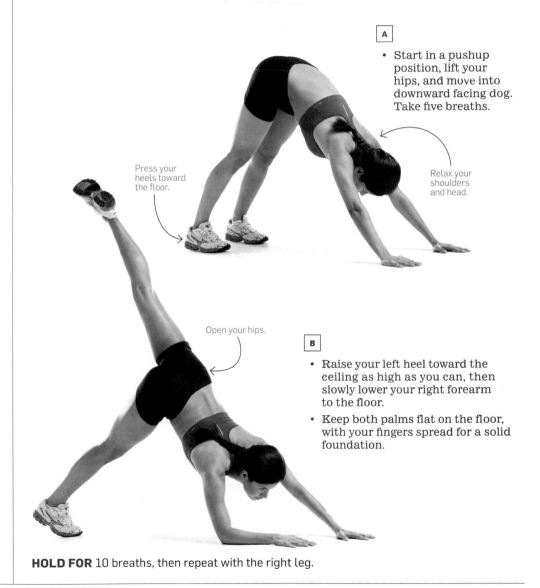

A

- Start in a pushup position, lift your hips, and move into downward facing dog. Take five breaths.

Press your heels toward the floor.

Relax your shoulders and head.

Open your hips.

B

- Raise your left heel toward the ceiling as high as you can, then slowly lower your right forearm to the floor.
- Keep both palms flat on the floor, with your fingers spread for a solid foundation.

HOLD FOR 10 breaths, then repeat with the right leg.

Mood-Lifting Workout

Warrior 3

It will be easier to square your hips if you flex this foot so your toes are pointing straight down.

Reach your arms straight forward past your ears.

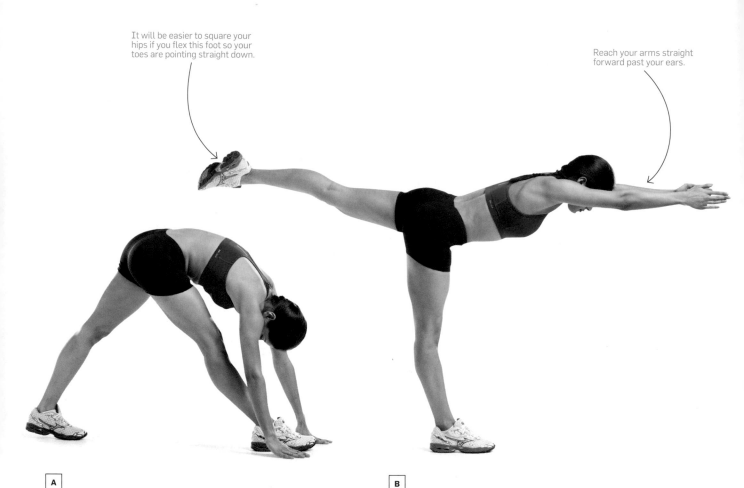

A

- From Modified Down-Dog Split, lower your leg, straighten your arm, and bring one foot between your hands.

B

- Shift your weight onto the foot between your hands as you raise your opposite leg.
- At the same time, raise your torso until it is parallel to the floor and reach your arms forward.

HOLD FOR 10 breaths, then repeat the pose while lifting your other leg.

Modified Half-Moon Arch

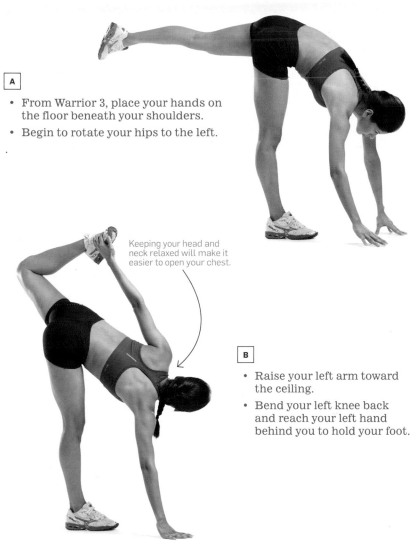

A

- From Warrior 3, place your hands on the floor beneath your shoulders.
- Begin to rotate your hips to the left.

Keeping your head and neck relaxed will make it easier to open your chest.

B

- Raise your left arm toward the ceiling.
- Bend your left knee back and reach your left hand behind you to hold your foot.

HOLD FOR 10 breaths, then repeat with your opposite leg and arm.

Tree

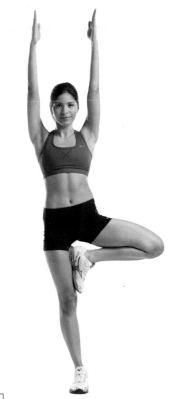

A

- From Modified Half-Moon Arch, turn your hips and shoulders back toward the floor, then use your core muscles to roll your body up to standing.
- Place the sole of your left foot on your right inner thigh.
- Lift your arms straight up above your shoulders.

HOLD FOR 10 breaths, then raise your right foot.

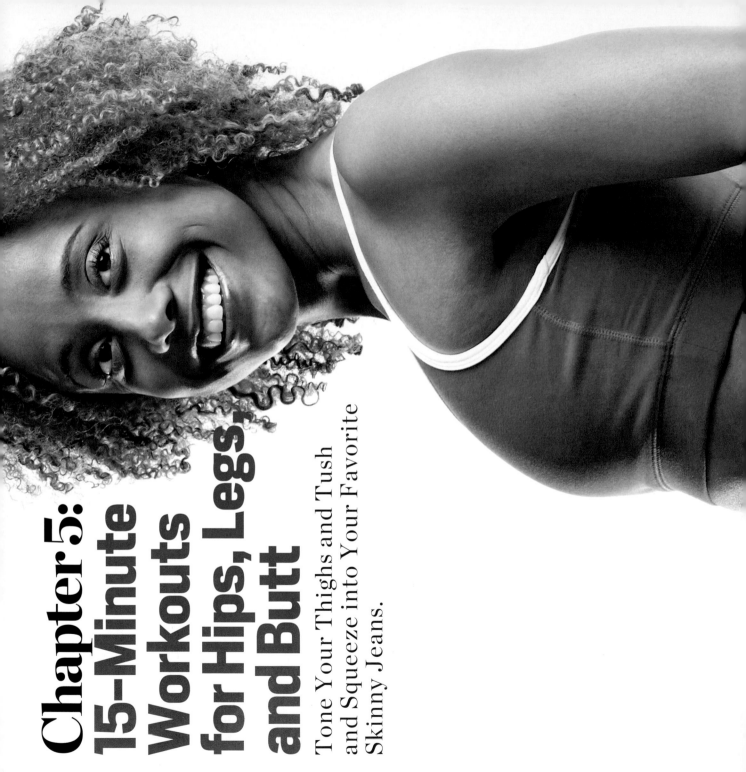

Chapter 5: 15-Minute Workouts for Hips, Legs, and Butt

Tone Your Thighs and Tush and Squeeze into Your Favorite Skinny Jeans.

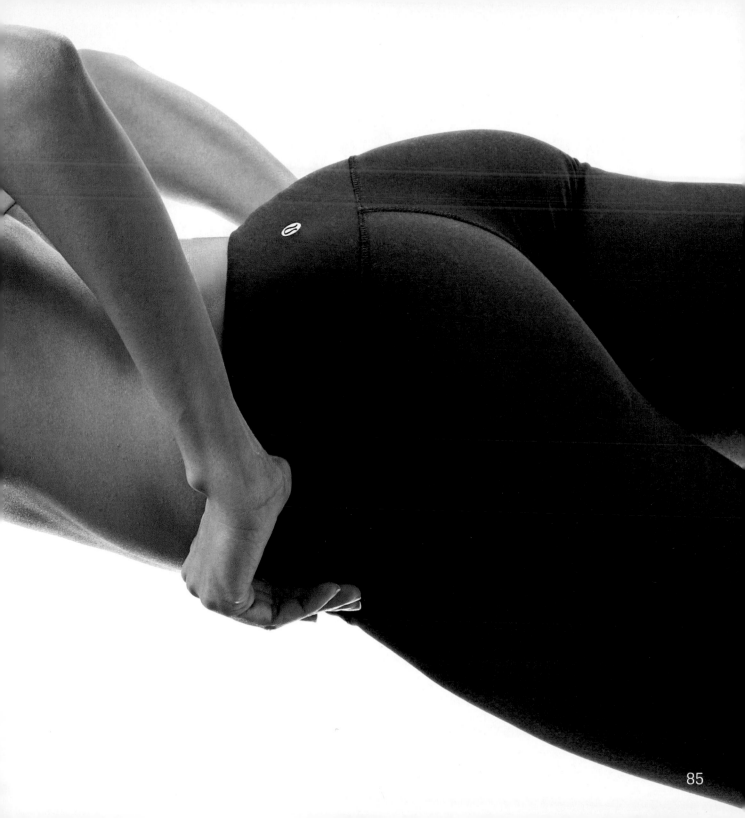

Superfast Love-Your-Lower-Body Workouts

It's the region most of us love to hate—our hips, thighs, backsides, even our calves. Not surprising, really, when you consider that as women we're predisposed to deposit fat below the belt so we have energy reserves in case of famine. Combine that with the fact that we spend so much time sitting on our God-given pantry, and is it any wonder we have to keep buying new pants? For a lower body you'll love in your skinny jeans, you need to do two things: burn fat, and target your tush with toning exercises to lift and firm it from every angle.

Begin with the basics...

For the best results from these workouts, choose one (or more) to do 2 days a week. Be sure to leave a day of rest between workouts so your muscles can recover. (And you can always piggyback any of these routines on another 15-minute workout for an überbody blast.) Do the prescribed number of reps and circuits while using a weight at which you can barely eke out the last rep of each exercise's final set with perfect form. If your form suffers, use a lighter weight until you become stronger.

Find It Quick: Your 15-Minute Legs and Butt Circuit Plan

MUSCLE MAGIC

Your legs do more than help you climb stairs and get out of a chair. Strengthening the muscles of the front of the thigh (quadriceps), inner thigh (hip adductors), the butt (the gluteus maximus, medius, and minimus), hamstrings, and calves can also help you lose weight and even girdle your tummy. For one, this is the largest muscle group of your body, and as such it burns a ton of calories. Squats and lunges are among the most efficient exercises for negating calories because they engage such a large area of tissue, including core muscles. And when you strengthen your glutes and lower back muscles you naturally pull your lower abdomen in, de-emphasizing that problematic pooch.

Tighter Tush Workout

If you're carrying a bit more junk in your trunk than you'd like, chances are good that you've got a few pounds to lose. There's no getting around eating right and scorching calories, and this workout will help. It puts your whole body in motion to crank your metabolism and hits those glutes from every angle to firm and shrink your bottom line.

START HERE: ▮

Do these moves one after another with no rest in between. Then repeat the circuit for a total of two rounds.

Grand Plié Squat

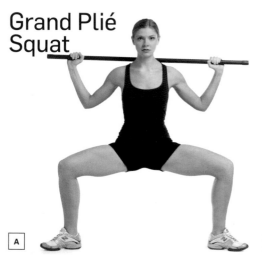

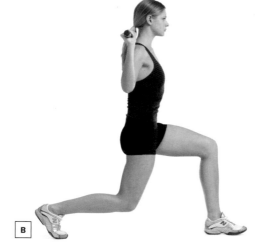

A

- Grab a 15- to 20-pound fitness bar with an overhand grip, your hands wider than shoulder-width apart.
- Rest the bar across your shoulder blades and position your legs wider than shoulder-width apart with your toes turned out.
- Squat until your thighs are parallel to the floor.

REPS: Do 12 to 15.

B

- From the squatting position rotate your entire body 90 degrees to the left by pivoting on the balls of both feet.
- Return to the center, stand, and squat again, this time rotating to the right. That's 1 rep.

Curtsy Squat Rear Leg Lift

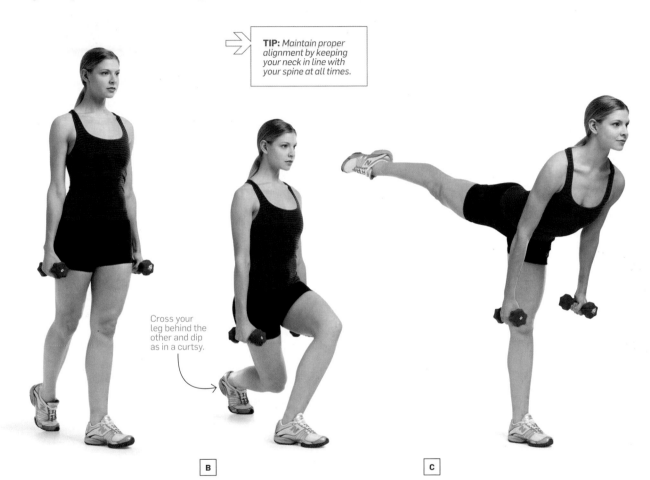

TIP: *Maintain proper alignment by keeping your neck in line with your spine at all times.*

Cross your leg behind the other and dip as in a curtsy.

A

- Grab a pair of dumbbells and stand with your feet hip-width apart, arms at your sides.
- Cross your right leg behind your left, slightly to the left of your left heel, and rest your toe on the floor about 2 feet behind you.

B

- Keeping your right heel up, squat down as far as you can without letting your left knee extend past your toes.

C

- Straighten your left leg and raise your right leg as high as possible behind you, lowering your torso toward the floor. Return to the starting position.

REPS: Do 12 to 15 and then repeat on the other side.

Tighter Tush Workout

Prone Hip Extension

A

- Lie facedown lengthwise over a bench or padded stool with your legs hanging off the edge.

Your hips should rest on the bench, your upper thighs hanging off.

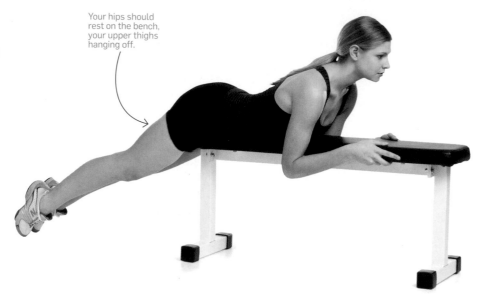

Squeeze your glutes.

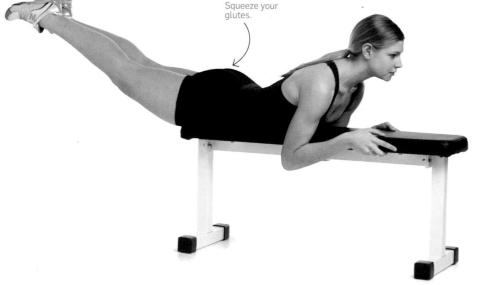

B

- Engage your abs and lift both legs until your body forms a straight line. Then slowly raise your legs higher, as comfort allows.

- Hold for 5 seconds, and then lower slowly. That's 1 rep.

REPS: Do 10 to 12.

Skater's Stepup

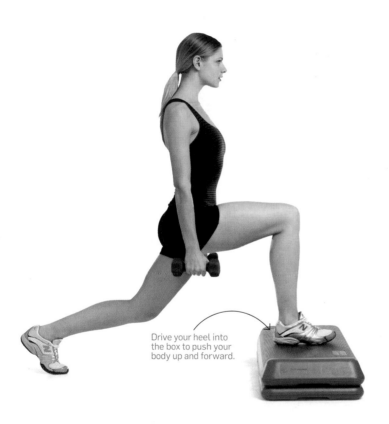

Drive your heel into the box to push your body up and forward.

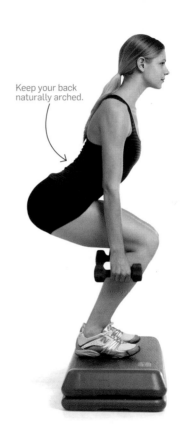

Keep your back naturally arched.

A

- Hold a pair of 5- to 15-pound dumbbells at hip level and stand facing a step with your right foot planted on the step.

- Leaning your chest forward slightly, lunge backward with your left leg, bending your right knee to 90 degrees.

REPS: Do 10 to 12 on each leg.

B

- From that position, bring your left foot up to meet the right on the step; squat and hold for 2 seconds.

- Stand and return to the starting position. That's 1 rep. Repeat with the other leg.

Tighter Tush Workout

Facedown Hip External Rotation

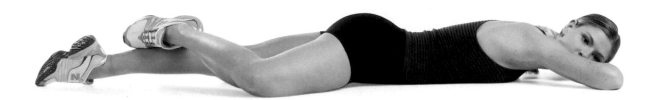

A

- Lie facedown on the floor with your arms folded under your head, legs extended straight behind you.
- Bend your right leg, knee pointed out and resting on the floor, and place your foot on the back of your left knee, keeping both hips on the floor.

TIP: *Don't let the look of this one fool you: It is one of the most challenging and effective moves for targeting your external hip muscles, which have a major impact on your glutes.*

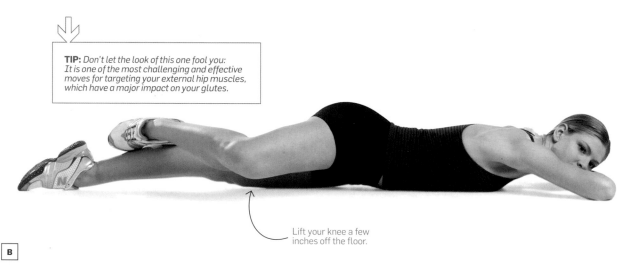

Lift your knee a few inches off the floor.

B

- Contract your right butt cheek and lift your right knee a few inches off the floor while trying to keep your hip down.
- Pause, then return to the starting position.

REPS: Complete 12 to 15 with each leg.

Squat Thrust

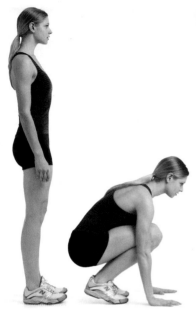

A
- Stand with your feet together, arms at your sides.

B
- Bend your knees and place your palms on the floor in front of your feet with your arms along the outsides of your knees and shift your weight onto your palms.

For more challenge, do a pushup here.

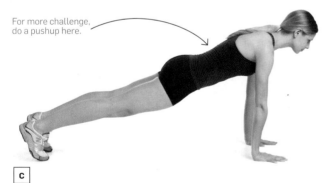

C
- Using your arms for support, jump both feet back and land in a plank position.
- Jump both feet forward, returning to the B position. Return to standing. That's 1 rep.

REPS: Do 12 to 15.

Dumbbell Straight-Leg Deadlift

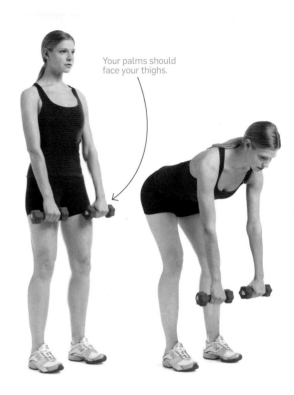

Your palms should face your thighs.

A
- Grab 5- to 8-pound dumbbells and hold them in front of your thighs, palms facing backward, feet hip-width apart, knees slightly bent.

B
- Bend at your hips to lower your torso until it's almost parallel to the floor. Allow the dumbbells to hang.
- Return to standing, keeping the weights close to your body (as if you're shaving your legs with the dumbbells). That's 1 rep.

REPS: Do 8 to 10.

I-Need-Some-Lift-in-My-Levis Workout

Are your apple cheeks a bit absent? Whether you have a naturally flat fanny or your seat is sagging from too much office chair sitting, you can round out your rear view with exercises that call all your butt muscles into action, from the beefy gluteus maximus to the often overlooked gluteus medius and minimus.

START HERE:

Do these moves one after another with no rest in between. Then repeat the circuit for a total of two rounds.

1 and ¼ Barbell Squat

A

- Place a barbell across your upper back and stand with your feet hip-width apart, palms facing forward.

B

- Lower your hips by bending at the knees until your thighs are parallel to the floor.
- Push back up a quarter of the way.
- Pause before going back down to parallel. Pause again, then return to start. That's 1 rep.

Pause here at a quarter of the way before both going lower and standing up straight.

REPS: Do 12 to 15.

Front Lunge Push Off

TIP: *Contract your glutes and look straight ahead to maintain your balance.*

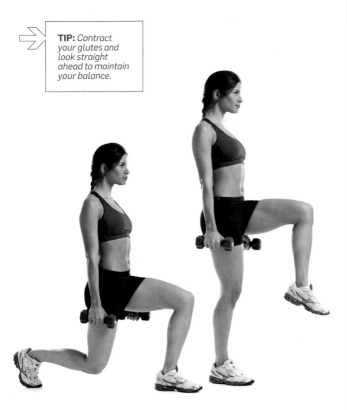

A

- Grab a pair of 10- to 15-pound dumbbells and stand with your feet together and your arms at your sides.
- Leading first with your left foot, lunge forward and lower your hips until both knees form 90-degree angles.

B

- With your right leg, pull yourself back to standing as you raise your left leg until your thigh is parallel to the floor.
- Balance on your right leg for 1 second, then return to the starting position.

REPS: Do 12 to 15 with each leg forward and lifted.

Sumo Squat and Leg Raise

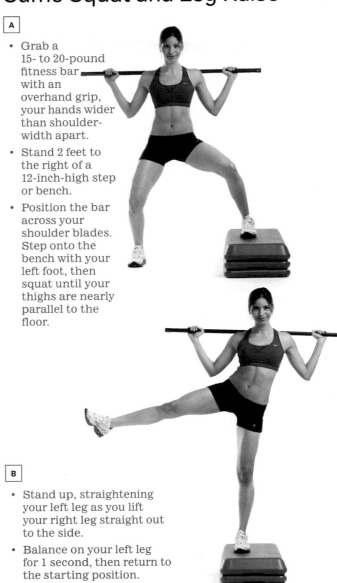

A

- Grab a 15- to 20-pound fitness bar with an overhand grip, your hands wider than shoulder-width apart.
- Stand 2 feet to the right of a 12-inch-high step or bench.
- Position the bar across your shoulder blades. Step onto the bench with your left foot, then squat until your thighs are nearly parallel to the floor.

B

- Stand up, straightening your left leg as you lift your right leg straight out to the side.
- Balance on your left leg for 1 second, then return to the starting position.

REPS: Do 12 to 15, then repeat on the other side.

95

I-Need-Some-Lift-in-My-Levis Workout

Hip Bridge and Heel Drag

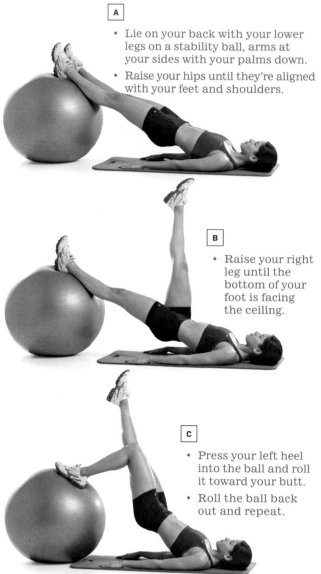

A
- Lie on your back with your lower legs on a stability ball, arms at your sides with your palms down.
- Raise your hips until they're aligned with your feet and shoulders.

B
- Raise your right leg until the bottom of your foot is facing the ceiling.

C
- Press your left heel into the ball and roll it toward your butt.
- Roll the ball back out and repeat.

REPS: Keeping your hips lifted, repeat the rolling motion 12 to 15 times. Repeat with the other leg.

Alternate-Leg Deadlift

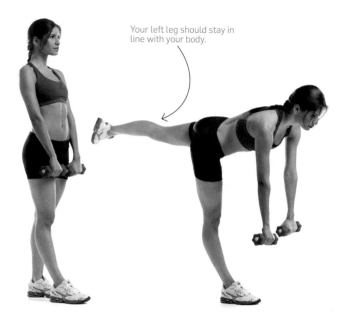

Your left leg should stay in line with your body.

A
- Hold a 5- to 15-pound dumbbell in each hand and stand with your right foot in front of your left.

B
- Lean forward from your hips and raise your left leg behind you until your body is almost parallel to the floor and the weights are in line with your shoulders.
- Return to the starting position. That's 1 rep.

REPS: Do 12, then repeat with the opposite leg lifted.

Dumbbell Stepup Press Back

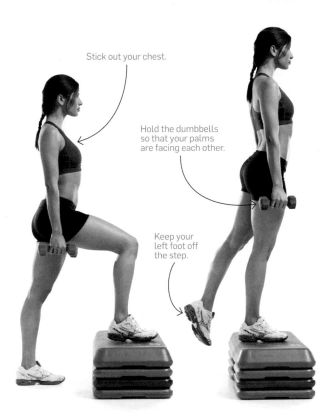

Stick out your chest.

Hold the dumbbells so that your palms are facing each other.

Keep your left foot off the step.

A

- Grab a pair of 5- to 10-pound dumbbells, stand in front of a bench or step, and place your right foot firmly on the step.

B

- Press down with your right heel and push your body up until your right leg is straight.
- Slowly lower back to the starting position. That's 1 rep.

REPS: Do 10 to 12 reps with the right leg, then repeat with the left.

Glute Bridge March

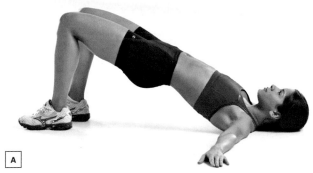

A

- Lie on your back with your knees bent and your feet flat on the floor. Rest your arms on the floor, palms down, at shoulder level.
- Raise your hips so your body forms a straight line from your shoulders to your knees.

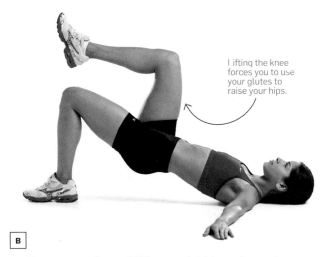

Lifting the knee forces you to use your glutes to raise your hips.

B

- Brace your abs and lift your right knee toward your chest.
- Hold for 2 counts, then lower your right foot. Repeat with the other leg. That's 1 rep.

REPS: Do 5 to 10.

So Long, Saddlebags Workout

If your butt looks a bit like a bleeding heart, spilling out too much on the sides, your outer thighs need some special attention. The following routine is specially designed to tighten, tone, and shrink those stubborn saddlebags for a sleek and sexy silhouette.

START HERE: ■

Do these moves one after another with no rest in between. Then repeat the circuit for a total of two times.

Rotation Lunge

A

- Grab a 5- to 15-pound dumbbell with each hand. Stand with your feet hip-width apart and your arms straight down at your sides.

B

- Take a big step forward with your left foot and, bracing your abs, twist your torso to the left as you bend your left knee and lower your body. Your left knee should form a 90-degree angle. Keep a slight bend in your right leg.

C

- Twist back to center, then push off your left foot, and stand back up.
- Repeat the move with the right foot. That's 1 rep.

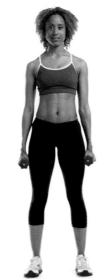

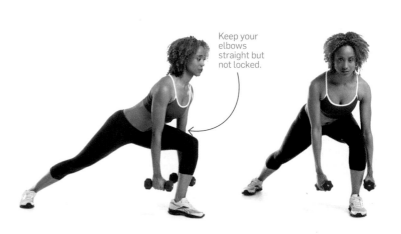

Keep your elbows straight but not locked.

REPS: Do 10 to 15.

Hydrant Extension

Keep your lower back as still as possible throughout the exercise.

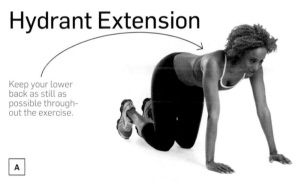

A

- Get on all fours with your knees directly beneath your hips and your hands under your shoulders.

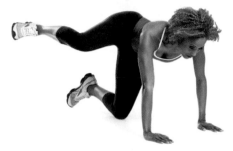

B

- Keeping your right knee bent, lift it up and out to the side as high as possible.

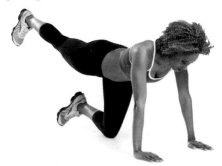

C

- Next, extend the right leg straight back so it's in line with your torso.
- Pause, then bring it back to the starting position. Repeat with your left leg. That's 1 rep.

REPS: Do 12 to 15.

Reverse Lunge Single-Arm Press

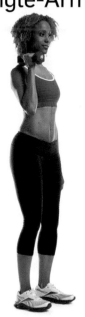

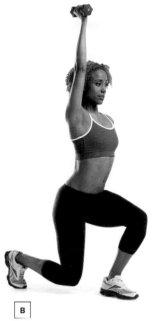

A

- Grab a 5- to 15-pound dumbbell in your right hand and hold it next to your right shoulder, palm facing in.

B

- Step backward with your right foot and lower your body until your knees are bent to 90 degrees (your right knee should nearly touch the floor) while pressing the dumbbell directly over your shoulder without bending or leaning at the waist.
- Lower the weight back to the starting position as you push quickly back to standing. That's 1 rep.

REPS: Do 10 to 15, then repeat the exercise with the weight in your left hand and stepping back with your left foot.

So Long, Saddlebags Workout

Lateral Shuffle

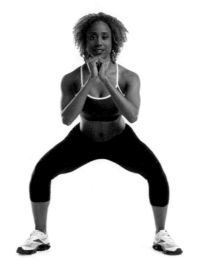
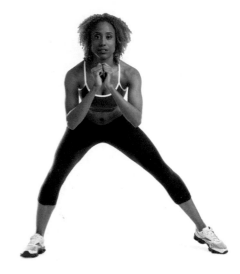

A

- Stand with your feet slightly wider than hip-width apart and turned out 45 degrees.
- Bend into a squat with your knees over your ankles.

B

- Step out with your left foot, keeping your knees bent in the squat position.
- Step left with your right foot to return to the starting position.
- Continue walking sideways, taking 10 steps to the left and then 10 to the right.

REPS: Do 10 to each side.

Plié Squat with Stability Ball

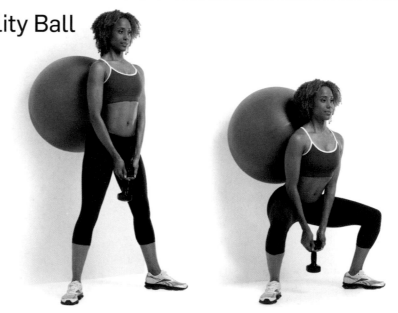

A

- With a stability ball between your lower back and the wall, hold a 10- to 20-pound dumbbell with both hands between your legs.
- Stand with your feet wider than your hips and turn your toes out.

B

- Contract your abs and lower to a 4-count until your knees are at 90 degrees.
- Hold for 4 counts, then slowly stand up to a 4-count.

REPS: Do 10 to 15.

45-Degree Lunge

A

- Stand with your feet hip-width apart, arms at your sides.

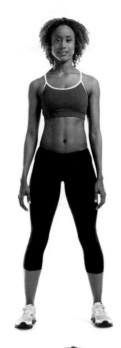

B

- Lunge 45 degrees to the left, keeping your hips facing forward and your right leg straight.
- Pause, then return to the starting position. That's 1 rep.

REPS: Do 10 to 12, then repeat on your right side.

Static Squat with Front Raise

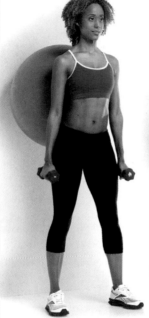
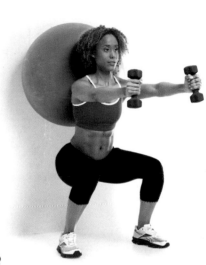

A

- With a stability ball between your lower back and the wall, hold a 3- to 8-pound dumbbell in each hand, palms in.
- Step forward and spread your feet hip-width apart. Lean back into the ball.

REPS: Do 8 to 10.

B

- Contract your abs and glutes, then lower your hips until your knees are at 90 degrees.
- In this position, slowly raise your arms in front of your body to shoulder height. Lower them, then raise them 7 to 9 more times.
- Rise to the starting position.

Killer Calves for Taller Boots Workout

Sculpted, sexy calves look killer in tall boots, kitten heels, shorts, capris, and skirts of every length. Strong calves protect your knees and can help you can say good-bye to a runner's worst nightmare, shin splints. This routine includes balance challenges that fire up the stabilizers throughout your lower legs as well as a few isolation exercises to really burn your calves.

START HERE:

Do these moves one after another with no rest in between. Then repeat the circuit for a total of three times.

Overhead squat

- Stand with your feet slightly wider than shoulder-width apart, toes turned out slightly.
- Grab a rolled-up towel with an overhand grip, hands shoulder-width apart, and raise it overhead so your shoulders are roughly in line with your heels.

- Squat down as far as possible without letting your knees jut out past your toes.
- Return to standing. That's 1 rep.

The towel helps keep your shoulders aligned. If you don't have a towel, raise your hands overhead—but keep your shoulders back and in line with your heels.

REPS: Do 10 to 15.

Toe Raise

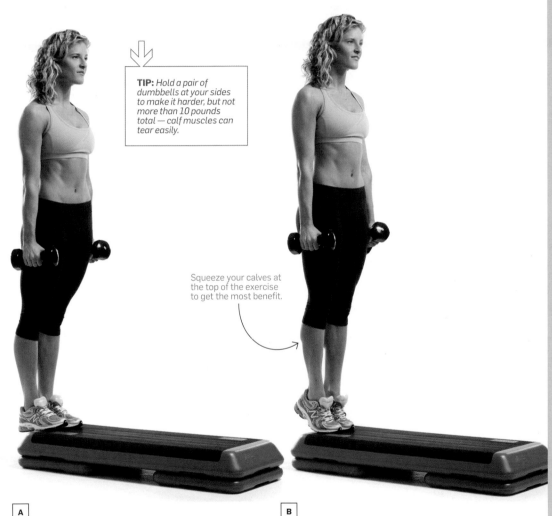

TIP: *Hold a pair of dumbbells at your sides to make it harder, but not more than 10 pounds total — calf muscles can tear easily.*

Squeeze your calves at the top of the exercise to get the most benefit.

A

- You can do a toe raise on pretty much any step or curb. Stand on a step with your feet slightly apart and drop your heels down below it.

REPS: Do 10 to 15.

B

- Then push straight up onto your tiptoes.
- Slowly lower your heels and repeat.

WATCH LESS, WEIGH LESS

Shed pounds with the press of a button—the one marked OFF on your TV's remote control. In a study, people who scaled back their daily viewing time by half (to 2½ hours, on average) burned 120 calories more per day by being more active than those who continued to watch their usual amount, according to the *Archives of Internal Medicine*. The average American clocks 5 hours of TV a day; halving that could help you lose 12 pounds or more in a year.

Killer Calves for Taller Boots Workout

Single-Leg Squat

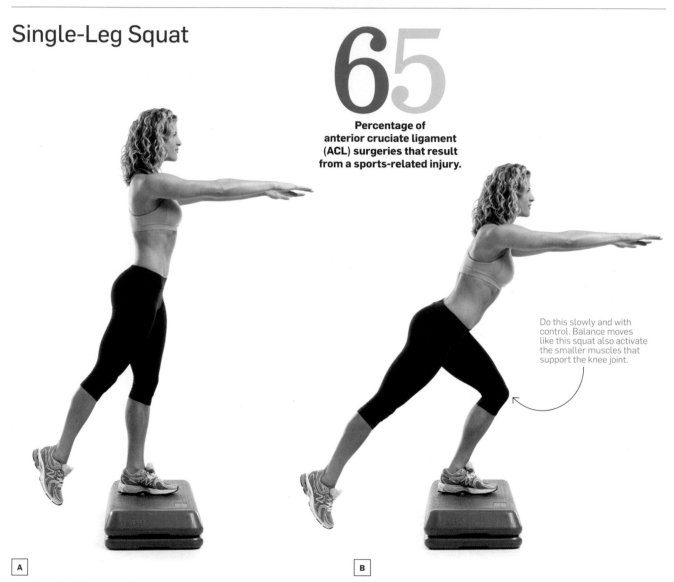

65

Percentage of anterior cruciate ligament (ACL) surgeries that result from a sports-related injury.

Do this slowly and with control. Balance moves like this squat also activate the smaller muscles that support the knee joint.

A

- Stand with your left foot on a step, with your right leg hanging behind you.

B

- Bend your left knee until your thigh is close to parallel to the ground, extending your arms for balance and pushing your hips and right leg back.

REPS: Do 12 to 15, then repeat the exercise with your right foot on the step.

Plié Heel Lift

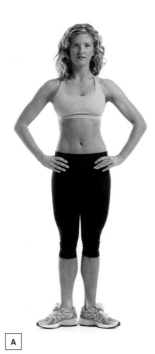

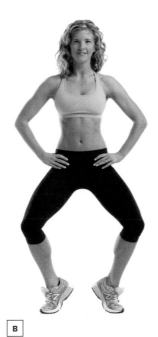

A

- Stand with your heels touching, toes turned out and hands on your hips.
- With straight legs, lift both heels up off the floor.

B

- Keeping your heels lifted, plié by bending both knees slightly.
- Next, drop your heels down to the floor and roll them back up, still in the plié.
- Continue lowering and lifting your heels until you you can't do any more.

REPS: Do as many as you can with good form.

Lunging Stepup

If you feel off balance, do the exercise without weights until you've nailed the form.

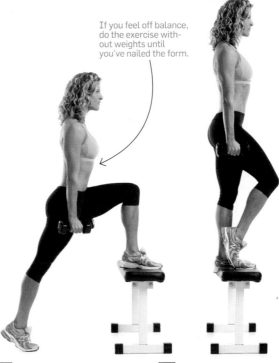

A

- Grab a pair of 5- to 10-pound dumbbells and stand 2 to 3 feet from an exercise bench.
- Place your left foot on the bench.

B

- Drive your left heel down and pull your right leg up.
- Allow only the toes of your right foot to touch the bench.
- Lower your right leg first and then your left.
- Repeat, lunging up with your right leg. That's 1 rep.

REPS: Do 10 to 12.

Thinner Inner Thighs Workout

The thighs are a common trouble spot for women. Like your booty, if they're bigger than you'd like, it might be a matter of buckling down and swearing off second helpings. Chances are, however, they're also in need of some toning, especially in the hard-to-hit inner thigh area, which tends to go a little soft from disuse. The following routine includes single-leg as well as isolation exercises.

START HERE: ■

Do these moves one after another with no rest in between. Then repeat the circuit for a total of two times.

Lateral Reverse Lunge-Reach Combo

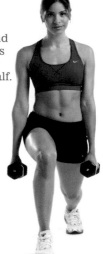

A

- Grab a pair of 10- to 15-pound dumbbells and stand with your feet together and your arms at your sides.

- Keeping your right leg straight and your toes facing forward, lunge to the left and lower your hips until your left thigh is parallel to the floor.

- Bend at the hips and lower the dumbbells so they're on either side of your left calf.

B

- Return to center.

- Next, perform a reverse lunge, stepping back with your left leg.

- Bend at the hips and lower the dumbbells so they're on either side of your right calf. Return to start.

REPS: Do 12 to 15 and then repeat, lunging with your right leg.

Offset Squat

Keep the dumbbell as far from your body as you can throughout the squat to work your glutes harder.

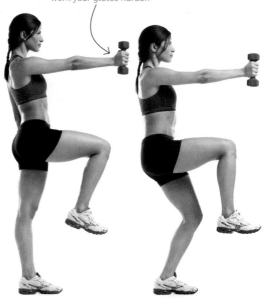

A

- Grab a 5- to 8-pound dumbbell in your right hand, hold it at your right side, and lift your right foot so you're balancing on your left.
- Raise your right arm straight out in front of you until it's at shoulder level.

B

- Squat down, bringing your left thigh as close to parallel to the floor as you can. (This is tough!)
- Pause for a second and then push back up to the starting position.

REPS: Do 12, then work the other leg and arm.

Quadruped Hip Extension

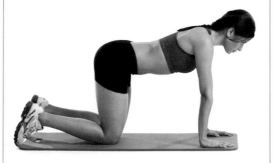

A

- Get on all fours.

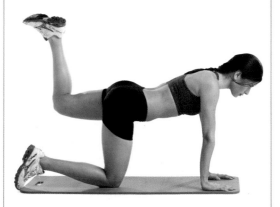

B

- Lift one leg behind you, keeping the knee bent at a 90-degree angle, until your sole faces the ceiling. Lower and repeat.

REPS: Do 12 to 15, then switch legs.

SAVE YOUR KNEES

Active women are more than eight times more likely than active men to tear the anterior cruciate ligament—or ACL—in the knee. But you can protect yourself: Exercises that test your balance, like the offset squat shown on this page, are the most effective way to help prevent ACL injuries. Add single-leg balance exercises to your routine to strengthen the muscles that support your knee joint. Try this: Stand on your left foot with your right knee slightly bent and your right foot a few inches off the floor. Keeping your back straight, bend from your hips and touch your left foot with your right hand. Your right leg should go back behind you as you bend forward. Stand up straight and repeat for 10 to 15 reps, then do the exercise while balancing on your right foot.

Thinner Inner Thighs Workout

Unilateral Lunge with Knee Balance

A

- Grab a pair of 12- to 15-pound dumbbells and stand with your back to a 12-inch-high step 2 to 3 feet away.
- Place your left toes on the bench and sink into a lunge.

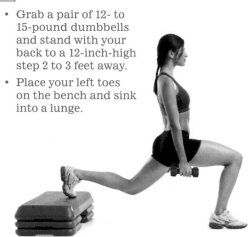

B

- Straighten your right leg as you bring your left knee in front and up until your left thigh is parallel to the floor.
- Balance on your right leg for 1 second, then return to the starting position.

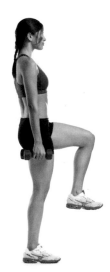

REPS: Do 12 to 15, then repeat on the other side.

Single-Leg Plank

Place your feet as wide as your shoulders.

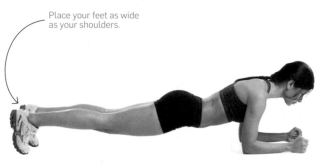

A

- Assume a plank position by propping yourself up on your forearms with your elbows directly below your shoulders and your toes flexed underneath you.

For a greater challenge, lift the arm opposite your raised leg straight out in front of you.

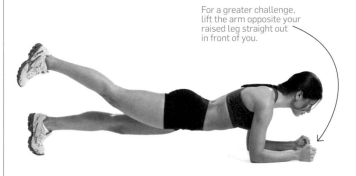

B

- Your body should form a straight line. Brace your abs and lift your right leg up about 10 inches.
- Balance your bodyweight on your forearms and the stabilizing leg. Hold for 5 to 10 seconds. Switch legs and repeat on the other side.

REPS: Do 10 to 12 on each side.

Side-to-Side Leg Swing

Modified Glute-Ham Raise

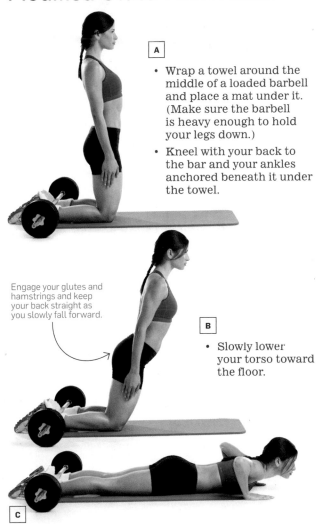

A
- Wrap a towel around the middle of a loaded barbell and place a mat under it. (Make sure the barbell is heavy enough to hold your legs down.)
- Kneel with your back to the bar and your ankles anchored beneath it under the towel.

Engage your glutes and hamstrings and keep your back straight as you slowly fall forward.

B
- Slowly lower your torso toward the floor.

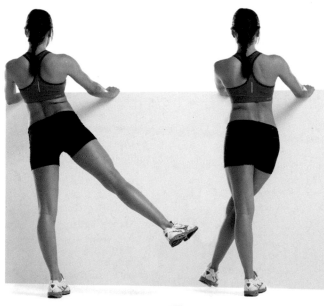

A
- Stand and grab a sturdy object such as a chair in front of you with both hands.
- Swing your right leg out to the right as high as you can.

B
- Then swing it back down and across the front of your left leg. That's 1 rep.

REPS: Do 12 to 20, then switch legs and repeat.

C
- Use your arms to catch yourself when your legs give out.
- Return to the starting position by pushing up forcefully with your arms.

REPS: Do 10 to 12.

Fit Into Your Skinny Jeans Workout

Buried in the back of your wardrobe is an old friend from whom you were once inseparable: the jeans you splurged on when you were at your skinniest. Now they're just languishing in your closet because it's too much effort to stuff yourself inside them. We've got a plan to fix that. This high-energy routine blasts calories while firming your lower-body muscles from every direction.

START HERE:

Do these moves one after another with no rest in between. Then repeat the circuit for a total of two times.

Squat-to-Lunge Leg Curl

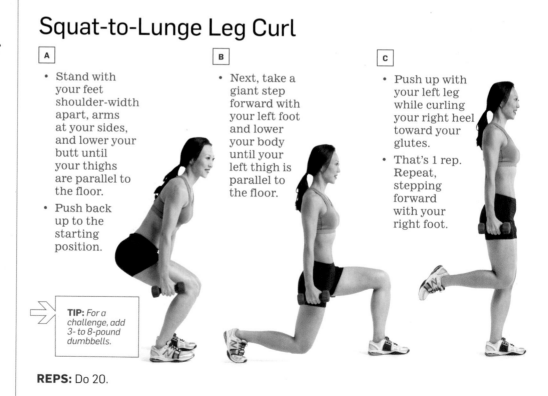

A

- Stand with your feet shoulder-width apart, arms at your sides, and lower your butt until your thighs are parallel to the floor.
- Push back up to the starting position.

TIP: For a challenge, add 3- to 8-pound dumbbells.

B

- Next, take a giant step forward with your left foot and lower your body until your left thigh is parallel to the floor.

C

- Push up with your left leg while curling your right heel toward your glutes.
- That's 1 rep. Repeat, stepping forward with your right foot.

REPS: Do 20.

Dumbbell Sumo Squat

Keep your torso as upright as you can for the entire movement, with your lower back naturally arched.

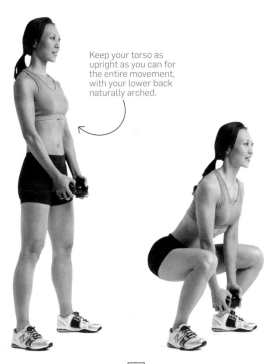

A

- Grab a heavy dumbbell and hold an end with each hand at arm's length in front of your waist.
- Set your feet about twice your shoulder-width apart, your toes turned out slightly.

B

- Lower your body as far as you can by pushing your hips back and bending your knees.
- Pause, then push yourself back to the starting position.

REPS: Do 10 to 12.

Stability Lunge

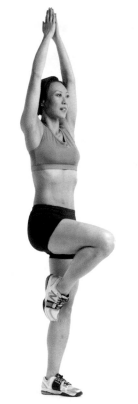

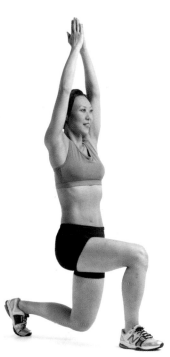

A

- Stand with your feet shoulder-width apart and your arms at your sides.
- Lift your right knee until your thigh is parallel to the floor as you raise your arms overhead, palms touching.

B

- Hold for 5 seconds, then slowly drop your right foot into a front lunge.
- Bring your left leg forward and return to standing. That's 1 rep.

REPS: Do 10 to 12 on each leg, alternating sides.

Fit Into Your Skinny Jeans Workout

Dumbbell Bent-Knee Deadlift

 TIP: *As you raise and lower the weights, keep the dumbbells as close to your body as possible.*

Don't round your back.

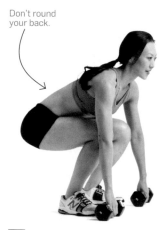

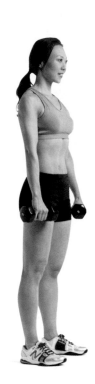

A

- Set a pair of 10-to 15-pound dumbbells on the floor in front of you.
- Squat, keeping your chest up, and grab the dumbbells with an overhand grip. Your arms should be straight and your lower back slightly arched, not rounded.

B

- Contract your glutes and stand up with the dumbbells, straightening your legs, thrusting your hips forward, and pulling your torso back and up.
- Slowly lower the dumbbells to the floor. That's 1 rep.

REPS: Do 10 to 12.

Single-Leg, Single-Arm Reach

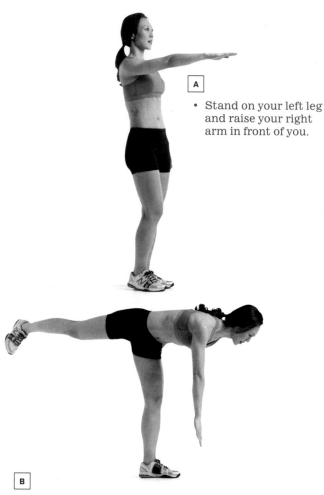

A

- Stand on your left leg and raise your right arm in front of you.

B

- Lower your torso and lift your right leg behind you until both are parallel to the floor.
- Contract your glutes and hamstrings to return to standing. That's 1 rep.

REPS: Do 10 to 12 reps, then switch sides and repeat.

Elevated Reverse Lunge

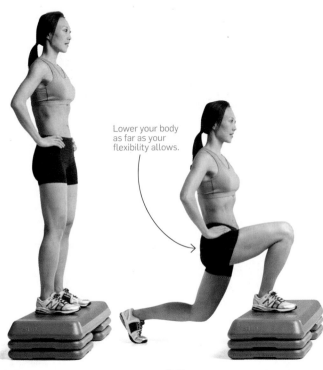

Lower your body as far as your flexibility allows.

A

- Stand on a 6-inch step or box, hands on your hips.

B

- Squeeze your left glute, step back with your left leg, and lower until your right knee is bent at least 90 degrees.
- Pause, then push through the right leg to return to the starting position. That's 1 rep.

REPS: Do 4 to 6, then repeat with the right leg.

Cable Pull-Through

TIP: *For a secure grip, use the rope or the handle attachment.*

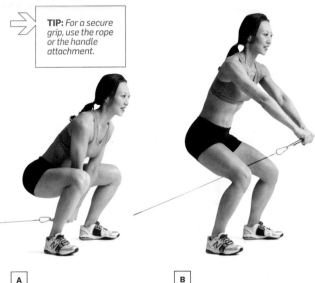

A

- Stand about 2 feet from a pulley station set at a very light weight (increase it only after you've nailed the form), with the cable on the lowest setting (the one closest to the floor).
- With your back to the station, position your feet shoulder-width apart, then bend from your hips as you squat until your thighs are nearly parallel to the floor.
- Reach back through your legs and grab the handle.

B

- Keeping your head up, drive your heels into the floor and straighten your legs to standing.
- Pause, then lower the weight and repeat.

REPS: Do 10 to 12.

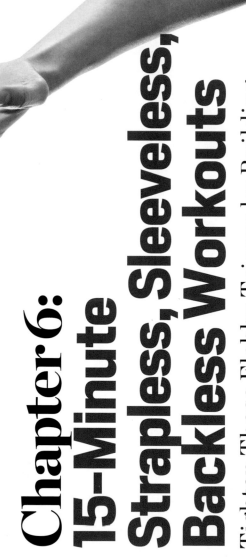

Chapter 6:
15-Minute
Strapless, Sleeveless, Backless Workouts

Tighten Those Flabby Triceps by Building Lean, Muscular Arms and Shoulders That You Will Want to Show Off.

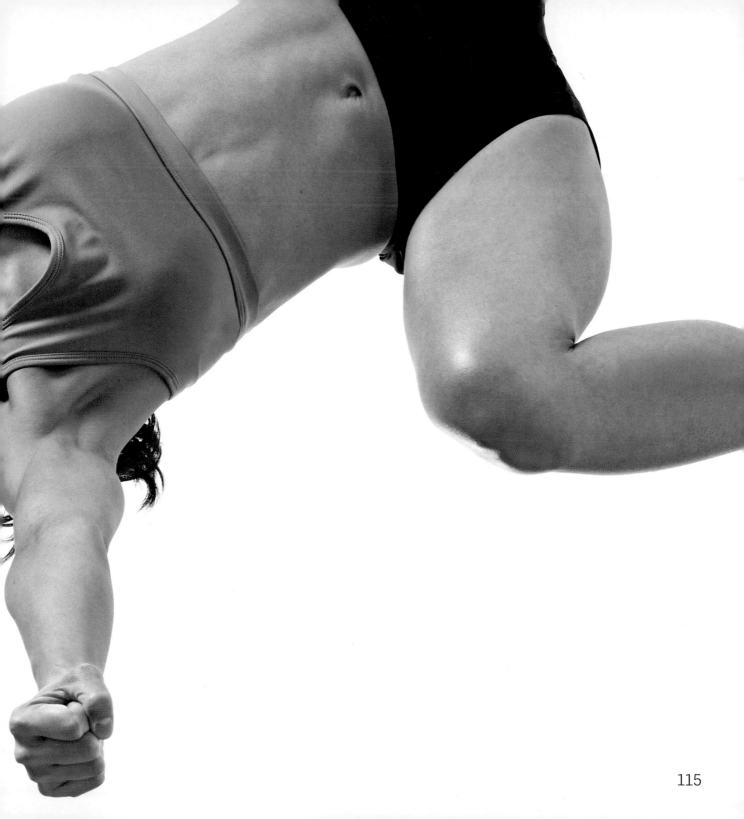

Superfast Strapless, Sleeveless, Backless Workouts

Your arms and shoulders make a big first impression. A well-defined upper body not only broadcasts strength and confidence, it literally makes you stand up straighter. You see, the muscles of your upper back help pull your shoulders down and back, so that you stand up tall, instead of slumped over. The added benefit, of course, is that this lifts your front up, too, for a perkier appearance, if you catch the drift. The result: You'll look great and feel confident in your most revealing tops.

Find It Quick: Your 15-Minute Upper-Body Circuit Plan

p.118
Tiny-Tank-Top Workout

Standing V Raise

Shoulder Press

Rotating Triceps Kickback

Pike Walk Pushup Combo

Airplane/ Superman Extension

Crescent Lunge and Row

T Pushup

p.124
Jiggle-Free Triceps Workout

Bench Dip

Balance Row

Triceps Leg Extension

The 1-Minute Hammer Curl

Pyramid Pushup

Chinup

Medicine Ball Rolling Pushup

p.130
Michelle-Obama-Arms Workout

Standing Lunge Shoulder Cross

Lateral Band Raise

Biceps Curl

Step Walk Over

Standing V Pull

Cobra Pushup

Triceps Pushdown with Grip Flip

p.136
Spread Your Wings Workout

Renegade Row

Floor Y Raise

Reverse Fly

Floor T Raise

Lying Lat Pullover

Floor I Raise

1 and $\frac{1}{4}$ Lat Pulldown

p.140
Pushup Bra Workout

Unilateral Pulsing Pushup

Standing One-Arm Press

Single-Arm Bench Press

Reverse Pushup

Incline Dumbbell Press

Scoop Hold

Triceps Dip and Reach

ANATOMY LESSON

Get to know the muscles that matter: All contribute to sexy arms and an attractive profile.

Pectorals: The muscles that pushups strengthen will give your bosom a lift

Deltoids: Three sections of lean muscle that make up your shoulders

Lats and traps: Build lovely latissimus dorsi to show off in backless dresses. You'll find them running from your lower back along the spine and hip to the inside of your upper arm. The trapezi-uses are the triangle-shaped muscles on the upper back that lift up your front.

Biceps: The two muscle groups on the front of your upper arms that help you curl those grocery bags

Triceps: The muscles opposite the biceps on the backs of the upper arms. Building and toning these will help reduce the flabby "chicken wing" look that so many women abhor. Don't worry about becoming too muscular by building your bis and tris with weights.

Start with the basics...

Here, you'll find plans to tackle your triceps (no more waving goodbye twice!), biceps, shoulders, upper back, and chest. Good news: Because women tend to carry less bodyweight in their upper bodies, you'll see results from these workouts fast.

Do one (or more) of these upper-body workouts 2 days a week, leaving a day of rest in between. You can piggyback any of these routines with another 15-minute workout for a total-body blast. Do the prescribed number of reps for each exercise, opting for a weight at which you can barely squeeze out the last rep of your final set with good form.

Tiny-Tank-Top Workout

The typical tank top exposes you 360 degrees, all the way around your upper back, shoulders, upper chest, and a bit of your sides. Looking great in one means toning those muscles from every angle. The following workout will shape up all those places that peek out from your spaghetti straps, and tighten and firm your core.

START HERE:

Do these moves one after another with no rest in between. Then repeat the circuit for a total of two times, with a minute of rest between circuits.

Standing V Raise

 A

- Grab a lightweight dumbbell in each hand and stand with your feet shoulder-width apart, arms at your sides, palms in.

 B

- With your arms straight but not locked, raise the weights in a V shape until your arms are parallel to the floor.
- Hold for 1 second, then return to the starting position.

REPS: Do 12 to 15.

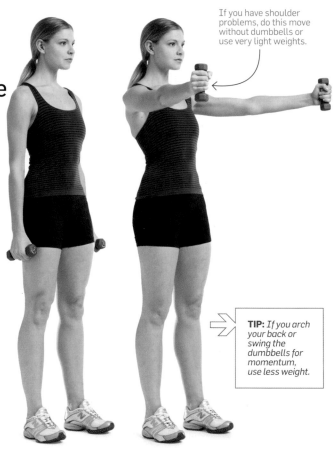

If you have shoulder problems, do this move without dumbbells or use very light weights.

TIP: If you arch your back or swing the dumbbells for momentum, use less weight.

Shoulder Press

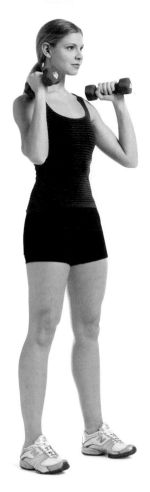

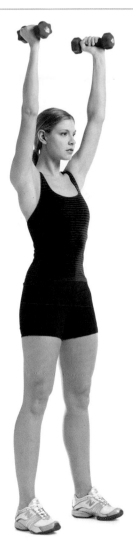

ONE DESSERT, TWO FORKS

A couple that diets together is more likely to lose weight. In a recent Israeli study, researchers taught couples about healthy eating, but assigned only the men to various kinds of eating plans. After 6 months, the women had also shed weight. The study authors say that sharing dishes and eating together helps dieters stick to their plans and resist temptation.

A

- Grab a dumbbell in each hand and stand with your feet shoulder-width apart, knees slightly bent.
- Hold the dumbbells just above your shoulders, palms facing each other.

REPS: Do 6 to 8.

B

- Press the weights up until your arms are straight overhead.
- Hold for 1 second, then take 3 seconds to lower the dumbbells back to your shoulders.

119

Tiny-Tank-Top Workout

Rotating Triceps Kickback

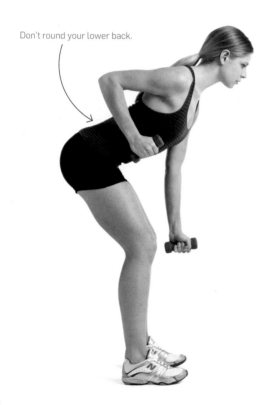

Don't round your lower back.

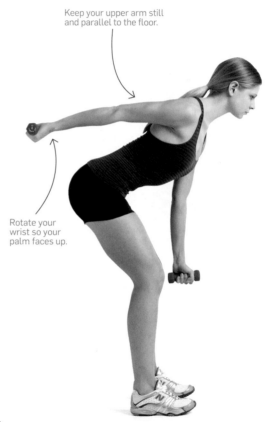

Keep your upper arm still and parallel to the floor.

Rotate your wrist so your palm faces up.

A

- Stand with your knees bent and lean forward slightly, holding a dumbbell in each hand, palms in.
- Bend your right elbow and bring the right dumbbell up by your side to make your upper arm parallel with the floor.

REPS: Do 12 lo 15 with each arm.

B

- Next, press the dumbbell back, and as you straighten your arm, rotate it so that your palm faces the ceiling.
- Rotate it back so that your palm faces in and return your arm to the bent position.

Pike Walk Pushup Combo

A

- Stand with your feet together, arms at your sides.

B

- Bend over (it's okay for your knees to be slightly bent) and place your hands or fingertips on the floor in front of you.

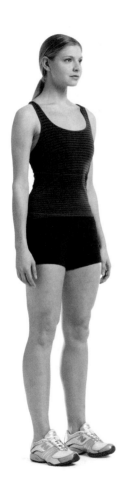

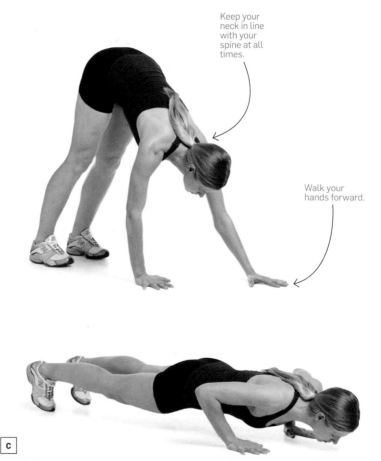

Keep your neck in line with your spine at all times.

Walk your hands forward.

C

- Walk your hands forward until you are in a pushup position and then do 1 pushup.
- Keeping your hands in place, walk your feet forward until they're as close to your hands as possible. That's 1 rep.
- Continue moving forward until you've done 5 or 6 pushups.

REPS: Do 5 or 6.

Tiny-Tank-Top Workout

Airplane/Superman Extension

A

- Lie facedown and extend your arms out at shoulder height, keeping your elbows slightly bent and your palms on the floor.

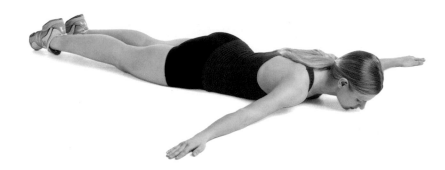

B

- Pull your shoulder blades together and lift your arms, torso, and legs off the floor.

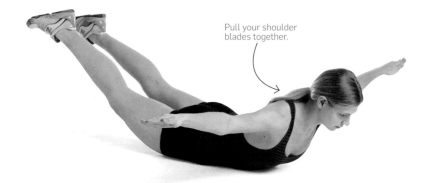

Pull your shoulder blades together.

C

- Holding that position, bring your arms in front of you, hold for 1 count, and then move them back to shoulder height.
- Lower yourself to the floor. That's 1 rep.

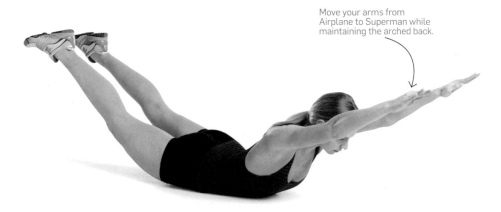

Move your arms from Airplane to Superman while maintaining the arched back.

REPS: Do 10 to 15.

Crescent Lunge and Row

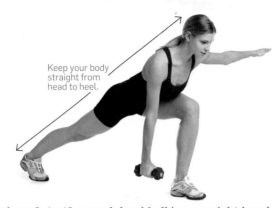

Keep your body straight from head to heel.

A

- Grab an 8- to 12-pound dumbbell in your right hand and stand with your feet together, arms at your sides.
- Lunge forward with your left leg until your left knee is bent to 90 degrees.
- Lower your torso as close as possible to your left knee as you raise your left arm out to the side to shoulder height, palm down. Allow the dumbbell to hang naturally.

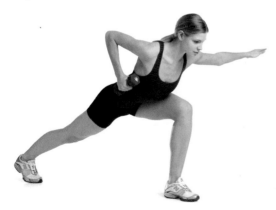

B

- Row the dumbbell straight up until your right elbow passes your torso. That's 1 rep.

REPS: Do 12 to 15, then reverse sides and repeat for the same number of reps.

T Pushup

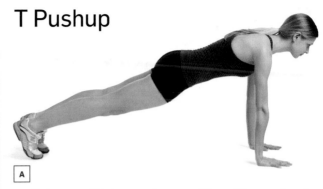

A

- Get yourself into a pushup position with your hands on the floor directly below your shoulders.
- Lower yourself to the floor.

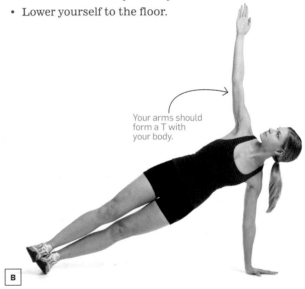

Your arms should form a T with your body.

B

- As you push yourself up, rotate the right side of your body upward, lift your right hand, and roll onto the outside of your left foot.
- Straighten your right arm so your fingertips point toward the ceiling. Hold for 1 second before returning to the down pushup position. Repeat, this time rotating left and reaching up with your left arm. That's 1 rep.

REPS: Do 5.

Jiggle-Free Triceps Workout

Women are particularly prone to "bingo wings," those flaps that hang down from the backs of our upper arms and wiggle when we wave. That's because unlike curling muscles (the biceps), which get regular use, our pushing muscles (the triceps), see very little action. Women also have a tendency to deposit fat in this area, which compounds the problem. The fix is in this workout.

START HERE:
Do these moves one after another with no rest in between. Then repeat the circuit for a total of two times, with a minute of rest between circuits.

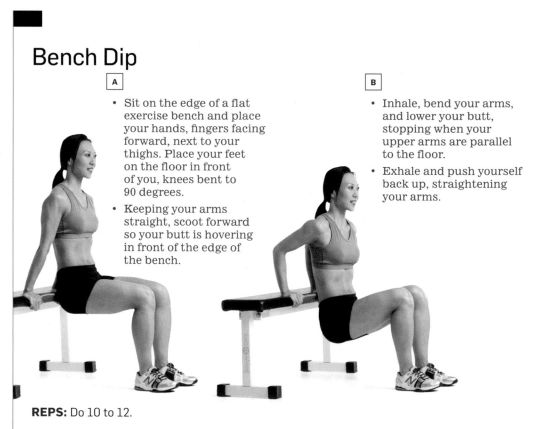

Bench Dip

A

- Sit on the edge of a flat exercise bench and place your hands, fingers facing forward, next to your thighs. Place your feet on the floor in front of you, knees bent to 90 degrees.
- Keeping your arms straight, scoot forward so your butt is hovering in front of the edge of the bench.

B

- Inhale, bend your arms, and lower your butt, stopping when your upper arms are parallel to the floor.
- Exhale and push yourself back up, straightening your arms.

REPS: Do 10 to 12.

Balance Row

KNEE THERAPY: *Exercises that test your balance are the most effective technique for preventing ACL injuries, according to Australian researchers.*

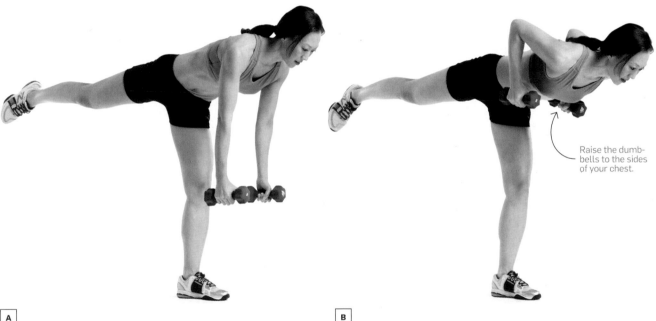

Raise the dumb-bells to the sides of your chest.

A

- Grab a dumbbell in each hand and let your arms hang at your sides, palms facing in. Stand with your feet hip-width apart.
- Bend forward while extending your right leg straight behind you until your body forms a T. Let your arms hang straight down, palms facing each other.

REPS: Do 5 or 6 on each leg.

B

- Squeeze your shoulder blades together and bring your elbows toward the ceiling, raising the weights to each side of your chest.
- After completing all the reps, stand on your right leg, lift your left and repeat the exercise.

Jiggle-Free Triceps Workout

Triceps Leg Extension

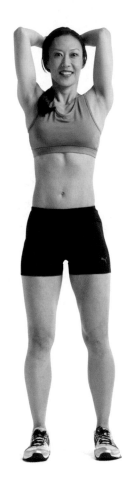

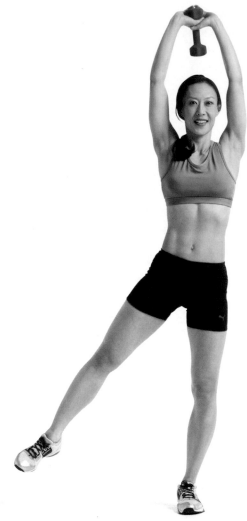

A

- Stand with your feet hip-width apart, holding an 8- to 12-pound dumbbell with both hands.
- Contract your abs, lift the dumbbell overhead, and slowly drop your hands behind your head, keeping your elbows next to your ears.

REPS: Do 8.

B

- Next, push the dumbbell toward the ceiling and simultaneously extend your right leg to the side. Release to the starting position and repeat, this time raising your left leg. That's 1 rep.

The 1-Minute Hammer Curl

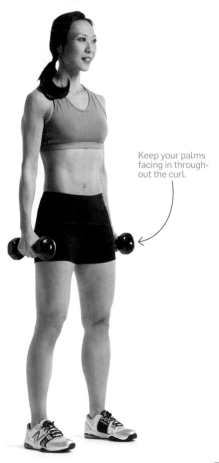

Keep your palms facing in throughout the curl.

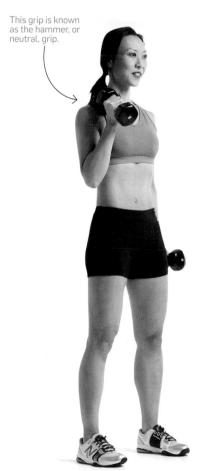

This grip is known as the hammer, or neutral, grip.

A

- Stand with your feet shoulder-width apart.
- Grab a pair of dumbbells and hold them next to your thighs, palms facing each other.

B

- Curl the weight in your right hand toward your shoulder without rotating your wrist.
- As you lower the dumbbell, curl the weight in your left hand.
- Alternate your arms rhythmically.

REPS: Do as many as you can with good form in 1 minute.

Jiggle-Free Triceps Workout

Pyramid Pushup

A

- From a regular pushup position, move your hands to form a triangle on the floor (with your thumbs and forefingers touching).
- Your hands should be centered between your shoulders and your nose.

TIP: *Do it on your knees for an easier version.*

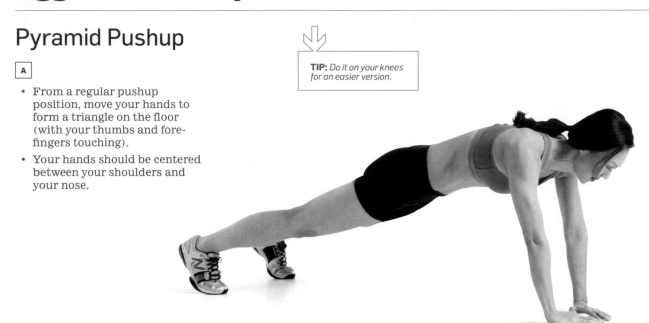

B

- Next, lower yourself until you're a few inches above your hands and pause for 2 seconds. Return to the starting position and repeat.

Squeeze your glutes and brace your abs to help keep your back stable and straight.

REPS: Do 8 to 12.

Chinup

TIP: *Chinups are tough. If you can't manage one yet, have a workout partner help you raise yourself by placing her hands beneath your ankles.*

A

- Using a wide, under-hand grip (palms facing you), hang from a bar with your elbows straight, knees bent back, and ankles crossed.

B

- Pull yourself up until your chin clears the bar and slowly lower yourself back to the starting position.

REPS: Do as many as you can.

Medicine Ball Rolling Pushup

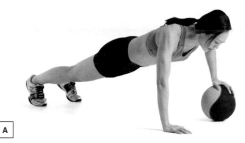

A

- Get in a pushup position with your left hand on top of a 5- to 8-pound medicine ball and your right hand on the floor.

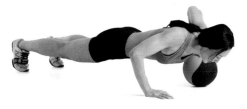

B

- Lower yourself until your chest is as close to the floor as possible.
- Press back up until your arms are fully extended.

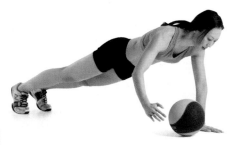

C

- Roll the ball to your right, then quickly place your weight on your left hand and place your right hand on top of the ball.
- Do another pushup, then roll the ball back to the left That's 1 rep.

REPS: Do 6 to 10, moving quickly.

Michelle-Obama-Arms Workout

Toss that baggy boyfriend hang-to-your-knees oversize XL T-shirt and get yourself a cute, fitted girl T that says, "I am a woman. And I kick butt." The following workout will give you Michelle Obama–style biceps, as well as sculpted shoulders and triceps and a toned upper back and chest. You'll never go shapeless again.

START HERE:

Do these moves one after another with no rest in between. Then repeat the circuit for a total of two times, with a minute of rest between circuits.

Standing Lunge Shoulder Cross

 A

- Hold a 5-pound dumbbell in your right hand and step forward with your left foot as if you're about to lunge.
- Bend your right elbow 90 degrees and raise it so it's in line with your shoulder, with your palm facing forward.

B

- Next, sink down until your left thigh is parallel to the floor. As you lunge, bring the dumbbell down and across your body to the outside of your left thigh.
- Stand up and raise your arm to the starting position. After 10, repeat with the weight in the left hand and your right foot forward.

REPS: Do 10 on each side.

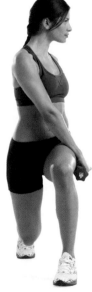
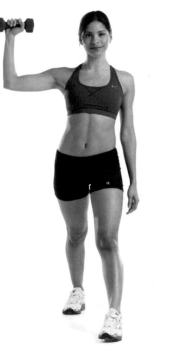

Lateral Band Raise

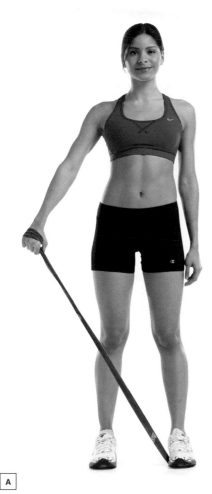

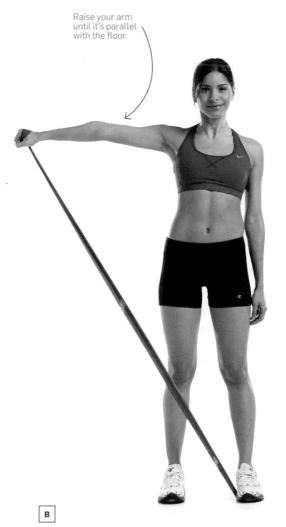

Raise your arm until it's parallel with the floor.

LOOSEN UP BY LIFTING

Lifting weights through a full range of motion can improve your flexibility better than stretching does, according to a University of North Dakota study. The likely reason? During resistance exercise, your muscles first contract and then stretch to their full range between each repetition. One way to make weight training even more effective for flexibility: Each time you reach the "down" position of the lift (where you feel the stretch), pause for 2 to 3 seconds without relaxing your muscles.

A

- Grab an exercise band and stand with your feet shoulder-width apart.
- Hold one end of the band with your right hand at your side with your elbow slightly bent, and step on the other end of the band with your left foot.

REPS: Do 10 on each side.

B

- Raise your right arm straight up to the side until it's in line with your shoulders, then lower it slowly. Repeat.
- After completing all reps, hold an end of the band under your right foot and extend the band with your left hand.

Michelle-Obama-Arms Workout

Biceps Curl

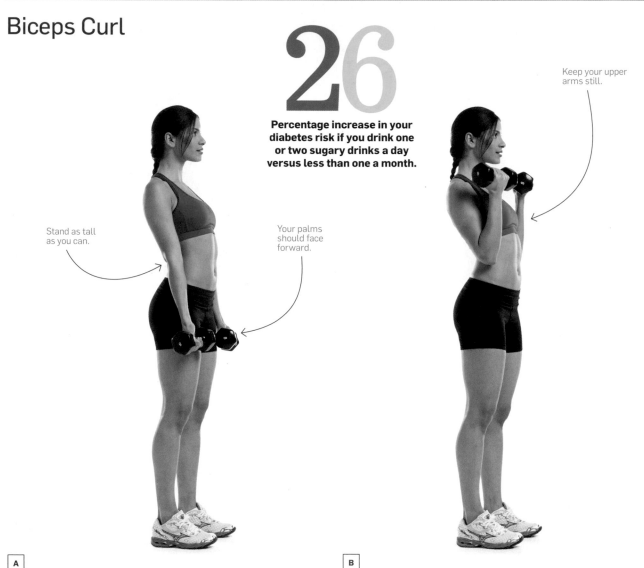

26

Percentage increase in your diabetes risk if you drink one or two sugary drinks a day versus less than one a month.

Stand as tall as you can.

Your palms should face forward.

Keep your upper arms still.

A

• Stand while holding a dumbbell in each hand, palms facing forward, with your feet shoulder-width apart and your arms hanging in front of you.

REPS: Do 10.

B

• Curl the weights toward your shoulders, hold for a second, then return to the starting position.

Step Walk Over

A

- Assume a pushup position with your palms on the narrow side of a 6- to 12-inch step.

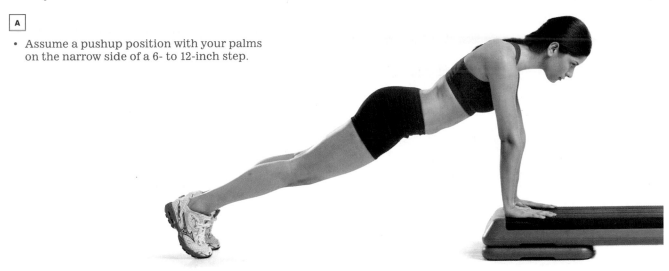

B

- Keeping your legs, spine, and neck aligned, shift your weight onto your left arm and place your right palm on the floor.
- Next, push up with your right hand and place your left palm on the floor next to your right hand.
- Now step onto the step with your left hand, then with your right. That's 1 rep.

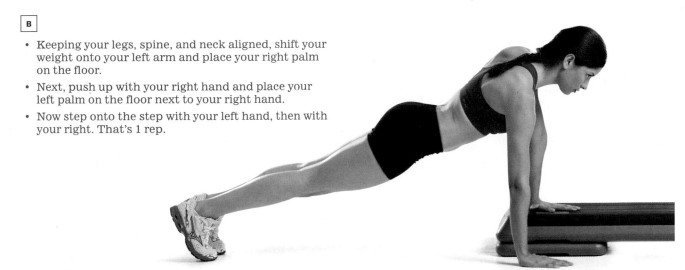

REPS: Repeat, stepping down to the opposite side, and continue alternating sides for 16 reps.

Michelle-Obama-Arms Workout

Standing V Pull

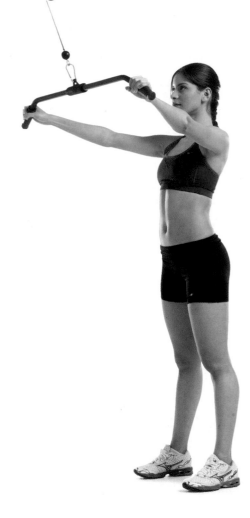

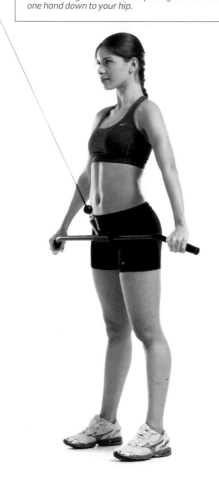

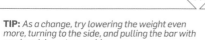

TIP: *As a change, try lowering the weight even more, turning to the side, and pulling the bar with one hand down to your hip.*

A

- Stand facing the lat pulldown cable station and grab the bar with your hands just outside of the curves, palms down.
- Step back about 2 feet.

REPS: Do 12 to 15.

B

- Keeping your arms straight, pull the bar to your hips.
- Use a light weight (about 20 pounds) to allow your back—and not your arms—to pull the bar.

Cobra Pushup

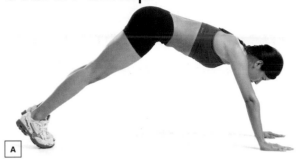

A

- Assume a standard pushup position, then walk your feet forward and raise your hips into a pike position, so your body almost forms an upside down V.

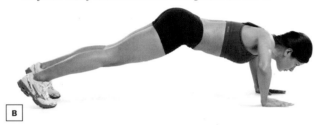

B

- Keeping your hips elevated, lower your body until your chin nearly touches the floor.

The final position resembles the Cobra pose in yoga. This pushup is also known as the Judo pushup.

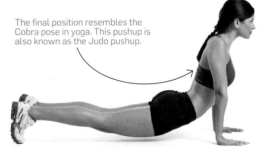

C

- Next, lower your hips until they almost touch the floor while simultaneously pressing up and raising your head and shoulders toward the ceiling.
- Reverse the movement back to the starting position and repeat.

REPS: Do 10.

Triceps Pushdown with Grip Flip

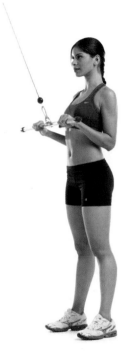
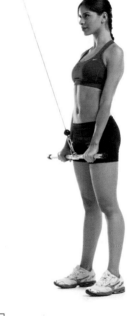

A

- Attach a straight bar to the high pulley of a cable station and grab the bar with an overhand grip, hands shoulder-width apart.
- Tuck your upper arms close to your sides and bend your elbows about 90 degrees.

B

- Without moving your upper arms, push the bar down until your arms are straight.
- Pause, then return to the starting position. That's 1 rep.

REPS: Do 15, then reverse your grip so you're grasping the bar with an underhand grip and immediately do another 15.

Spread Your Wings Workout

Check out the red carpet at any Hollywood event, and you'll see the starlets make as graceful an exit as they do an entrance with their defined shoulder blades and muscular backs. A toned, strong back also helps you stand up straight (and look instantly slimmer) and leaves an impression when you dare to go "bareback." This routine also builds muscles that support the spine.

START HERE:

Do these moves one after another with no rest in between. Then repeat the circuit for a total of two times, with a minute of rest between circuits.

Renegade Row

 A

- Grab dumbbells and assume a pushup position with your hands on the weights, arms extended, and feet slightly wider than hip-width apart.

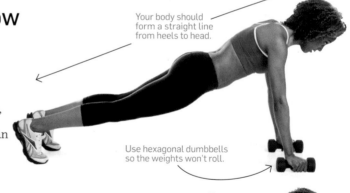

Your body should form a straight line from heels to head.

Use hexagonal dumbbells so the weights won't roll.

B

- Bend your right arm and raise the dumbbell to chest level, pressing the left dumbbell into the floor for balance.

- Lower the weight to the floor, then repeat the move by rowing the left dumbbell. That's 1 rep.

REPS: Do 6 to 8.

Floor Y Raise

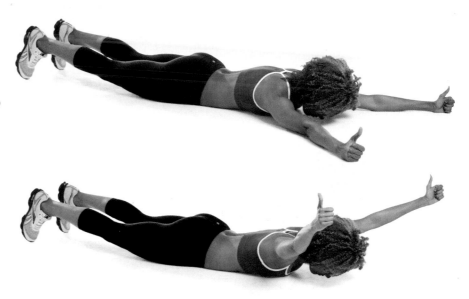

 A

- Lie facedown with your arms resting on the floor beyond your head, completely straight and at 30-degree angles to your body, so your body forms a Y.
- Your palms should be facing each other.

 B

- Raise your arms as high as you comfortably can.
- Lower back to the starting position.

REPS: Do 12.

Reverse Fly

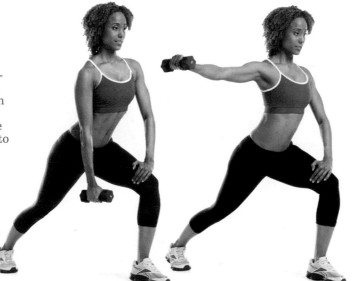

 A

- Grab a lightweight dumbbell with your right hand. Place your feet wider than your shoulders and turn your toes and torso to the left, which will put you into a staggered stance.
- Lean forward, with your left hand on your thigh.

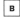 **B**

- Lift the weight out to the side to shoulder height, then lower it.

REPS: Do 12 to 15. Then repeat with the left hand.

ROCK YOUR WORKOUT

Studies show that listening to motivational music can boost your endurance by as much as 15 percent.

Spread Your Wings Workout

Floor T Raise

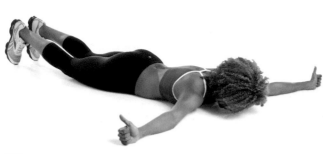

A

- Lie facedown on the floor and spread your arms out to your sides so your body forms a T.
- Form a light fist with both hands and turn your thumbs up toward the ceiling.

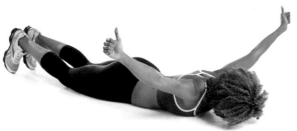

B

- Now slowly raise your arms as high as you comfortably can.
- Lower them back to the starting position.

REPS: Do 12.

Lying Lat Pullover

Before pulling the dumbbells back over your chest, squeeze your shoulder blades together.

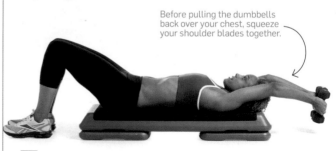

A

- Grab a pair of 5- to 8-pound dumbbells and lie faceup on a 6- to 12-inch high aerobic step, knees bent and feet flat on the floor.
- Hold the weights behind your head so that your arms are in line with your body and your elbows are slightly bent.

Palms should remain facing each other throughout the move.

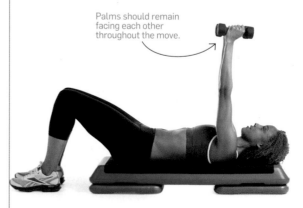

B

- Raise the dumbbells toward the ceiling until your arms are perpendicular to your torso.
- Then, in one fluid motion, lower them behind your head (as far as possible without touching the floor).

REPS: Do 15.

Floor I Raise

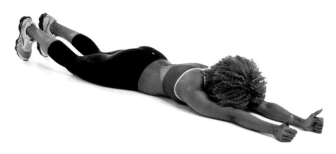

A

- Lie facedown on the floor with your arms extended forward so that your body forms a straight line from your feet to your hands.

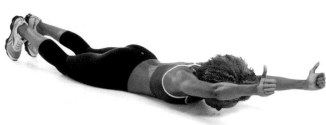

B

- With your hands forming loose fists and your thumbs pointing toward the ceiling, slowly raise your arms as high as you comfortably can.
- Lower them back to the starting position.

REPS: Do 12.

1 and ¼ Lat Pulldown

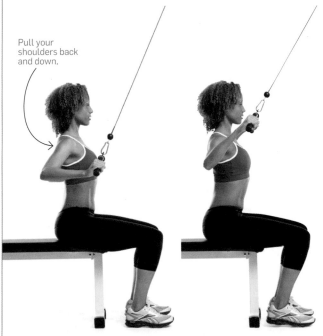

Pull your shoulders back and down.

A

- Sit facing a lat pulldown cable station. Grab the bar with a wide overhand grip.
- Lean back slightly and pull down on the bar until it touches your sternum.

B

- Slowly allow the bar to rise to mouth level, then pull it back down. That's 1 rep.

REPS: Do 12.

Pushup Bra Workout

Let's be clear: You can't affect the shape (or size) of your boobs by lifting weights. But you can give them a boost by strengthening and building the muscles that sit beneath your breasts. The following routine will create strong, sexy cleavage and give you a little lift for a look that would make Victoria's Secret proud.

START HERE:

Do these moves one after another with no rest between them. Then repeat the circuit for a total of two times, with a minute of rest between circuits.

Unilateral Pulsing Pushup

A

- Assume a pushup position, keeping your hands beneath your shoulders, and pull your abs tight.
- Lower your body until it's about an inch from the floor and pulse down for 3 counts.

B

- Next, push back to the starting position, and as you rise, cross your right hand over your left.
- Then move your left hand out to the left and do another pushup, pulsing down again for 3 counts.
- When you push up, cross your left hand over your right and repeat to the right. That's 1 rep.

REPS: Do 5.

28

Percentage increase in muscle endurance after consuming caffeine, according to a study in the journal *Medicine and Science in Sports and Exercise*.

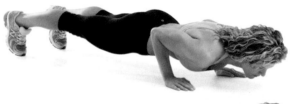

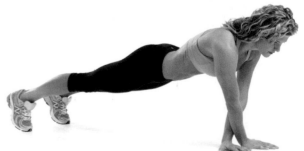

Standing One-Arm Press

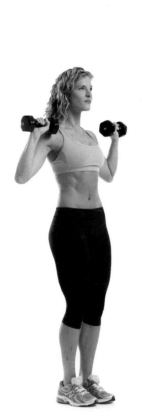
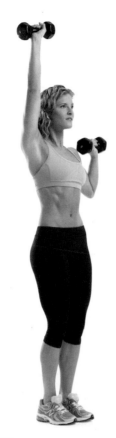

A

- Grab a pair of dumb-bells and stand straight, knees slightly bent.
- Raise the dumbbells in front of your shoulders, palms facing forward.

B

- Press the right dumb-bell overhead, keeping your arm in line with your ear.
- Slowly lower your right arm to shoulder height, then press the left dumbbell overhead. That's 1 rep.

REPS: Do 14.

Single-Arm Bench Press

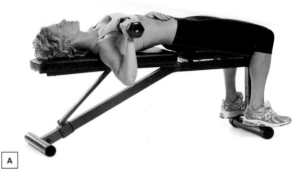

A

- Grab a dumbbell in your right hand and lie on your back on a flat bench, holding the dumbbell at the side of your chest. Your palm should be facing your lower body, but turned slightly inward.
- Place your left hand on your abs.

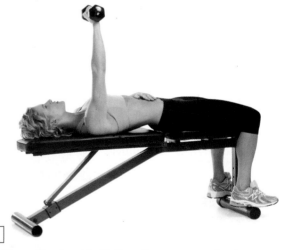

B

- Press the dumbbell directly over your chest, straightening your arm completely.
- Pause, then press the weight back to the starting position.

REPS: Do 12 to 15, then repeat the exercise with the dumbbell in your left hand.

Pushup Bra Workout

Reverse Pushup

A

- Set a chinup bar or the bar on a Smith machine to 3 to 4 feet from the floor. Lie on your back with your chest directly below the bar.
- Reach up and grab the bar with a shoulder-width, underhand grip so you're hanging from the bar and your body forms a straight diagonal line from your heels to your shoulders.

B

- Keeping your core tight, pull yourself up until your chest meets the bar.

REPS: Do 10 to 12.

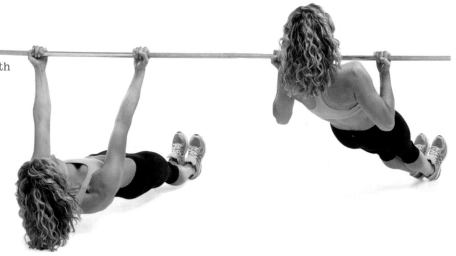

Incline Dumbbell Press

A

- Lie on your back on an incline bench set at about 45 degrees holding a dumbbell in each hand at your shoulders, palms facing forward.

B

- Push the dumbbells up until your arms are fully extended, then lower them to the starting position.

REPS: Do 10 to 12.

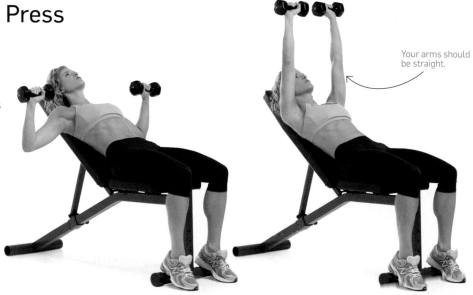

Your arms should be straight.

Scoop Hold

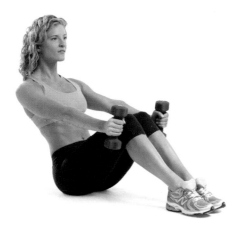

A

- Grab a 5-pound dumbbell in each hand, palms facing in. Sit with your knees bent, feet together flat on the floor, and arms extended outside your knees.

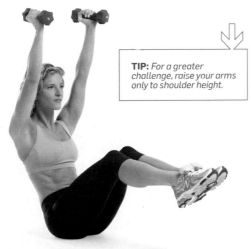

> **TIP:** *For a greater challenge, raise your arms only to shoulder height.*

B

- Raise your feet 6 to 12 inches and, keeping your arms straight, lift the weights over your head, pressing them together at the top.

REPS: Hold this position for as long as you can.

Triceps Dip and Reach

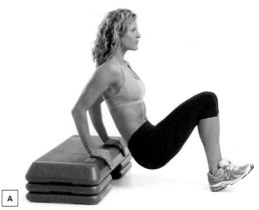

A

- Sit on the floor with your knees slightly bent and your back as close as you can get it to a 12-inch-high step. Grab the edge of the step with your hands slightly more than hip-width apart.
- Push your heels into the floor as you straighten your arms. Perform a dip.

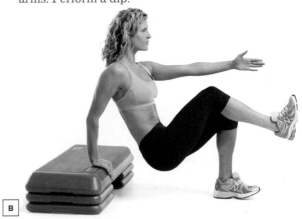

B

- Straighten your arms, then reach your left arm straight out in front of your body at shoulder height while lifting your right leg.
- Hold for a few seconds, then repeat, lifting the opposite arm and leg. That's 1 rep.

REPS: Do 12 to 15.

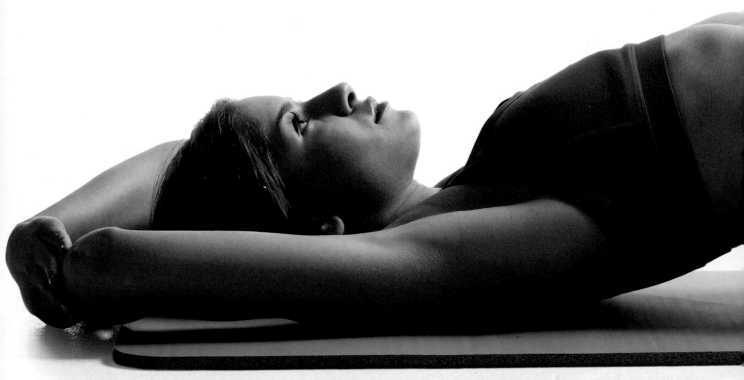

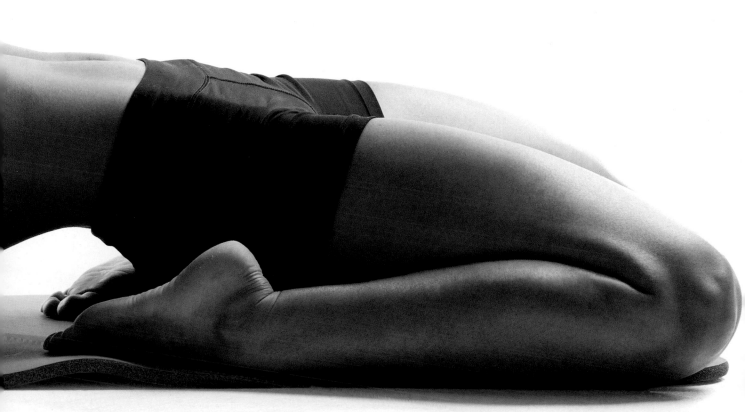

Chapter 7:
15-Minute Core Workouts

Injury-Proof Your Back, and Tighten
and Tone Your Middle.

Superfast Core Workouts

First, let's make one thing abundantly clear: Your core is more than your abs. Somewhere along the way, well-intentioned exercisers (and, indeed, even fitness instructors) started using the two terms, "core" and "abs," synonymously. The abdominals are essential players in your core muscle group, but they have an equally important supporting cast—namely all the muscles that run from your hips to your shoulders, including the muscles of your back and your obliques, which run down the sides of your torso. Mark Verstegen, the trainer and author of the book *Core Performance* who brought the concept of core training to the mainstream, likens strengthening this whole system of muscles to giving yourself a full-body makeover. You'll feel younger, stronger, and even smarter in the long run.

Abs with Benefits

HERE'S WHAT THESE WORKOUTS PROMISE:
STRAIGHTER, STRONGER POSTURE Your core muscles are the scaffolding that hold you upright. The stronger and more balanced they are, the straighter (and taller and thinner) you'll look.
BULLET-PROOF BACK (AND MORE) Studies show that much common back pain can be alleviated by strengthening the supporting muscles that run up and down your spine, as well as the deep abdominal muscles that create a corset for your midsection.
LIGHTNING FAST REACTIONS "Stabilizing your core hones your fine motor skills, so you can react quickly and stay balanced on unstable surfaces," says Verstegen.

Find It Quick: Your 15-Minute Core Circuit Plan

ANATOMY LESSON

YOUR CORE, the girdle of muscles that stabilize the spine, is made up of more than two dozen muscles. Get to know the key players:

Rectus abdominis: The six-pack muscles in front of your belly that are activated when you do crunches

Transverse abdominis: Deep muscles under the six-pack that pull your abdominal wall inward

Obliques: The abs muscles on the sides of your torso that help you bend to the side and resist rotation

Hip flexors: The muscles that allow you to flex your hips and raise your upper legs to walk and run

Lower back: The many muscles here play a critcal role in core mechanics by keeping your spine stable when you bend backward

IMPROVED MENTAL FUNCTION Your spine is the messenger between your brain and your body. "Having a stable and aligned spine allows your brain to receive your body's messages more efficiently," Verstegen says.

A FLATTER BELLY Training your core will indeed give you a flatter belly as you strengthen the soft and sagging muscles around your midsection.

Start with the basics...

The following workouts are designed to strengthen your entire core with a variety of moves that challenge your balance, stability, and rotational strength. For the best results, do one (or more) of these core workouts 2 days a week. You can do more, just be sure to leave a day of rest between workouts so your muscles can recover. Do the prescribed number of sets and reps for each exercise.

Each workout also lets you hone in on a special problem area, whether it be a lower-belly pooch or upper-back bra bulge. Pick the superfast workouts that hit your problem areas and you'll start seeing results in as little as 4 weeks!

Flat Belly Without a Single Crunch Workout

I remember when crunches became "the" ab-toning exercise du jour. Everyone was doing dozens of crunches a day; there were even special crunch devices to save the strain on your neck. Though the crunch is an effective move, there's more than one way to firm a midsection. Like this crunchless workout of dynamic exercises that will streamline your silhouette fast.

START HERE:

Do these moves one after another with no rest in between. Rest for 60 seconds at the end. Then repeat the circuit once more.

Reverse Wood Chop

A

- Squat, holding a medicine ball next to your left hip with both hands.

B

- Keep your arms straight and raise the ball up and across your body until you're standing and the ball is above your right shoulder.
- Lower back to the starting position. That's 1 rep.

REPS: Do 10, then start with the ball next to your right hip and raise it to your left shoulder 10 times.

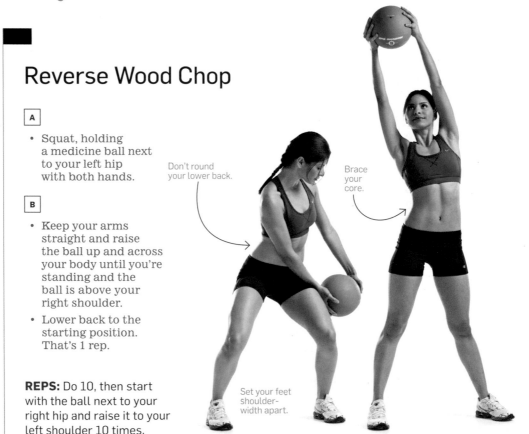

Don't round your lower back.

Brace your core.

Set your feet shoulder-width apart.

Single-Arm Lunge

A

- Hold a dumbbell and raise your left arm, keeping your elbow close to your ear.

B

- Step forward with your right foot, lowering until your thigh is parallel to the floor.
- Push off your right foot to stand. That's 1 rep.

REPS: Do 8 to 10 with each leg and arm.

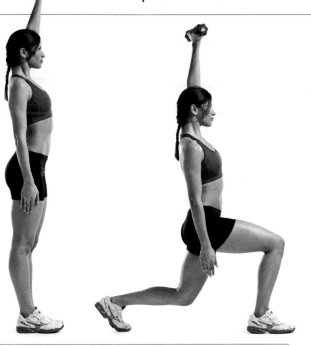

Reverse Plank with Leg Raise

A

- Assume a reverse plank position with legs outstretched, hands behind your butt, fingers forward.

B

- Press up onto your hands and lift your right leg, keeping your hips raised.
- Hold for 3 seconds. Then lower your leg.

REPS: Do 10 times on each side.

TIP: *Weak glutes contribute to unflattering belly bulge. These moves will fix that.*

DO MORE STABILITY EXERCISES

Don't like crunches? Fine with us. You'd be better off doing stability exercises—like planks, chops and mountain climbers. Those moves work the muscles that stabilize your spine, which is your core's more important job. If you didn't have these muscles, your torso would flop over like a limp stalk of boiled asparagus instead of staying straight upright. Crunches and situps work the abdominal muscles that flex the spine. But rounding your lower back repeatedly with these exercises can contribute to lower-back problems. So make the most of your core with stability exercises while adding occasional moves that rotate and flex the trunk, exercise the hip flexors, and work the obliques for a solid, stable core.

Flat Belly Without a Single Crunch Workout

Single-Arm Bent-Over Row

Don't round your lower back.

Don't rotate or lift your torso as you row the weight.

Bend your knees slightly

A

- Hold a dumbbell in your right hand, bend your knees, and lean forward from your hips.

B

- Brace your abs and pull the weight up to chest height without rotating your torso.
- Return to the starting position. That's 1 rep.

REPS: Do 10 to 12 with each arm.

Half-Seated Leg Circle

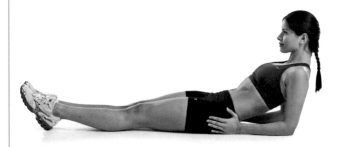

A

- Sit on the floor with your legs fully extended, leaning back on your elbows, your fingers cupping the sides of your hips.

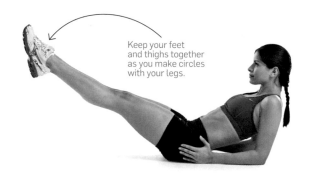

Keep your feet and thighs together as you make circles with your legs.

B

- Engage your core and lift your legs about 45 degrees.
- Point your toes, press your thighs together, and trace 12 large clockwise circles, then 12 counterclockwise circles.

REPS: Do 12 each way.

Rock 'n' Roll Core

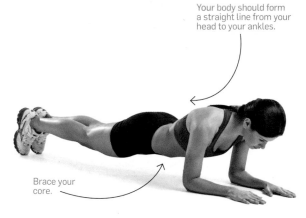

Your body should form a straight line from your head to your ankles.

Brace your core.

A

- Assume a plank position with your forearms flat on the floor and your palms down.

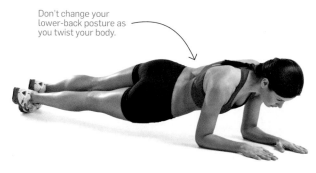

Don't change your lower-back posture as you twist your body.

B

- Keeping your hands in place and using your feet as the pivot point, twist your body to the left as far as possible without losing your balance.
- Repeat to the right. That's 1 rep.

REPS: Do three sets of 8 to 10, resting for 30 seconds between sets.

Hammer Toss

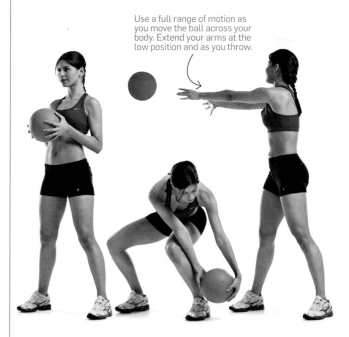

Use a full range of motion as you move the ball across your body. Extend your arms at the low position and as you throw.

A

- Grab a 5-pound medicine ball and stand with your feet shoulder-width apart, knees slightly bent.
- Hold the ball with both hands in front of your chest.

B

- Lower your hips and touch the ball outside your left foot.

C

- Stand up quickly, bringing the ball across the front of your body, and toss it to a partner, releasing to the right at about shoulder height.
- Have the partner toss it back. That's 1 rep.

REPS: Do 10, then repeat to the other side.

151

The Sidewinder Workout

If you're pouring out over the waistband of your pants, you've got muffin top going on. Firming your obliques can shrink the spillage.

START HERE: ■

Do these moves one after another with no rest between them. Then repeat the circuit for a total of two times.

Prone Oblique Roll

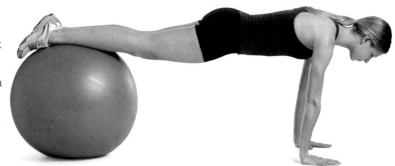

A

- Assume a plank position with your shins about hip-width apart on a stability ball and your hands shoulder-width apart on the floor.

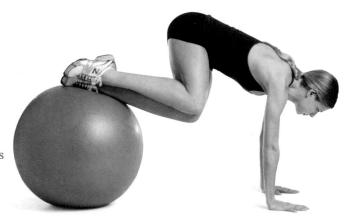

B

- Draw your knees toward your right shoulder.
- Return to the center, then draw your knees toward your left shoulder. That's 1 rep.

REPS: Do 12 to 15.

Walk-the-Plank and Rotate

A

- Assume a plank position with your hands on a 12- to 18-inch high step.

B

- With your weight on your left arm, rotate your body while raising your right arm toward the ceiling.

Brace your core throughout the movement.

Transfer your weight to your arm and hand when moving the opposite hand on and off the step.

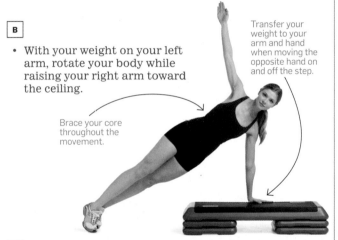

C

- Return to the plank position and step your hands, right then left, to each side of the bench. Step back up, leading with your left hand. That's 1 rep.

REPS: Do 8 to 10, then repeat the exercise, this time raising your left arm toward the ceiling.

Side-Lying Double-Leg Lift

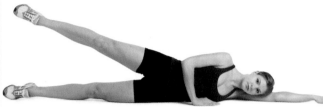

A

- Lie on your left side with your legs stacked, your head resting on the bottom arm, your right hand on the floor.
- Lift your right leg to 45 degrees, hold for a breath and return.

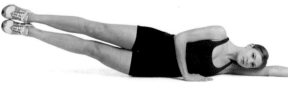

B

- Next, squeeze your legs together and lift both off the floor. Hold for a breath, then lower them.

REPS: Do 8 to 10, then repeat the moves while lying on your right side.

The Sidewinder Workout

Side Imprint

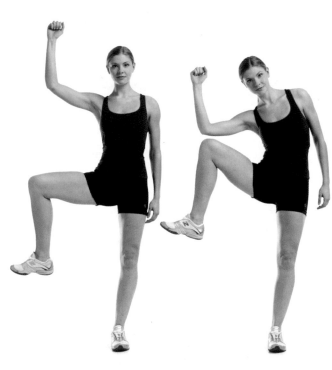

A

- Stand with your shoulders in line with your hips and raise your right arm. Shift onto your left leg and lift and rotate your right leg at the hip, turning your toes out.

B

- Crunch your right elbow and right knee together, pinching your waist. Return to the starting position.

REPS: Do 10 to each side.

Canoe

A

- Stand with your feet about 3 feet apart, knees slightly bent and hands clasped around a 2- to 5-pound dumbbell held in front of your chest.

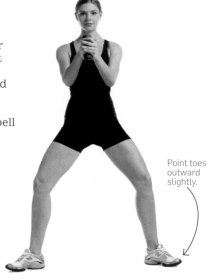

Point toes outward slightly.

B

- Keeping your hips still, bring your hands down to your right hip, "paddling" backward. Next, raise your hands up to chest level and then paddle them to the left hip.

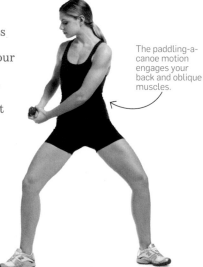

The paddling-a-canoe motion engages your back and oblique muscles.

REPS: Do 20 alternating from side to side.

Side Plank with Rotation

Before attempting this exercise, you should be able to hold the side plank for 60 seconds.

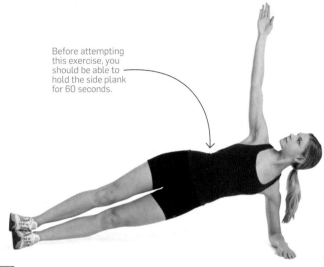

A

- Assume a left-side plank position, your left elbow directly under your shoulder.
- Brace your abs and reach your right hand toward the ceiling.

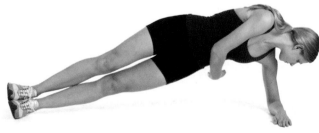

B

- Slowly tuck your right arm under your body and twist forward until your torso is almost parallel to the floor. Return to the side plank. That's 1 rep.

REPS: Do 5 to 10 on each side.

Ab Chopper

TIP: *This rotational exercise helps your abs work with your lower back and hip muscles to rotate your body with more power for explosive sports moves.*

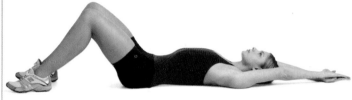

A

- Lie on your back with your hands together straight overhead.

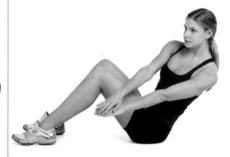

B

- Contract your abs and crunch up, bringing your hands over to the outside of your left thigh. Return to the starting position and repeat to the right. That's 1 rep.

REPS: Do 15. As you get stronger, grab a 3- to 5-pound dumbbell with both hands and do 10.

Banish Bra Bulge Workout

Nothing wrecks a good look in a tight-fitting top faster than two flabby rolls spilling out over your bra straps. Working the back and sides of your core as well as the abdominal muscles in the front will give you smooth, sleek lines even in your clingiest clothes.

START HERE:

Do these moves one after another with no rest between them. Then repeat the circuit for a total of three times.

Back Extension Leg Raise

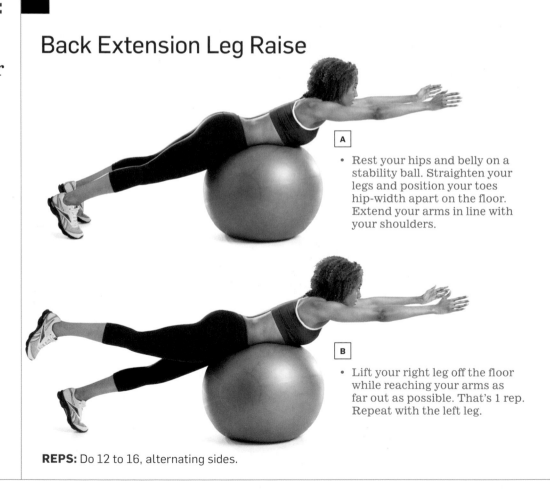

A

- Rest your hips and belly on a stability ball. Straighten your legs and position your toes hip-width apart on the floor. Extend your arms in line with your shoulders.

B

- Lift your right leg off the floor while reaching your arms as far out as possible. That's 1 rep. Repeat with the left leg.

REPS: Do 12 to 16, alternating sides.

Double-Leg Stretch

A

- Lie on your back on the floor, bend and hold onto your shins, and curl your shoulders up off the floor.

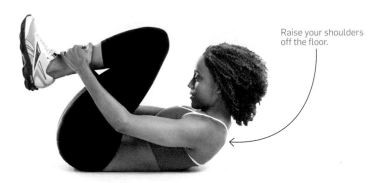

Raise your shoulders off the floor.

B

- Keeping your hips down and your lower back pressed into the floor, extend your legs up and out at a 45-degree angle to the floor as you reach your arms straight up (biceps near ears), forming a wide U shape with your body.

- Hold this position, pressing your ribs down toward the floor.
- Use your abs to bring your legs and arms back to the starting position, with your knees bent.

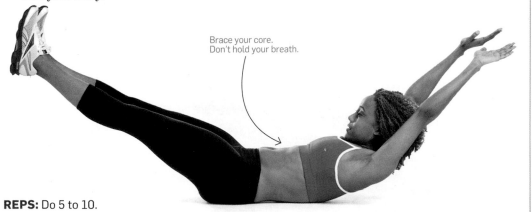

Brace your core. Don't hold your breath.

REPS: Do 5 to 10.

Banish Bra Bulge Workout

T-Stabilizer

A

- Assume a pushup position with your hands on the floor directly under your shoulders.

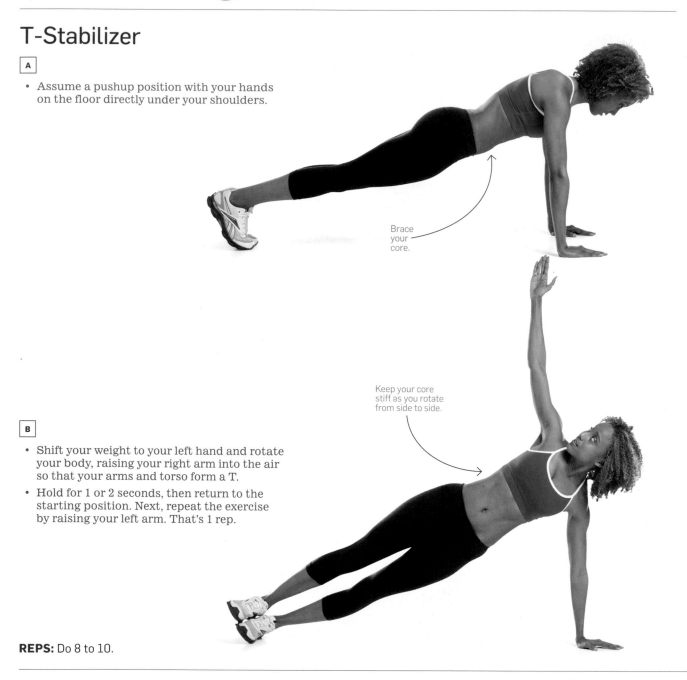

Brace your core.

Keep your core stiff as you rotate from side to side.

B

- Shift your weight to your left hand and rotate your body, raising your right arm into the air so that your arms and torso form a T.

- Hold for 1 or 2 seconds, then return to the starting position. Next, repeat the exercise by raising your left arm. That's 1 rep.

REPS: Do 8 to 10.

Alternating Dumbbell Row

As you lift one dumbbell, lower the other.

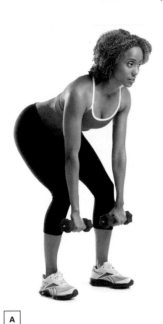
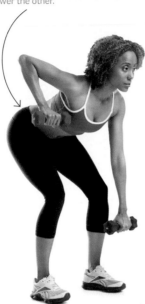

A

B

- Grab a pair of dumbbells with an overhand grip and stand with your feet shoulder-width apart and your knees slightly bent. Bend at your hips, keeping your lower back naturally arched, and lower your torso until it's almost parallel with the floor. Let the dumbbells hang at arm's length from your shoulders.

- Now pull the dumbbell in your right hand to the side of your torso by raising your upper arm, bending your elbow, and squeezing your shoulder blade toward your spine.

- As you lower that dumbbell, row the dumbbell in your left hand to the side of your torso. That's 1 rep.

REPS: Do 8 to 10.

Double-Arm Reach

You can also do this move without a dumbbell in your hands.

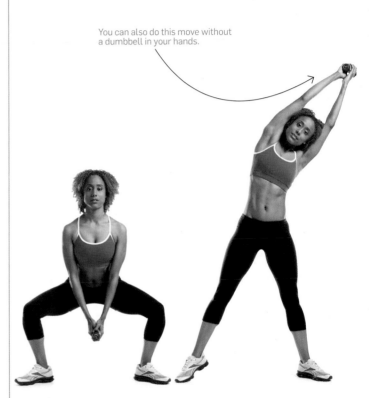

A

B

- Stand with your feet about 3 feet apart and clasp a 2- to 5-pound dumbbell in front of you with both hands.

- Contract your abs and perform a plié keeping your hands toward the floor.

- As you push up, raise your arms to the left.

- Next, lower your hands with another plié and then lift them to the right. That's 1 rep.

REPS: Do 20.

Belly Pooch Workout

Even otherwise slender, fit women can end up with a sway belly due to underworked lower-abdominal muscles. Runners and other cardio junkies are notorious for letting their midsections go soft while they spend hours on their legs. This workout is designed to tap into the deep abdominal muscles—the transverse abdominis—that pull in your waistline like a natural corset.

START HERE: ▬

Do these moves one after another with no rest in between. Then repeat the circuit for a total of two times.

Stability Ball Pelvic Tilt Crunch

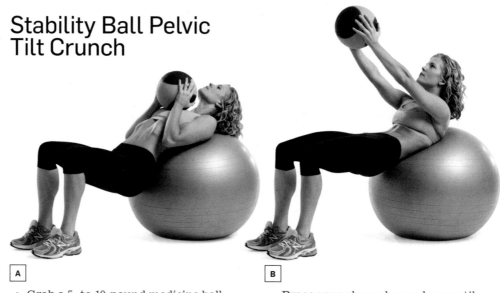

A

- Grab a 5- to 10-pound medicine ball. Lie faceup on a stability ball with your back and head pressed into the ball, your feet together on the floor, and the medicine ball positioned against your chest.

REPS: Do 12 to 15.

B

- Brace your abs and crunch up until your shoulders are off the ball.
- Then reach the medicine ball toward the ceiling.
- Lower it down and return to the starting position.

Nose to Knee

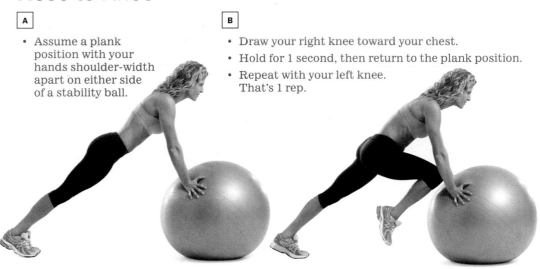

A

- Assume a plank position with your hands shoulder-width apart on either side of a stability ball.

B

- Draw your right knee toward your chest.
- Hold for 1 second, then return to the plank position.
- Repeat with your left knee. That's 1 rep.

REPS: Do 12 to 15.

HAVE A BALL!

People who add stability ball exercises to their ab workouts build midsections that are four times more stable than those who do no stability ball moves, according to a study published in the *Journal of Strength and Conditioning Research.*

The Matrix

A

- Grab a 5- to 10-pound medicine ball and kneel on the floor with your knees hip-width apart.
- Lengthen your spine and press the ball against your abs.

B

- Slowly lean back as far as possible, keeping your knees planted.
- Hold the reclined position for 3 seconds, then use your core to slowly come up to the starting position.

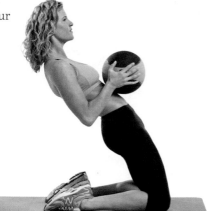

REPS: Do 12 to 15.

Belly Pooch Workout

Arm Pullover Straight-Leg Crunch

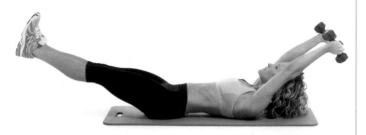

A

- Grab a pair of 10- to 12-pound dumbbells and lie on your back with your arms extended behind you.
- Extend your legs at a 45-degree angle.

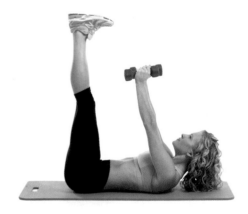

B

- Bring your arms up over your chest and lift your shoulders off the mat while raising your legs until they're perpendicular to the floor.
- Return to the starting position (don't let your legs touch the floor).

REPS: Do 12 to 15.

Knee Cross Crunch

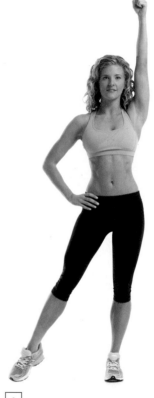
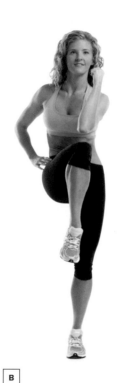

A

- Stand with your shoulders in line with your hips and extend your left arm up and your right leg to the side, toes pointed.

B

- Next, lower your left elbow and raise your right knee, crunching them together on a diagonal line.
- Return to the starting position.

REPS: Do 12 to 15 on each side.

The Sprinter

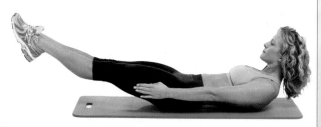

A

- Lie on your back with your arms at your sides, your legs straight, and your heels hovering 6 to 12 inches off the floor.

Control your movement through the entire exercise, bracing your core to keep pressure off your back

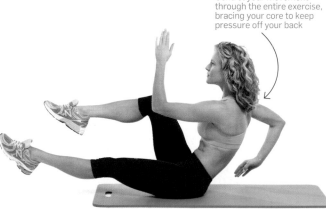

B

- Start sitting up while elevating your left arm with the elbow bent so it resembles a sprinter's pumping motion. At the peak of the situp, bring your right knee to your chest.
- Return to the starting position, keeping your legs raised, and repeat with the opposite arm and leg. That's 1 rep.

REPS: Do 10 to 12.

Wall Crunch and Twist

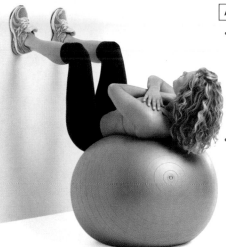

A

- Sit on a stability ball facing a wall, then lie back so the middle to small of your back is resting on the ball.
- Place your feet hip-width apart on the wall with your knees bent to 90 degrees; cross your hands over your chest.

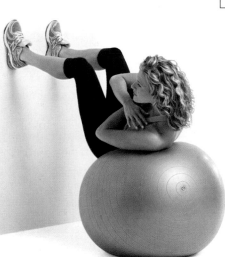

B

- Curl up and twist through the waist to the left.
- Return to center and curl down.
- Alternate to twist right. That's 1 rep.

REPS: Do 10 to 12.

Belly Blast Workout

To blast away belly fat while firming all those key core muscles, you need to crank up your calorie burn. This action-packed routine that includes moves from Kurt, Brett, and Mike Brungardt, brothers and authors of *The Complete Book of Core Training*, hits every body muscle needed to form a flat belly and raises your heart rate to burn belly fat fast.

START HERE:

Do these exercises in order. Between exercises, don't rest; instead, jump rope (or do high-intensity calisthenics) for 60 seconds. Perform the entire circuit once and you're done!

Sun Salute with Cross

A

- Stand with your legs hip-width apart, arms extended overhead with hands just touching.

B

- Bending forward at the waist, reach down with both hands and touch your right foot, keeping your torso straight and moving as one unit.
- Straighten back to the starting position. Repeat on the opposite side to complete 1 rep.

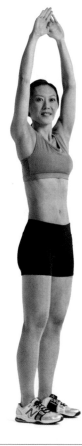
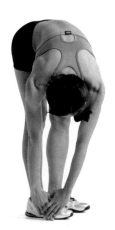

REPS: Do 10 to 20.

Ankle Reach

- Lie on your belly with your legs straight and your toes touching the floor.
- Bend your arms with your palms on the floor in line with your ears.

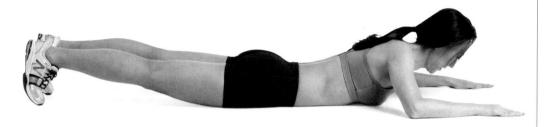

B

- Reaching both arms back and up, bend your right leg, reaching your heel toward your butt as you touch your hands to your right ankle.
- Slowly lower your arms and leg to the starting position. Repeat with your left leg to complete 1 rep.

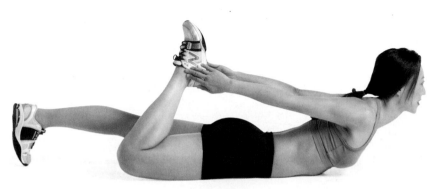

REPS: Do 10 to 20.

PROTECT YOUR NECK

Put your tongue on the roof of your mouth when you do crunches or other ab moves where you lift your upper body. "It will help align your head properly, which helps reduce neck strain," says Michael Mejia, CSCS, *Men's Health* exercise advisor and a strength and conditioning specialist in Long Island, New York.

Belly Blast Workout

Double Side Jackknife

- Lie on your left side, your legs stacked and straight.
- Wrap your left arm in front of your torso, placing it on your right hip, and put your right hand behind your head.

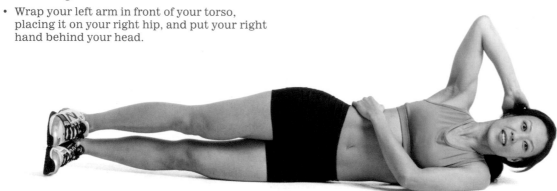

B

- Simultaneously raise your torso and legs, bringing your shoulders toward your hips.
- Return to the starting position in a controlled motion and repeat for all reps, then switch sides and repeat the same number of reps to complete one set.

TIP: *If the exercise is too hard, start by lifting only your legs.*

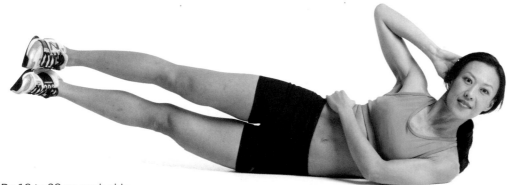

REPS: Do 10 to 20 on each side.

Dynamic V Crunch

A

- Lie faceup with your legs straight and in line with your hips and perpendicular to your torso.
- Extend your arms in front of you, keeping them in line with your shoulders. Contract your abs and lower your legs so they're at a 45-degree angle with your hips.

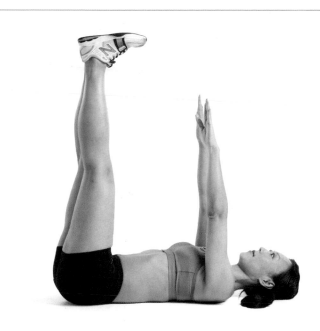

B

- Bring your hands together and reach toward your left leg, simultaneously raising it in line with your hips.
- Lower your left leg to the 45-degree position. Repeat with the right leg to complete 1 rep.

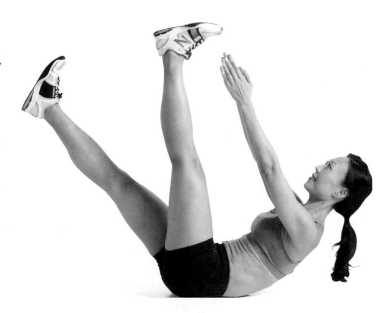

REPS: Do 10 to 20.

GIVE YOUR CORE A WALKOUT

Canadian researchers found that the plank walkout achieves 100 percent activation of your rectus abdominis (the six-pack muscles). Add this move to your workouts to help carve your core.

1. Assume the up position of a pushup, with your hands just past shoulder-width and your body in a straight line.

2. Brace your abs and hold them that way for the entire exercise.

3. Slowly walk your hands out in front of your head until your back begins to "collapse"—in other words, the point at which your hips start to sag.

4. Walk your feet forward so your body is back in the starting position of a pushup, and then repeat.

5. Complete a total of 6 to 10 repetitions.

Belly Blast Workout

Raised Hips Crunch

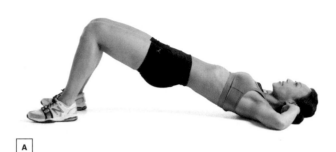

A

- Lie faceup with your knees bent and your feet flat on the floor, your hands behind your head, and your fingers unclasped.
- Press your hips off the floor into a bridge position, keeping your hips level.

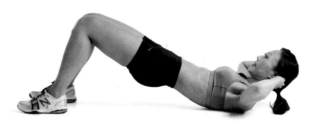

B

- Maintaining the bridge, contract your abs and then raise your head, neck, and shoulders off the floor as one unit. (You'll be supported by your feet and upper back.)
- Pause, then lower yourself and repeat. For more of a challenge, lift one foot slightly while you perform half of your reps, then lift the other foot for the other half.

REPS: Do 10 to 20.

Side Double Crunch

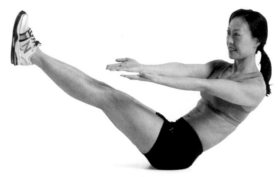

A

- Lie balanced on your left buttock, with your legs straight but not locked, and your arms straight, palms up.

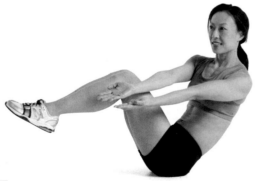

B

- Simultaneously crunch your legs and torso together, bending your knees toward your chest while still balancing on your left buttock.
- Return to the starting position.

REPS: Do 10 to 20, then switch sides and repeat.

Bosu Reverse Hyperextensions

The Perfect Crunch
Circle Crunch

TIP: *To make this exercise harder, raise your legs with your knees bent at 90 degrees and your calves parallel to floor as you perform each rep.*

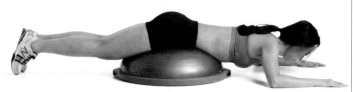

A

- Lie facedown with your belly on a Bosu, your legs fully extended, and your palms flat on the floor.

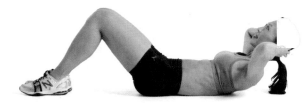

A

- Lie faceup with your knees bent, your feet flat on the floor, and your hands behind your head with your fingers lightly touching.
- Lift your shoulders off the floor until you feel a tight contraction.

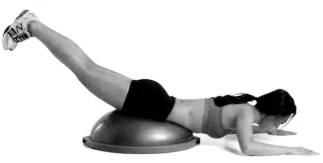

B

- Squeeze your lower back and glutes to raise your legs, holding the contraction for as long as you can at the top of the movement.
- Lower your legs until they lightly touch the floor.

REPS: Do 10 to 20.

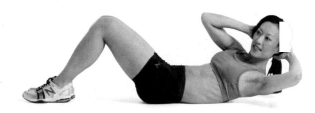

B

- Curl your torso around in a small, clockwise circular motion (starting from 6 to 9 to 12 to 3 and back down to 6).
- For the next rep, repeat in the opposite, counter-clockwise direction.

REPS: Do 10 to 20.

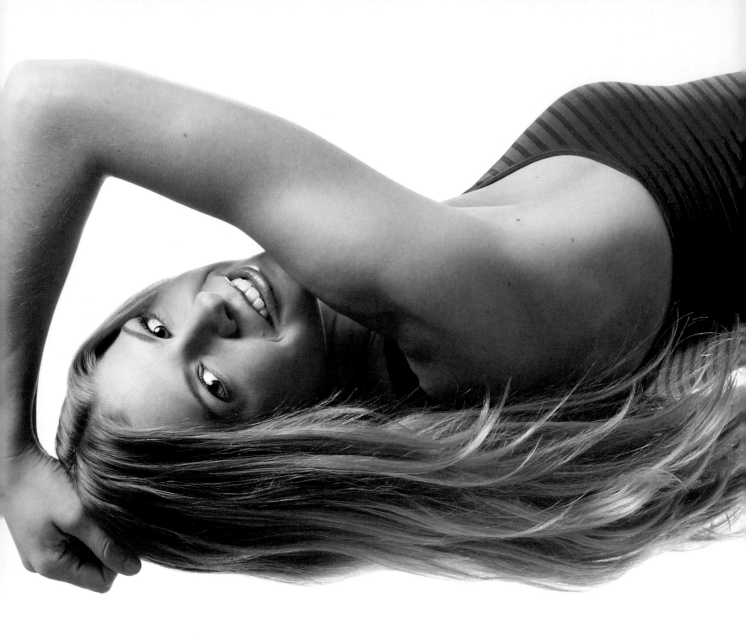

Chapter 8: 15-Minute Fat-Burning HIIT Workouts

High-Intensity Interval Training, or HIIT, Is Your Weekly Secret Weapon for Trimming and Tightening Your Body.

Superfast Interval Training Workouts

The next time you're in the gym, look at the dashboard of your treadmill (or elliptical or stationary bike). You see that colored bar chart showing what your heart rate should be to put you in the "fat-burning zone?" Ever wonder why reaching that rate was so easy (or why it seemed to take an endless amount of time to burn a decent amount of calories)? That type of training, where you slog along slowly for hours on end in the hopes of burning more stored fat, is like cooking a roast in a slow cooker—great if you have all day to do it, but nowhere near as efficient as firing up the grill and searing the sucker. And that's exactly what you'll be doing to your fat with our superfast fat-burning workouts, which use high-intensity interval training (HIIT).

Find It Quick: Your 15-Minute High-Intensity Interval Training Plan

SPRINT AWAY FROM DIABETES

A study in Norway found that a high-intensity interval exercise program can reverse metabolic syndrome, the precursor to type 2 diabetes. Researchers compared 45 minutes of moderate exercise to an interval training program in which participants performed four 4-minute bouts at 90 percent of their maximum heart rate and found that HIIT workouts are more beneficial than the longer, slower exercise routines at preventing obesity, diabetes, and cardiovascular problems.

As you learned in Chapter 1, HIIT workouts are built for speed. So they tap into every single muscle fiber, scorch tons of calories, and rev up your metabolism for hours (even days) afterwards. With these workouts you'll be burning fat almost from the get-go by going faster and harder than your normal cardio rate. Sound intimidating? Don't worry. You'll only be doing these "sprints" briefly, for 30 seconds to 2 minutes. Then you'll slow down to a normal speed. It's an incredibly efficient way to get rid of extra pounds, explains Jason Talanian, PhD, who researched HIIT at the University of Guelph, Ontario. "HIIT elicits rapid skeletal muscle remodeling and increases your total exercise capacity—the ability to use oxygen and burn fat—in a fraction of the time than if you work out less intensely," he says. That means you also make more muscle tissue and generate more fat-burning enzymes and hormones.

We've taken the HIIT principles and applied them to all of your favorite forms of cardio to create our superfast fat-burning workouts. Do one a week as the plan (see page 21) recommends. If you're inspired, you can do more, but remember, these workouts are strong medicine, so cap them at three times a week, allowing a day of recovery in between. During the exercise, alternate between short high-intensity bursts, where you're exerting yourself at, say, level 8 or 9 on a 1 to 10 scale, and longer medium-intensity sessions, where your effort will be more like a 6 on that same scale.

Treadmill Workouts

There are two ways to turn up the intensity on the treadmill: push the pace or jack up the incline. Here are two HIIT workouts to get it done whichever way you like best.

Workout #1: The Speed Demon

The Speed Demon uses sprints to fry fat, but we still recommend putting the incline at 1 (when it's 0, it's like you're running downhill.) As you get fitter, you can increase the speed even more to make the workout harder, or add a percent or two to the incline. If you're a beginner, you can lower the speeds by 1 mph, or as much as you need to stay within the recommended effort range.

TIME	ACTIVITY	SPEED (MPH)	EFFORT (1–10)
0:00 – 3:00	Warmup walk	3.5–3.8	4–5
3:00 – 3:45	Sprint!	7+	9–10
3:45 – 4:30	Brisk jog	4.5–6.5	7
4:30 – 5:30	Sprint!	7+	9–10
5:30 – 6:30	Brisk jog	4.5–6.5	7
6:30 – 8:00	Sprint!	7+	9–10
8:00 – 9:00	Brisk jog	4.5–6.5	7
9:00 – 10:15	Sprint!	7+	9–10
10:15 – 11:15	Brisk jog	4.5–6.5	7
11:15 – 12:00	Sprint!	7+	9–10
12:00 – 12:45	Brisk jog	4.5–6.5	7
12:45 – 15:00	Cooldown walk	3.5–3.8	4–5

Workout #2: HIIT the Hills

This workout uses the treadmill's incline to simulate the challenge of hills. If you find it a little too high to start, simply take each one down by 1. As you become fitter and stronger, crank up the incline to conquer mountains (of calories!).

TIME	ACTIVITY/EFFORT (1-10)	SPEED (MPH)	INCLINE %
0:00 – 3:00	Warmup walk/4–5	3.5–3.8	1
3:00 – 4:00	Small hill jog/8–9	4–5	4–5
4:00 – 6:00	Brisk flat jog/7	4.2–6.5	0
6:00 – 7:00	Medium hill jog/9	4–5	6
7:00 – 9:00	Brisk flat jog/7	4.2–6.5	0
9:00 – 10:00	Big hill jog/10	4–5 (if possible)	7–8
10:00 – 12:00	Brisk flat jog/7	4.2–6.5	0
12:00 – 13:00	Peak! Fast walk/10	3.5–4	10
13:00 – 15:00	Cooldown/4-5	3.5–3.8	1–0

Running Workouts

When you run long distances, your body actually becomes more efficient, so you burn fewer calories. These hard-hitting workouts help you shed pounds with minimal mileage by forcing your body out of its comfort zone and making it work in ways it rarely does. It not only boosts your speed and fitness, but also takes a quarter of the time! These workouts are designed to be done on a track (try your local high school or college).

Workout #1: Dash It Off

The 200-meter dash (that's halfway around the track) is the perfect leg-searing distance because you don't have to hold back to finish. It's just flat-out full throttle the whole time, followed by a recovery jog for one lap. Seasoned runners will be a little quicker; novice runners may take a little longer.

TIME	SPEED	DISTANCE
0:00 – 5:00	Easy jog to warm up	About 2 laps
5:00 – 5:30	Dash	Aim for ¼ to ½ lap
5:30 – 7:00	Jog	Aim for about 1 lap
7:00 – 7:30	Dash	Aim for ¼ to ½ lap
7:30 – 10:00	Jog	Aim for about 1 lap
10:00 – 10:30	Dash	Aim for ¼ to ½ lap
10:30 – 13:00	Jog	Aim for about 1 lap
13:00 – 13:30	Dash	Aim for ¼ to ½ lap
13:30 – 15:00	Cooldown jog to walk	

MISERY LOVES COMPANY

If you're finding that HIIT workouts are a real pain in the butt, recruit some friends. Researchers at the University of Oxford found that people who train in groups can boost their pain tolerance more than those who work out alone. The scientists speculate that group dynamics during exercise may contribute to an underlying endorphin surge. We think people feed off the energy of others, which may be the same thing.

Workout #2: Flying Laps

These one-lap wonders will challenge all your energy systems to the max. Unlike the half-laps, where you're going full steam from the get-go, for these keep a little energy in reserve, just enough so that you don't find yourself flagging at the end of the interval, but rather can finish a little stronger than you started. Seasoned runners will be a little quicker; novice runners may take a little longer.

TIME	SPEED	DISTANCE
0:00 – 5:00	Easy jog to warm up	About 2 laps
5:00 – 7:00	Dash	Aim for about 1 lap
7:00 – 8:00	Easy jog	Aim for about ½ lap
8:00 – 10:00	Dash	Aim for about 1 lap
10:00 – 11:00	Easy jog	Aim for about ½ lap
11:00 – 13:00	Dash	Aim for about 1 lap
13:00 – 15:00	Jog easy to cool down	

Cycling Workouts

Whether you ride indoors or out, a bike is the perfect tool for superfast fat burning since there's no pounding on your joints, just pure, unabated eye-popping effort. These workouts are designed for both a spin or stationary bike and a road bike. On a spin or stationary bike you'll just be increasing the resistance. On a road bike you'll be shifting into a larger gear.

Workout #1: The Lance Armstrong

These workouts get your calorie-burning motor running by becoming progressively harder until you're at your ceiling (then you just hang on!). Gauge your intensity on a 1 to 10 scale. If you're outside, you can use the average speeds as a guide. More experienced riders may pedal faster.

TIME	ACTIVITY	LEVEL (1–10)	SPEED (MPH)
0:00 – 3:00	Warmup	6	10–15
3:00 – 5:00	Fast pedaling	8	16–17
5:00 – 6:00	Chase pace	9	18–19
6:00 – 6:30	Sprint!	10	20+
6:30 – 9:30	Easy pedaling	6	10–15
9:30 – 11:30	Fast pedaling	8	16–17
11:30 – 12:30	Chase pace	9	18–19
12:30 – 13:00	Sprint!	10	20+
13:00 – 15:00	Cooldown	6	10–15

Workout #2: Rolling Hills

If you're outside and have access to hills, you can ride up them for a prescribed amount of time and then cruise back down and repeat. If not, or if you're using a stationary bike, simply click into a bigger gear to increase the resistance. The goal is to make those pedals hard to turn during each effort while keeping the pedals turning around smoothly. Your speed will drop as the resistance increases, but you should be able to keep your pedal stroke fluid, not choppy. When the workout calls for a standing climb, rise off the seat for the duration of the interval. For seated climbs, stay planted in the saddle and increase your pace to pedal as quickly as you can.

TIME	ACTIVITY	LEVEL/GEAR	INCLINE/RESISTANCE
0:00 – 3:00	Warmup	6	0–3%/Light
3:00 – 4:00	Fast seated climb	7	4–6%/Medium
4:00 – 5:30	Seated climb	8	6–8%/Hard
5:30 – 6:00	Standing climb	9	8–10%/Very hard
6:00 – 8:00	Fast and flat	6	0–3%/Light
8:00 – 9:00	Fast seated climb	7	4–6%/Medium
9:00 – 10:30	Seated climb	8	6–8%/Hard
10:30 – 11:00	Standing climb	9	8–10%/Very hard
11:00 – 13:00	Fast and flat	7	0–3%/Light
13:00 – 15:00	Cooldown	6	0–3%/Light

Elliptical Workout

This perennial gym favorite provides a sweat-breaking, impact-free platform for high-intensity intervals. The following workout will push you through the machine's toughest settings for a full-body burn. You'll be increasing your speed, measured by the strides per minute indicator on the machine's dashboard, and ratcheting up the resistance at the same time, getting a little faster and tougher with each effort until you are maxed out. Remember, don't hold on to the rails, but rather pump your arms to keep your feet turning over as quickly as you can. If you have access to a machine with an incline feature, you also can add intensity by simulating some hill climbs. Just use the HIIT the Hills workout on page 175.

NOT A WALK IN THE PARK

While the elliptical has always been known as a great tool for injury rehab, lately it has developed an unfair reputation as the machine for those who would rather read than sweat. True, you can take it easy on this device by hanging on to the handrails and allowing pedal momentum to do the work—but used properly, it can kick your metabolism into high gear. A new study from the University of Nebraska found that exercising on an ellipitcal trainer burns as many calories as running on a treadmill at the same level of effort. Oxygen consumption was also equivalent on both machines, but people's average heart rates were actually higher when working out on the elliptical, possibly because the newness of the motion requires your muscles to do more balancing work. To keep your body guessing, alternate between both cardio machines.

Ramp It Up!

TIME	ACTIVITY	SPM*/EXERTION (1–10)	RESISTANCE
0:00 – 2:00	Warmup	130–140/5–6	3–5
2:00 – 4:00	Ramp (medium pace)	150–180/7–8	7–8
4:00 – 5:00	Sprint!	190/9–10	8–9
5:00 – 6:00	Steady	150/6–7	7
6:00 – 8:00	Ramp (medium pace)	160–190/7–8	7–8
8:00 – 9:00	Sprint!	200/10	9–10
9:00 – 10:00	Steady	150/6–7	7
10:00 – 12:00	Ramp (medium pace)	170–200/7–8	7–8
12:00 – 13:00	Sprint!	210/10	9–10
13:00 – 15:00	Cooldown	130–140/5–6	3–5

*Strides per minute.

Swimming Workout

Water is 800 times denser than air, so doing the equivalent of sprinting across a pool burns fat like nothing else. This workout will shed inches off your body. Do the workout as prescribed, swimming the recommended stroke for the prescribed number of lengths and at a range of effort from 1 to 10. (Note: The workout is based on a standard 25-meter lap pool; Olympic-size pools are 50 meters. If you're unsure of the size of your pool, ask the pool manager or lifeguard. One length is across the pool. One lap is across the pool and back.

FREESTYLE POINTERS

Better form means a better workout. Practice these fine points when learning to crawl.

1. Look at the bottom of the pool. Lifting your head causes your hips to drop and slows you down.

2. Be a fish. Practice swimming smooth and quietly without slapping the water, a sign of wasted energy.

3. When extending your leading hand, let is sink 8 inches before starting your pull. Imagine you're wrapping your arm over a barrel and pushing it behind you.

4. Roll, baby, roll. Developing good body roll allows you to use your strong lats, core, and back muscles to drive your stroke and it helps you cut through the water efficiently. And breathing becomes easier. To learn proper rotation, practice kicking on your side with a pair of flippers and one arm stretched in front of you.

A STROKE OF GENIUS

To get the most from your swimming intervals, build a more efficient (longer and faster) stroke. Try this drill: Take two strokes with your right arm, one with your left, one with your right, and then two with your left. Next, take one stroke each with your right and left, two with your right, then two with your left. Continue this pattern for 5 minutes. This helps you even out your stroke and find a good rhythm, says Keith Bell, PhD, of the American Swimming Association.

The Uptempo Medley

If you're an experienced swimmer, add lengths or laps; if you're a beginner, subtract lengths or laps.

TIME	STROKE	LENGTH	EFFORT
0:00 – 3:00	Freestyle/mixed kicking	About 2 laps	4–5
3:00 – 5:00	Freestyle	About 2 laps	6–7
5:00 – 5:45	Freestyle	About 1 lap	9
5:45 – 7:00	Freestyle/mixed kicking	About 1 lap	6
7:00 – 7:45	Freestyle	About 1 lap	9
7:45 – 9:00	Freestyle/mixed kicking	About 1 lap	6
9:00 – 9:45	Freestyle	About 1 lap	9
9:45 – 11:00	Freestyle/mixed kicking	About 1 lap	6
11:00 – 11:30	Breast	About 1 length	8–9
11:30 – 13:00	Freestyle	1 lap + 1 length	8–9
13:00 – 15:00	Back/mixed kicking	About 1 lap	4–5

Jump Rope Workout

If you haven't skipped rope since you watched *Sesame Street*, you'll soon see why boxers, who use this simple tool to enhance their footwork all the time, never seem to have an ounce of fat on their bodies. This workout mixes different kinds of jumps—alternating right and left feet, doing high double jumps, where the rope goes under your feet twice—to give your body different challenges between the fast bursts. In general, jump about 2 inches off the floor—just enough to allow the rope to skim the floor beneath your feet. Keep your elbows close to your body and stay on the balls of your feet.

CASH FOR SWEAT

Nothing motivates like material rewards. Promise yourself a splurge for not missing a workout session for 1 month. Or it may be even more effective to set up a penalty for missing them. "People will work twice as hard when money is at stake," says Ian Ayres, economist and professor at Yale Law School and author of *Carrots and Sticks: Unlock the Power of Incentives to Get Things Done*.

How to Try It: Register your goal and credit card info at stickk.com. If you don't do a predetermined number of workouts, the charity of your choice gets a payday that gets charged to your plastic. "This is even more effective if you give money to something you don't like," adds Ayres. Diehard liberal? Set up your account to donate to a conservative group, and watch the pounds melt away.

Skipping School

TIME	JUMP STYLE	SPEED	EFFORT
0:00 – 1:00	Two-Foot Jump	Moderate	5–6/medium
1:00 – 1:30	Single-Foot Hop	Moderate	7/medium high
1:30 – 2:30	Two-Foot Jump	Moderate	5–6/medium
2:30 – 3:00	Single-Foot Hop	Moderate	7/medium high
3:00 – 5:00	Two-Foot Jump	Fast	8–9/high
5:00 – 6:00	Two-Foot Jump	Moderate	5–6/medium
6:00 – 7:30	Double Jump*	Fast	9–10/highest
7:30 – 8:30	Two-Foot Jump	Moderate	5–6/medium
8:30 – 10:30	Jumping Jacks**	Moderate to fast	8/high
10:30 – 11:30	Two-Foot Jump	Moderate	5–6/medium
11:30 – 13:30	Run Through***	Moderate to fast	8–9/high
13:30 – 15:00	Two-Foot Jump	Moderate	5–6/medium

*   *Jump high enough to pass the rope under your feet twice before landing.*

** *Jump over the rope and land with your feet wide apart. Then on the next jump, land with your feet together.*

*** *Run in place while swinging the rope up and around.*

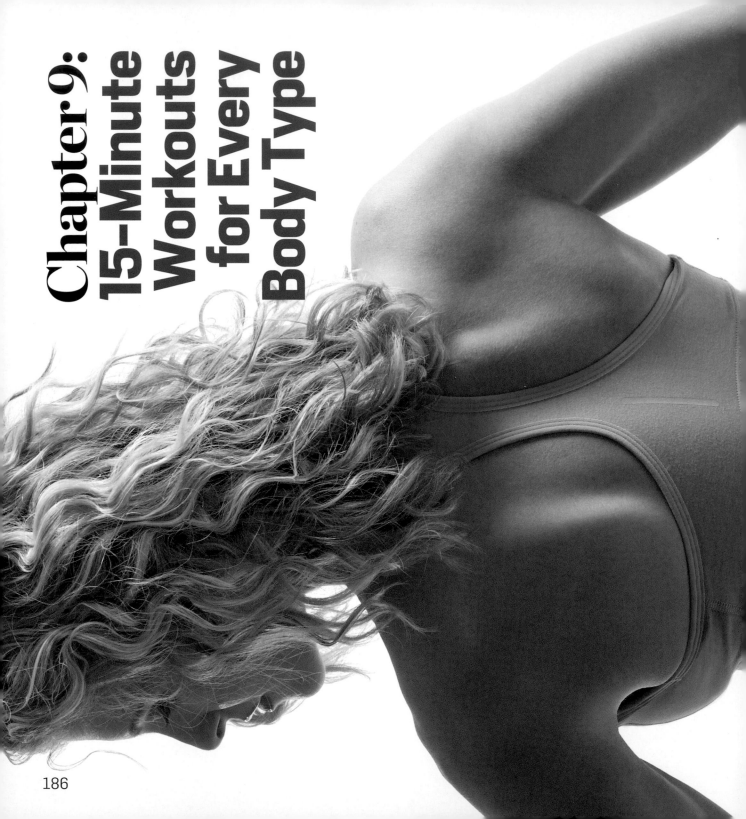

Chapter 9: 15-Minute Workouts for Every Body Type

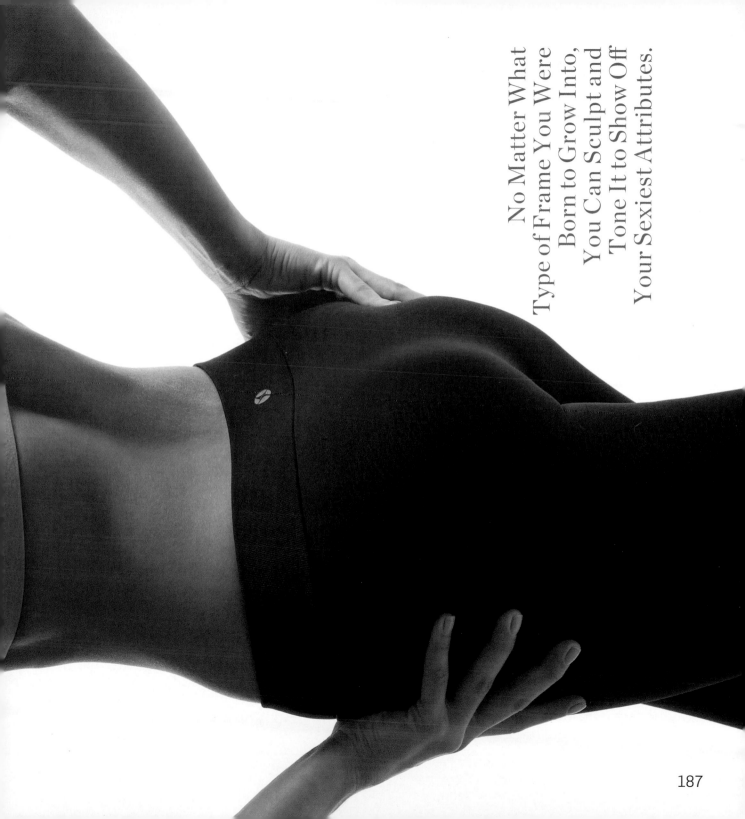

No Matter What Type of Frame You Were Born to Grow Into, You Can Sculpt and Tone It to Show Off Your Sexiest Attributes.

187

Superfast Body-Type Workouts

Most workouts are like off-the-rack dresses, made to suit most female forms fairly well, but if you want a true fit, you need to have it tailored. These workouts were custom-designed to address problems common to a particular body type, such as broad shoulders or a bottom-heavy build that can make you look imbalanced. So whether you're pear shaped, straight, curvy like an hourglass, or athletic, these superfast routines will help you look hot with what you've got.

Start with the basics...

You'll notice that each circuit workout below begins with the same four exercises: Lift-Off Lunge; Pushup and Leg Raise; Hundred on the Ball; and Mermaid. That's intentional because these moves are effective no matter what your particular body shape (find them starting on page 190).

Then we customize each program with four moves that are hand picked to show off your best attributes and tackle your problem spots. Now find your body type (don't worry, we have hints to help you) and get ready to get in shape. Do the workouts three times a week or mix in other 15-minute workouts.

WATCH YOUR FORM

Do your workout in front of a mirror. "This provides instant feedback; you'll know if your form is off, which is what a trainer would tell you," says Carla Sottovia, PhD, a senior personal trainer at the Cooper Fitness Center in Dallas. Look for these common mistakes: not keeping your neck in line with your spine and letting knees jut out past your toes when doing squats. Another mirror plus: A study at the University of Illinois at Urbana-Champaign found that seeing yourself sweat can give you the motivation you need to eke out more reps when you feel like giving up and going home.

Find It Quick: Your 15-Minute Circuits for Specific Body Types

p.194

Pear-Shaped-Body Workout

Lift-Off Lunge
Pushup and Leg Raise
Hundred on the Ball
Mermaid
Scissors Jump
Boat Curl and Press
Triangle Lateral Raise
Dip and Knee Raise

p.198

Hourglass-Body Workout

Lift-Off Lunge
Pushup and Leg Raise
Hundred on the Ball
Mermaid
Tai Chi Lunge
Side Planks with Moving Knee
Lateral Stepups
Glute Bridge with Triceps Extension

p.202

Boyish-Body Workout

Lift-Off Lunge
Pushup and Leg Raise
Hundred on the Ball
Mermaid
Crossover Crunch
Stacked Pushup
Plyo Plank
Squat and Overhead Press

p.206

Athletic-Body Workout

Lift-Off Lunge
Pushup and Leg Raise
Hundred on the Ball
Mermaid
Curtsy Hammer Raise
Swivel Squat
Tip and Row
Alternating Lateral Lunge

Main Moves

This chapter kicks off with four terrific exercises that we want everyone to do. Why? Because they'll ensure that you hit all the major muscle groups and put extra emphasis on your core region in every workout. Plus, these exercises are excellent for revving your metabolism.

START HERE: ⬛

The following four exercises are designed to complement every body type, so they are included in each of the four workouts.

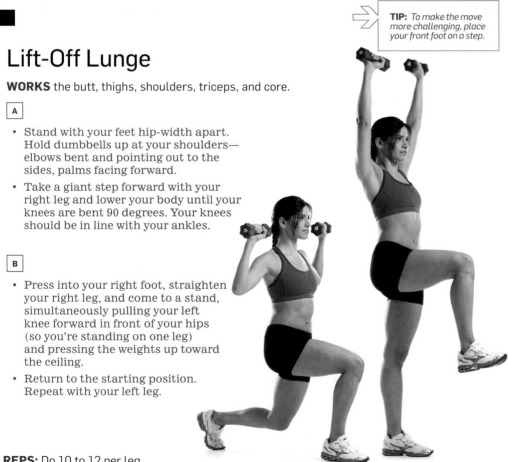

TIP: *To make the move more challenging, place your front foot on a step.*

Lift-Off Lunge

WORKS the butt, thighs, shoulders, triceps, and core.

A

- Stand with your feet hip-width apart. Hold dumbbells up at your shoulders—elbows bent and pointing out to the sides, palms facing forward.
- Take a giant step forward with your right leg and lower your body until your knees are bent 90 degrees. Your knees should be in line with your ankles.

B

- Press into your right foot, straighten your right leg, and come to a stand, simultaneously pulling your left knee forward in front of your hips (so you're standing on one leg) and pressing the weights up toward the ceiling.
- Return to the starting position. Repeat with your left leg.

REPS: Do 10 to 12 per leg.

Pushup and Leg Raise

WORKS the shoulders, triceps, chest, and core.

- Lie facedown on a stability ball, with both hands on the floor.
- Walk your hands out, allowing the ball to roll beneath your body until it is under your shins. Your hands should be directly below your shoulders, so it looks like you're ready to do a pushup.
- Keeping your torso straight and your abs contracted, bend your elbows and lower your chest toward the floor.
- Stop when your upper arms are parallel to the floor.

- Return to start, and immediately contract your glutes as you lift your left leg off the ball.
- Lower your left leg to the ball, then lift the right leg. That's 1 rep.

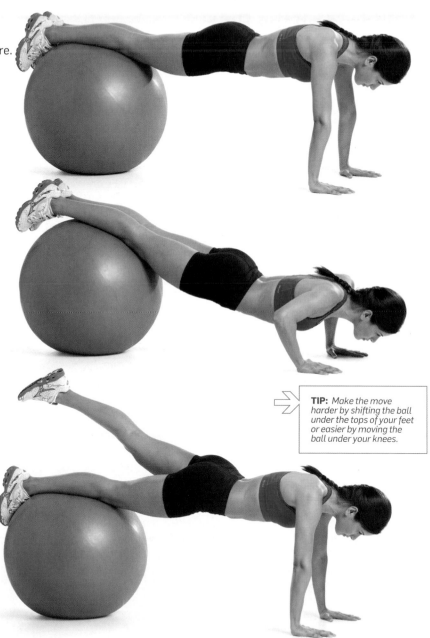

TIP: *Make the move harder by shifting the ball under the tops of your feet or easier by moving the ball under your knees.*

REPS: Do 8 to 12.

Main Moves

Hundred on the Ball

WORKS your core.

- Lie on your back with your arms by your sides. Bend your knees to 90 degrees and place your calves on a stability ball.

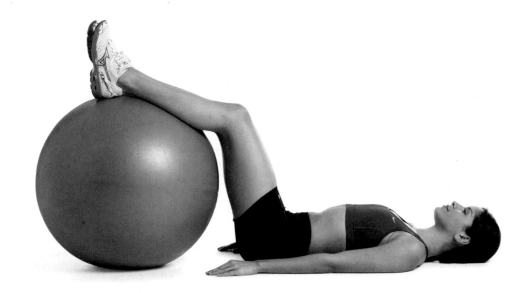

- Lift your head and shoulders off the floor, making sure to keep your head, neck, and shoulders relaxed. (Put your head down at any time if you feel stress in the upper body.)
- Lift your arms off the mat and, with your palms facing down, pulse your arms in unison with your breath: Take 5 short, consecutive inhales, followed by 5 short, consecutive exhales. That's 1 rep.

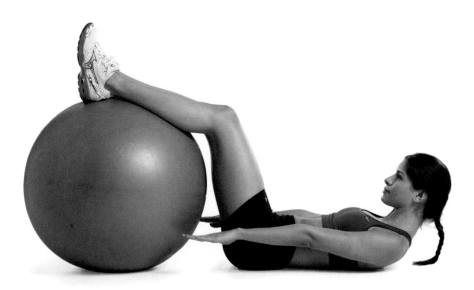

REPS: Do 10 (100 short inhales and exhales).

Mermaid

WORKS your core (especially obliques) and shoulders.

A

- Assume a side plank position, with your left elbow on the floor directly beneath your shoulder.
- Stagger your feet so your right foot is in front of your left foot.

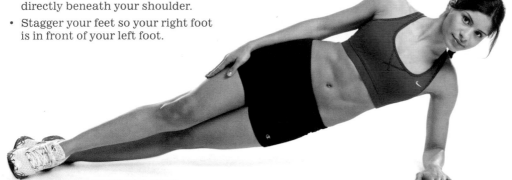

SICK? TAKE A DAY OFF

Don't exercise when you're sick—unless your symptoms are above the neck. And even then you might do better taking a day off. "Your body needs its resources to heal itself, not build muscle and endurance," says Alwyn Cosgrove, CSCS, a trainer in Santa Clarita, California.

B

- Raise your right arm directly overhead—biceps next to your ear, arm extended, and with your palm facing the floor—so your arm is in line with your body.
- Arch your left arm toward the floor as you raise your hips up.
- Return to the starting position and repeat.

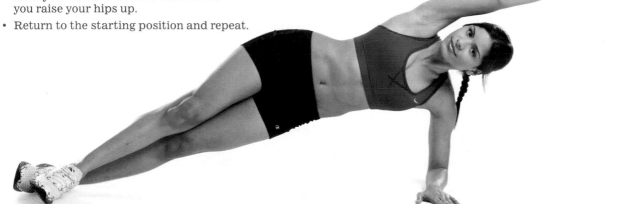

REPS: Do 8 to 10 on each side.

Pear-Body Workout

Pears often bemoan their bottom-heavy shape, but they also populate a roster of bombshell beauties including J-Lo, Alicia Keys, and Jennifer Love Hewitt. As the name implies, pears are smaller on top and easily pack weight onto their lower bodies. For pears, the goal should be body balance. You need to pay attention to the muscles above your belt, especially your shoulders, for nice, even body lines.

START HERE: ■

Complete the four basic moves starting on page 190 before doing the Scissors Jump. Perform the moves one after another, at the prescribed number of reps, with no rest between exercises. Repeat the circuit twice.

Scissors Jump

WORKS your butt and thighs; boosts your heart rate to burn calories.

A

- Stand with your left leg forward and your right leg extended behind you, toes on the floor. Bend your left knee and dip your right knee toward the floor, so you're in a lunge position.
- Place your arms straight out in front of you or out to the sides.

B

- Swiftly jump up and switch legs in midair, in a motion like a scissor.
- Land softly, your right leg forward and left leg back, then lower into a lunge position. When your back knee nearly grazes the ground, jump again.
- Keep jumping without resting.

REPS: Do 10 to 20.

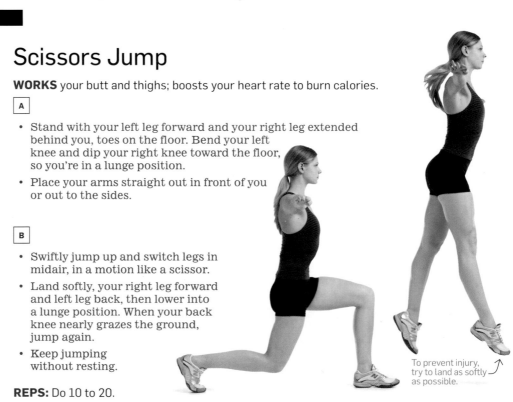

To prevent injury, try to land as softly as possible.

Boat Curl and Press

WORKS your core, biceps, and shoulders.

A

- Hold a lightweight dumbbell in each hand, with your arms extended at your sides and your palms facing forward. Sit on a bench and lean back slightly, pulling your knees to chest height, so you're balancing on your tailbone.
- Curl the weights to your shoulders.

B

- Immediately rotate your wrists so your palms face forward, and press the weights straight overhead.
- Return to the starting position. Each dumbbell extension is 1 rep.

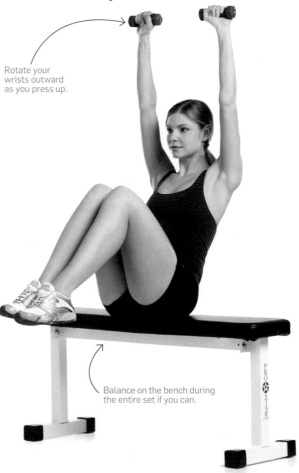

Rotate your wrists outward as you press up.

Balance on the bench during the entire set if you can.

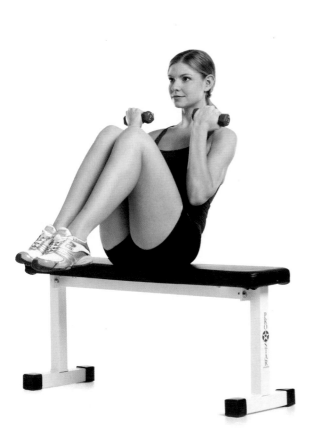

REPS: Do 8 to 10.

Pear-Body Workout

Triangle Lateral Raise

WORKS your butt, thighs, back, and shoulders.

Squeeze your shoulder blades together.

Your back leg should be straight.

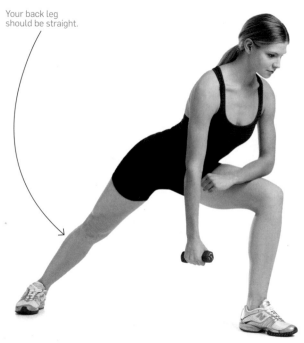

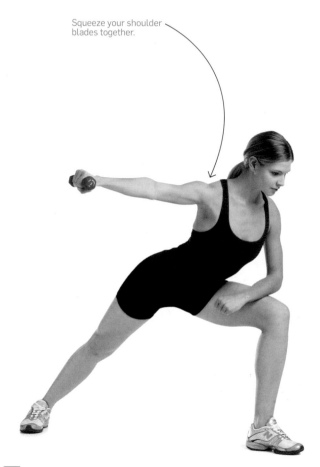

A

- Hold a dumbbell in your right hand and lunge forward with your left leg. Taking a cue from the triangle pose in yoga, turn your left foot out—so it's perpendicular to your leg—and rest your right forearm on your left thigh.
- Extend your right arm straight down, with your palm facing in.

REPS: Do 10 to 12 per arm.

B

- Keeping your right arm extended, squeeze your shoulder blades together and raise your right arm straight out to the side until it reaches shoulder height.
- Return to the starting position and repeat. After doing all reps, lunge forward with the right leg and complete the lateral raise with your left arm.

Dip and Knee Raise

WORKS your triceps, shoulders, upper back, and hip flexors.

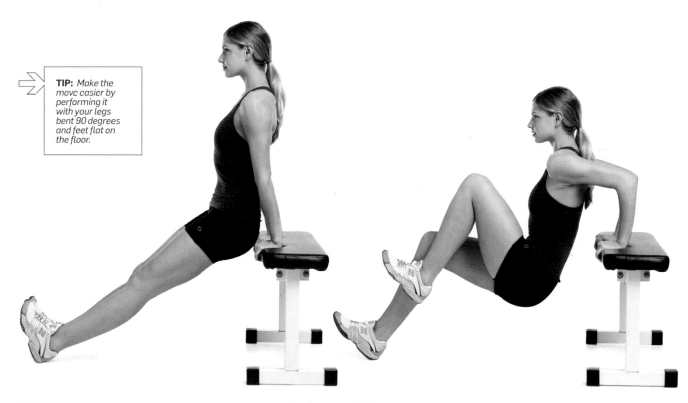

TIP: *Make the move easier by performing it with your legs bent 90 degrees and feet flat on the floor.*

A

- Sit on the edge of a bench. Grasp the seat on either side of your butt, making sure your fingers are facing forward, palms backward.
- Walk your feet out so you can inch yourself off the seat.

B

- Bend your arms, keeping your elbows pointed straight back, as you dip your butt toward the ground.
- Simultaneously contract your abs and pull your left knee toward your chest.
- Return to the starting position. Concentrate on using your arms to raise your body, rather than pushing up with your legs. Next, dip and raise your right leg. That's 1 rep.

REPS: Do 6.

Hourglass-Body Workout

Voluptuous gals like Beyoncé or Scarlett Johannson have balanced upper and lower bodies and slim midsections but tend to lack muscle tone. Curvaceous women run the risk of popping out a little bit too much in the thighs and arms, so they need to focus on their extremities.

START HERE:

Complete the four basic moves on page 190 before doing the lunges. Perform the moves one after another, at the pre-scribed number of reps, with no rest between exercises. Repeat the circuit twice, resting briefly between circuits.

Tai Chi Lunge

WORKS your butt, thighs, and core.

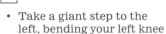

A

- Stand with your arms extended straight out in front of you, with your palms facing down.

B

- Take a giant step to the left, bending your left knee until it's 45 to 90 degrees
- Pause in this side-lunge position and rotate your torso and outstretched arms to the right, rotating at the waist.

C

- Rotate back to the center and return to the starting position. Repeat the move to the opposite side. That's 1 rep. Continue alternating for a full set.

TIP:
To make the move more challenging, hold a medicine ball.

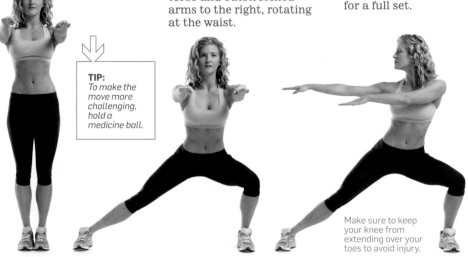

Make sure to keep your knee from extending over your toes to avoid injury.

REPS: Do 10 to 12.

Side Planks with Moving Knee

WORKS your core (especially obliques) and butt.

A

- Assume a plank position with your toes and forearms on the floor, elbows directly beneath your shoulders.

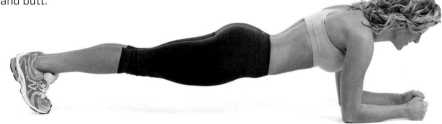

B

- Roll up to the left by lifting your right arm. Rotate your left arm, so your upper body is propped up on your left forearm, elbow directly beneath shoulder and forearm perpendicular to your body.
- Stack your right foot on top of your left.

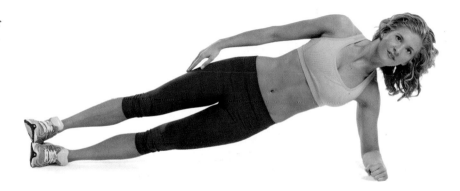

C

- Put your right hand on your hip, elbow pointing toward the ceiling.
- Raise your right leg and bend that knee toward your right elbow.
- Return to the starting position. Repeat, this time rolling to the right. That's 1 rep.

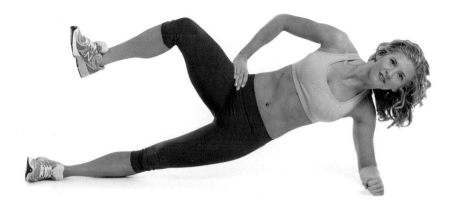

REPS: Do 8 to 10.

Hourglass-Body Workout

Lateral Stepups

WORKS your butt and thighs, plus raises heart rate to burn extra calories.

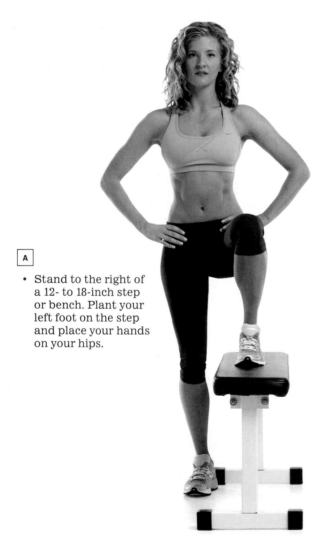

A

- Stand to the right of a 12- to 18-inch step or bench. Plant your left foot on the step and place your hands on your hips.

REPS: Do 10 to 12.

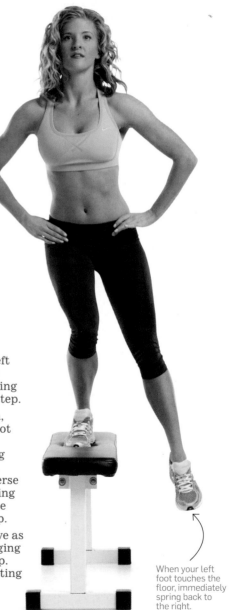

B

- Press into your left foot, extend your right leg, and spring up and over the step.

- On the way down, plant the right foot on the step and extend the left leg into a side lunge. Immediately reverse the move, springing up and over to the right. That's 1 rep.

- Think of this move as your feet exchanging places on the step. Continue alternating for a full set.

When your left foot touches the floor, immediately spring back to the right.

Glute Bridge with Triceps Extension

WORKS your butt, core, and triceps.

- Holding a dumbbell in each hand, lie on your back with your knees bent. Bend your elbows so the weights are positioned at either side of your head, palms facing your ears and elbows pointed toward the ceiling.

Keep your upper arms still when you raise the weights.

B

- Simultaneously contract your glutes and raise your hips—so your body forms a straight line from your shoulders to your knees—while you extend your arms, so the weights are lined up with your chest. Return to the starting position.

Contract your glutes.

REPS: Do 10 to 12.

Boyish-Body Workout

Straight-body women tend to be a little boyish (yet still plenty sexy) in build, like Cameron Diaz (see, we said sexy) and have a tough time gaining muscle tone. To add a little shape, women with straight builds should focus on tightening their abdominal muscles, which pull in the belly. Lower-body training will put a little pop in their hips, and upper back exercises will help broaden their top.

START HERE:

Complete the four basic moves on page 190 before doing the Crossover Crunch. Perform the moves one after another, at the prescribed number of reps, with no rest between exercises. Repeat the circuit twice.

Crossover Crunch

WORKS your core.

 A

- Lie on your back with arms and legs outstretched so your body forms an X.
- Contract your abs and raise your head, arms, and legs a few inches off the floor.

 B

- Keeping your limbs extended, simultaneously bring your arms and legs up and toward each other over your abdomen.
- Lower your limbs back to the starting position. That's 1 rep.

REPS: Do 10 to 12.

To make the move more challenging, keep your head, arms, and legs raised throughout the exercise. To make it a little easier, bring only one arm and leg off the floor each time.

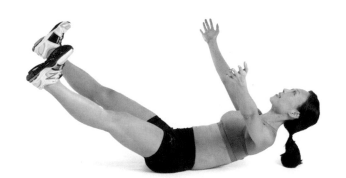

Stacked Pushup

WORKS your chest, shoulders, triceps, and core.

TIP: *The unbalanced nature of this exercise puts more stress on your lower arm and also adds a core rotation that exercises your abs, low back, and obliques.*

 A

- Assume a pushup position (resting either your knees or your toes on the floor), with your hands on the floor directly beneath your shoulders.

- Place your left hand on a thick book, yoga block, or aerobic step with no risers.

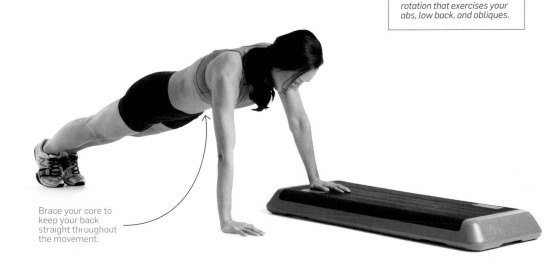

Brace your core to keep your back straight throughout the movement.

B

- Bend your arms and lower your chest until your arms are bent 90 degrees. Straighten your arms and press up. That's 1 rep.

- Do 4 to 6 reps, then switch sides, bringing your right hand up onto the book or step and your left hand down to the floor on the left side of the step.

- Repeat, this time crossing up and over to the right for 4 to 6 reps.

Try to keep your elbows close to your body as you descend.

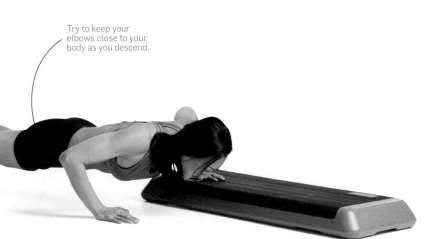

REPS: Do 10 to 12.

Boyish-Body Workout

Plyo Plank

WORKS your total body and raises heart rate to burn extra calories.

- Assume a standard pushup position, with your feet extended wider than shoulder-width apart.

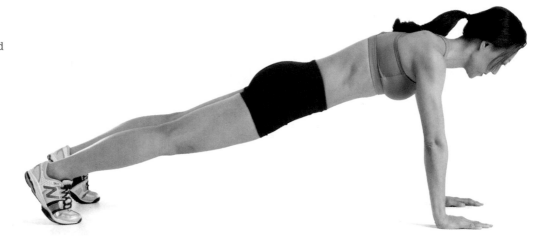

- Quickly hop your feet together and up toward the right.
- Hop back to the starting position. Then repeat to the left side. That's 1 rep.

Bend your knees as you hop to the right.

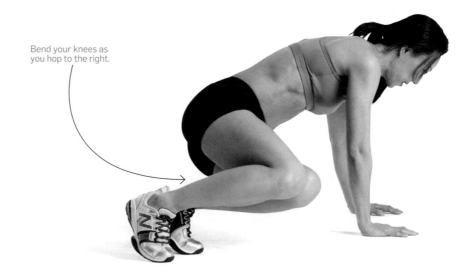

REPS: Do 10 to 12.

Squat and Overhead Press

WORKS your butt, thighs, shoulders, triceps, and core.

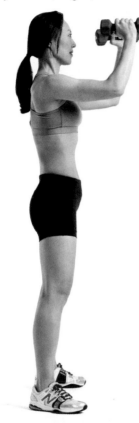

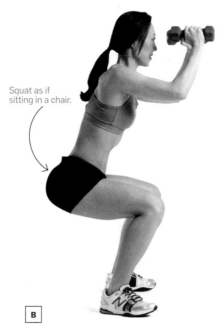

Squat as if sitting in a chair.

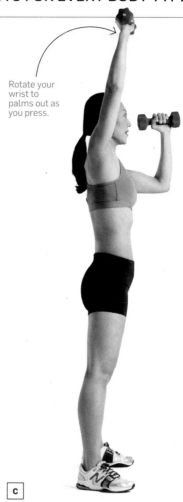

Rotate your wrist to palms out as you press.

A

- Hold a dumbbell in each hand, elbows bent in front of your torso, weights in front of your shoulders, palms facing in. Stand with your feet in a wide straddle stance, toes turned out.

B

- Bend your knees and squat back, keeping your knees from extending over your toes.

C

- Press back to the start position, turning your right palm forward and pressing the weight directly overhead.
- Immediately lower into another squat, pulling your right arm back to the starting position.
- Stand again, this time pressing the left weight overhead. That's 1 rep.

REPS: Do 10 to 12.

Athletic-Body Workout

The athletic body type is broad across the back and shoulders and narrow through the hips. Think Hayden Panettiere or Jessica Biel. Athletic builds tend to have relatively low body fat, but also cut more square silhouettes, as they can be a bit wide waisted. Athletic shapes don't need much toning, but some tummy-tightening and lower-body moves for glutes and thighs will complement an already strong build.

START HERE:

Complete the four basic moves on page 190 before doing the Curtsy Hammer Raises. Perform the moves one after another, at the prescribed number of reps, with no rest between exercises. Repeat the circuit twice.

Curtsy Hammer Raise

WORKS your butt, thighs, and shoulders.

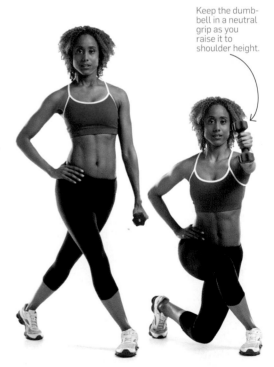

Keep the dumbbell in a neutral grip as you raise it to shoulder height.

A

- Stand with your feet hip-distance apart, holding a lightweight dumbbell in your left hand and resting your right hand on your hip.
- Take a giant step back and to the right with your left leg, so if you were standing on a clock facing 12, your left toes would end up at the 5 o'clock position.

B

- Bend your knees and lower your hips toward the floor until your right thigh is parallel to the floor.
- At the same time, raise your left arm (the one with the dumbbell in it) straight out in front of you to shoulder height.
- Return to the starting position. Complete a full set; then switch sides.

REPS: Do 10 to 12 per side.

Swivel Squat

WORKS your butt, thighs, and core.

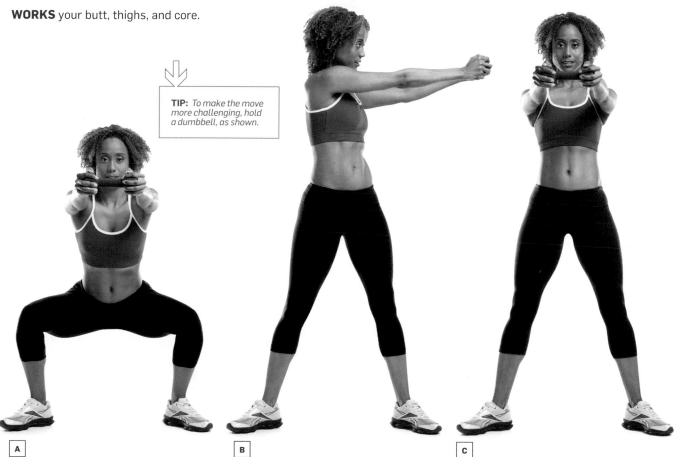

TIP: *To make the move more challenging, hold a dumbbell, as shown.*

A

- Stand with your feet hip-width apart, and extend your arms straight out in front of you.
- Bend your knees and sit back until your legs are bent 45 to 90 degrees; make sure to keep your knees from extending over your toes.

REPS: Do 10 to 12.

B

- Press back to a standing position as you rotate your torso and outstretched arms to the left.

C

- Rotate back to the center and immediately perform another squat, this time rotating to the left as you stand.
- Both sides make 1 rep. The sequence is this: Squat, stand—while simultaneously twisting to the side—then twist back to the center.

Athletic-Body Workout

Tip and Row

WORKS your butt and back.

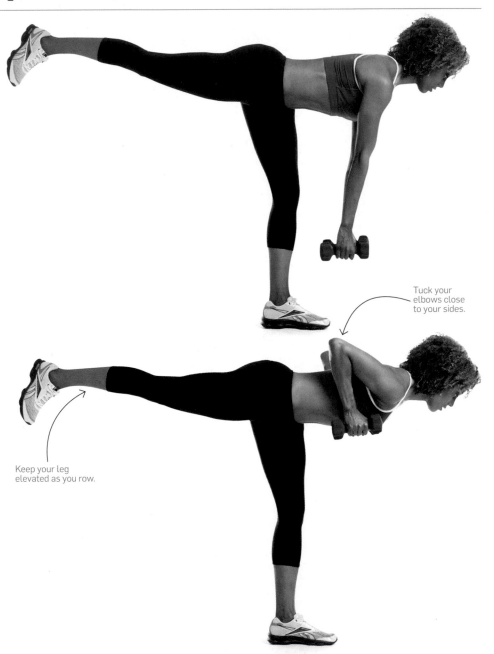

- Stand with your feet hip-width apart, arms by your sides holding weights.
- Lift your right leg straight up behind you as you bend from the hips to lower your upper body forward. Your torso and right leg should be parallel to the floor and your arms hanging straight down, palms facing each other.

Tuck your elbows close to your sides.

B

- Bend your elbows and pull the weights straight up to the sides of your chest.
- Lower the weights and return to a standing position. Repeat, this time lifting the left leg behind you as you tip forward. That's 1 rep.

Keep your leg elevated as you row.

REPS: Do 10 to 12.

Alternating Lateral Lunge

WORKS your thighs, butt, and core.

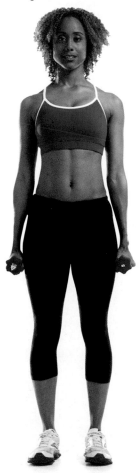

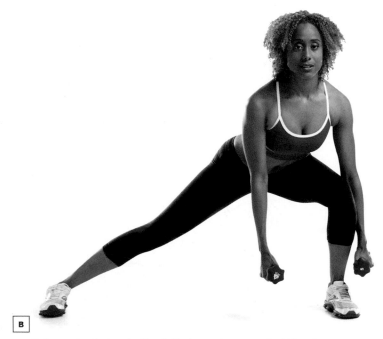

A

- Stand with your feet about hip-width apart, holding dumbbells at your sides.

B

- Take a giant step to the left, dropping your butt back (keeping your knee from extending over your toes) and pretending to place the weights on either side of your foot.
- Press back to the starting position. Then immediately repeat the move to the right. That's 1 rep.

REPS: Do 10 to 12.

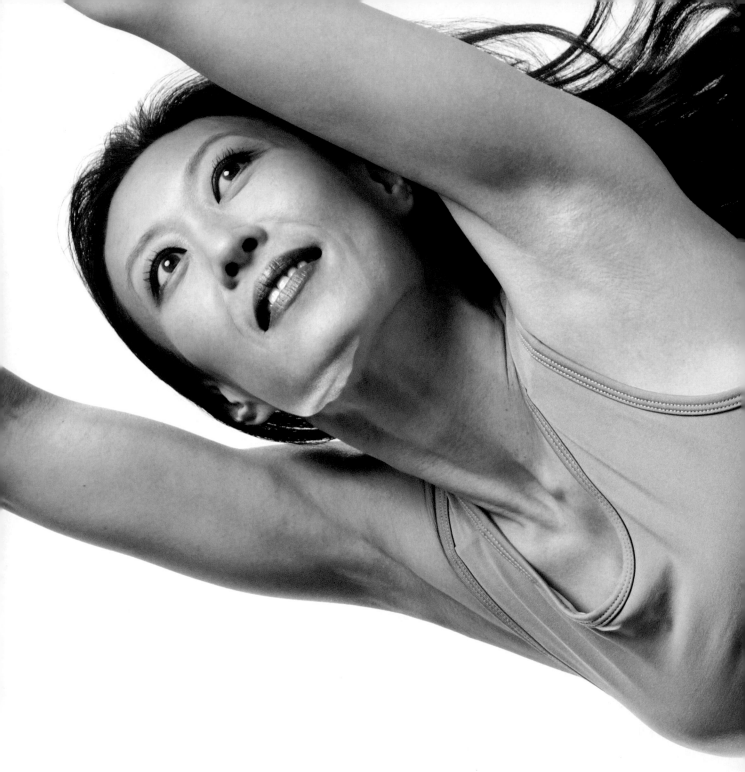

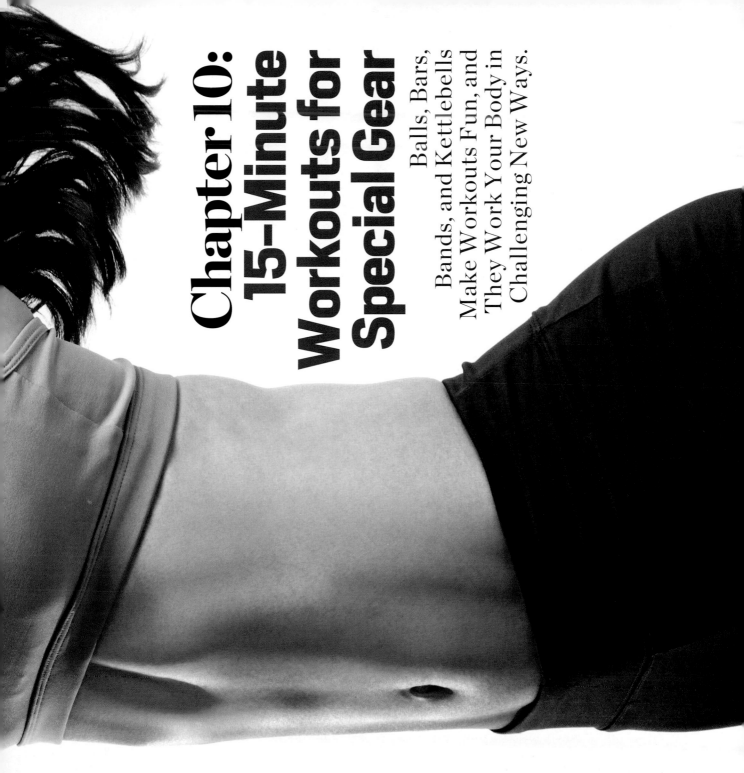

Chapter 10: 15-Minute Workouts for Special Gear

Balls, Bars, Bands, and Kettlebells Make Workouts Fun, and They Work Your Body in Challenging New Ways.

Superfast Special-Gear Workouts

I love gear. Balls, bands, foam rollers, and bells are like spices. You can use them to add pizzazz to your usual routine or you can build an entire workout around them. If you've been avoiding gear, perhaps out of fear of the unknown, I'd encourage you to expand your horizons. The beauty of gear is that each item lets you work your muscles in a fresh way, activating new fibers and taking your fitness and strength to another level. After all, that's why the stuff got invented in the first place.

Begin with the basics ...

In this chapter, you'll find moves using more than a half dozen pieces of unique equipment. Gear workouts, particularly those using kettlebells, can be a little tougher than your standard strength-training routine. If you're just starting a fitness routine, work up to these gradually. On the other hand, the fresh challenge of these routines make them an excellent option to jumpstart the benefits for seasoned lifters who may have hit a plateau. So grab your gear and let's go.

Find It Quick: Your 15-Minute Gear-Specific Circuit Plan

NEVER MISS A WORKOUT

Work travel can really mess up your ability to stick with an exercise program even if you're staying at a hotel with a gym. It's just a hassle to get down there sometimes. Exercise bands, which stow easily in a suitcase and can be used in your room, eliminate that excuse. Another piece of special gear to consider packing is a suspension training system such as the TRX, which consists of two nylon straps with loops at one end. The straps anchor to something sturdy, such as a door frame for many different bodyweight exercises: dips, pullups, triceps presses, shoulder extensions, and more.

Kettlebell Workout 1

Kick up your metabolism with kettlebells. Working out with these asymmetrical cannonball-like weights absolutely scorches calories. Researchers from the University of Wisconsin found that doing kettlebell snatches (a move where you simply squat and swing the bell, like the move on page 221) burns 20 calories a minute. That's more than spinning, rowing, elliptical training, stair stepping, or swimming! The two 15-minute kettlebell workouts in this chapter can each burn close to 300 calories. And that's just for starters. Factor in the muscle-building impact and the afterburn (the calories you burn after you exercise as your body repairs), and the total energy expenditure could shoot up by 50 percent.

Anatomy of a Kettlebell

The sculpting power of the kettlebell comes from its unique shape. The weight is asymmetrical, so your muscles have to work harder to balance and move it. That's why you should start with a light weight (no more than 10 pounds) until you get used to the unweildy shape, and master ideal form.

HANDLE: For most moves, you hold onto the handle, so you can swing the bell and pass it from hand to hand.

HORNS: The sides of the handle are called the horns. For some moves, especially if you're holding the bell upside down, you'll hold on here.

BASE (OR BELL): The main part of the weight, which is round with a flat base.

START HERE:

Do these moves one after another with no rest between them. Rest for 60 seconds at the end of the circuit. Then repeat the circuit twice more.

Around-the-Body Pass

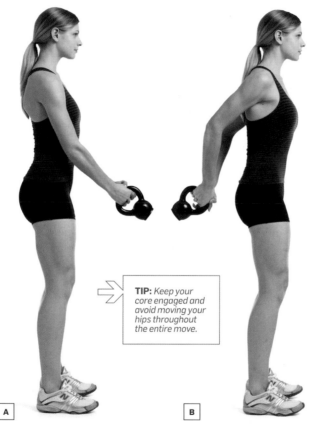

TIP: *Keep your core engaged and avoid moving your hips throughout the entire move.*

A
- Hold the kettlebell with both hands in front of your torso and stand with your feet hip-width apart.

B
- Release the kettlebell into your right hand and move both arms behind your back. Grab the bell with your left hand and bring it back to the front (completing a full circle around your body). That's 1 rep.

REPS: Do 10, then switch directions and repeat without stopping to rest.

DO WHAT YOU LOVE

The bottom line to being fit for life: Find what you really enjoy and what gets you going, says Kristen Dieffenbach, PhD, an assistant professor of athletic coaching education at West Virginia University. "Try as many classes, running paths, and exercise machines as you can. Somewhere between swimming and spinning, you will click with an activity or two." Spend your workout hours doing these types of exercise and you'll find excuses to get out more often instead of skipping sessions.

Kettlebell Workout 1

Swing

TIP: *If you have any back problems, do this move without using a weight.*

Keep your lower back slightly arched.

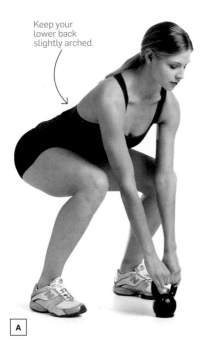

Push your hips back.

Swing the kettlebell between your legs.

A

- Grab a kettlebell with both hands and stand with your feet wider than hip-width apart.
- Squat down until your thighs are nearly parallel to the floor.

REPS: Do 15 to 20.

B

- Immediately stand and swing the kettlebell up to shoulder height.

C

- As the kettlebell begins to arc back down, bend your knees and squat, swinging the kettlebell between your legs. Then swing it back to shoulder height as you stand.

Bent-Knee Dead Lift

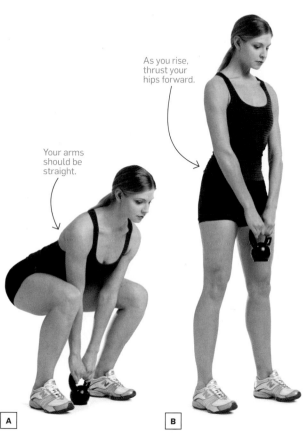

Your arms should be straight.

As you rise, thrust your hips forward.

A

- Stand with your feet hip-width apart, the kettlebell on the floor between your feet.
- Squat down and grab the handle with both hands, keeping your back flat.

B

- Brace your abs, squeeze your glutes, and slowly push down into your heels as you stand up, keeping your arms extended. That's 1 rep.

REPS: Do 10 to 12.

Halo

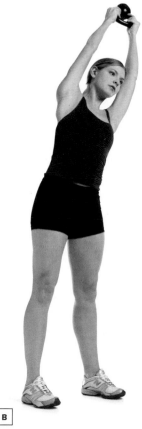

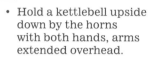

A

- Hold a kettlebell upside down by the horns with both hands, arms extended overhead.

B

- Keeping shoulders down, chest forward, and abs tight, rotate your torso from the waist in a circle to the left.
- The kettlebell should make small, controlled halos overhead.

REPS: Do 6 circles, then switch directions.

Kettlebell Workout 2

Kettlebells bring cardiovascular, strength, and flexibility training together into one efficient workout. Here are four more classic kettlebell exercises. Alternate this circuit with workout 1, or combine the two when you have more time.

START HERE: ▐

Do these moves one after another with no rest between them. Rest for 60 seconds at the end of the circuit. Then repeat the circuit twice more.

Split Squat Kettlebell Pass

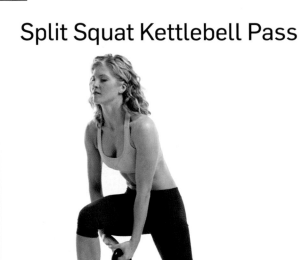

A

- Hold a kettlebell by the handle in your right hand, arms at your sides, palms facing in. Stand with your right foot 2 to 3 feet in front of the left, toes pointing forward, your back heel off the floor.
- Bend your knees, lowering your hips toward the floor, as you pass the bell under your right leg to your left hand.

B

- Then pass it over your right leg to your right hand as you straighten your legs
- * Continue for 8 passes, then reverse arms directions and repeat. Next, repeat the exercise with your left leg forward.

REPS: Do 16 under each leg, switching directions every 8 reps.

Figure 8

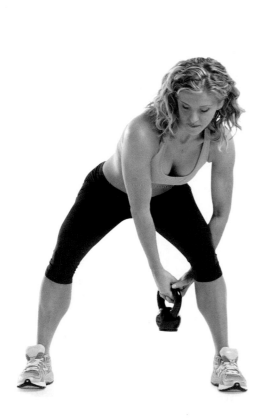

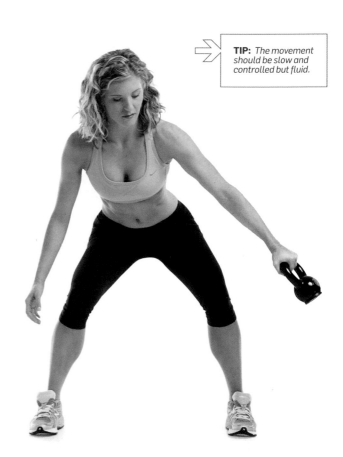

> **TIP:** *The movement should be slow and controlled but fluid.*

A

- Stand with your feet wider than hip-width apart, knees bent into a quarter-squat position, back straight, and chest up. Hold the kettlebell behind your left leg with both hands, one arm on each side of your leg.

REPS: Do 10.

B

- Grab the bell with your left hand and swing it in front of your left leg, between your legs, and behind your right leg in a figure-8 pattern.
- Grab it with your right hand and swing it in front of your right leg, between your legs, then behind your left leg. That's 1 rep.

Kettlebell Workout 2

Half Get Up

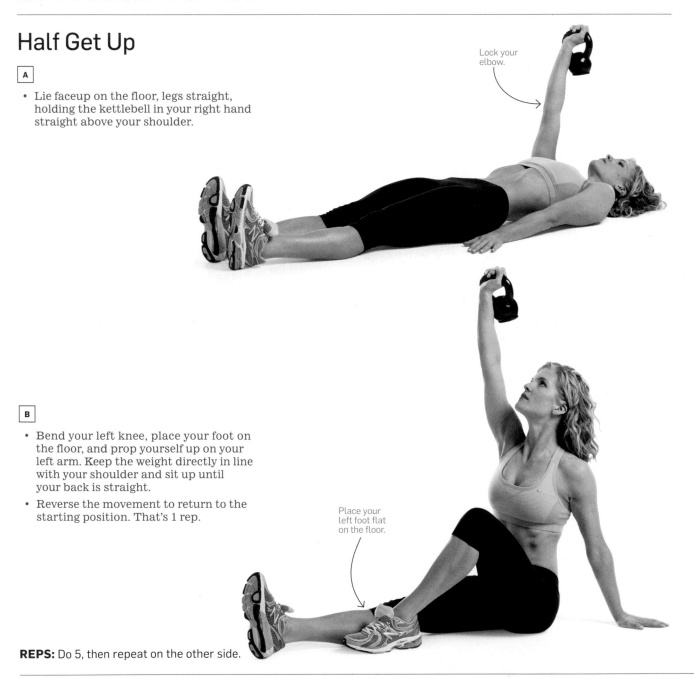

A

- Lie faceup on the floor, legs straight, holding the kettlebell in your right hand straight above your shoulder.

Lock your elbow.

B

- Bend your left knee, place your foot on the floor, and prop yourself up on your left arm. Keep the weight directly in line with your shoulder and sit up until your back is straight.

- Reverse the movement to return to the starting position. That's 1 rep.

Place your left foot flat on the floor.

REPS: Do 5, then repeat on the other side.

Snatch, Pull, and Push Press

A

- Grab a kettlebell and stand with your feet wider than shoulder-width apart, toes turned out about 45 degrees. Place the kettlebell on the floor between your feet.

REPS: Do 10.

B

- Stand up and lift the weight to chest height.

C

- Grab the sides of the handle and push the kettlebell straight overhead.
- Lower it to your chest and then to the floor. That's 1 rep.

Exercise Band Workout 1

It's easy to dismiss exercise bands or tubes as lightweight tools for girls who don't like to sweat. Nothing could be further from the truth. Despite their pretty colors and featherweight feel, exercise bands challenge your muscles with constant tension through a full range of motion, targeting parts that are often missed by free weights. And you can buy both the band style and rubber tube style in different resistance strengths to vary your exercise. The result is a powerful workout that you can take anywhere.

The first few times you do band exercises, you may feel more wobbly than usual. That's because unlike free-weight lifting, where the resistance is toughest midlift and easier in both the starting and final positions, a band's resistance becomes progressively more difficult from beginning to end and doesn't ease up in the final position.Concentrate on keeping your movements slow, smooth, and controlled throughout.

START HERE:

Move from one exercise to the next without rest. When you complete the last move, rest for 30 seconds, then repeat the entire circuit two more times.

■

Resistance Pushup

- Start in a pushup position, with your legs extended straight behind you and your hands shoulder-width apart. Position the band across your shoulder blades with tight resistance, each end tucked under a hand.

TIP: *If you find this too difficult, start in a modified pushup position, resting on your knees.*

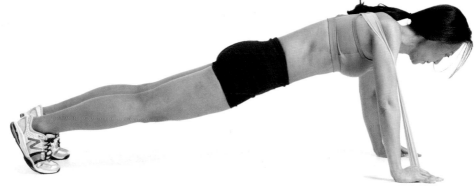

B

- Lower your body until your upper arms are parallel to the floor, then push back to the starting position. That's 1 rep.

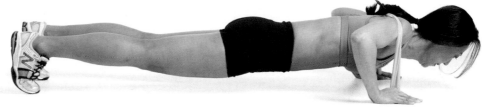

REPS: Do 10 (or as many as you can).

Exercise Band Workout 1

Squat with Side Kick

TIP: *Use exercise tubing with handles for this exercise.*

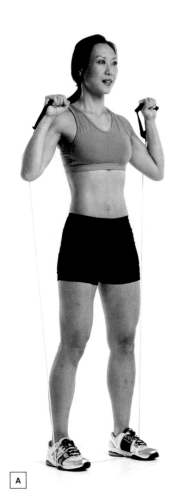

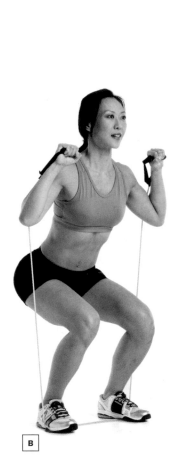

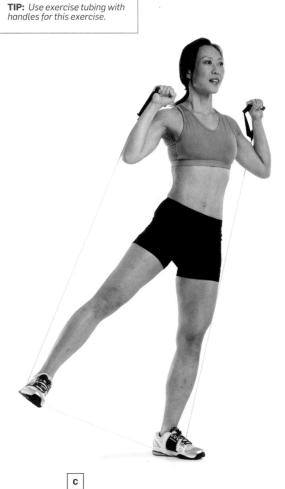

A

- Stand with your feet hip-width apart, abs tight, band under both feet. Grasp the ends and raise your hands to shoulder height.

REPS: Do 10 to 12.

B

- Bend your knees and hips and sit back as though sitting in a chair, keeping your knees in line with your ankles.

C

- Push through your heels and return to the starting position, immediately lifting the right leg out to the side as you stand. Repeat to the opposite side. That's 1 rep.

Seated Row

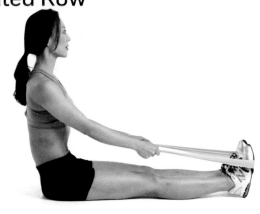

A

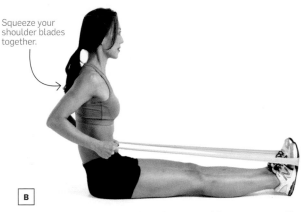

Squeeze your shoulder blades together.

B

- Sit on the floor with your legs straight and loop the resistance band securely around your feet, holding an end in each hand, arms extended in front of you. Keep your back straight and shoulders square.

REPS: Do 10 to 12.

- Tuck your elbows close to your sides as you pull the band to each side of your torso, squeezing your shoulder blades together.
- Pause, then slowly return to the starting position. That's 1 rep.

Frog Press

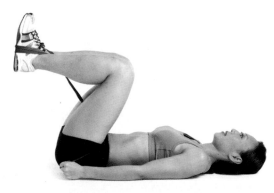

A

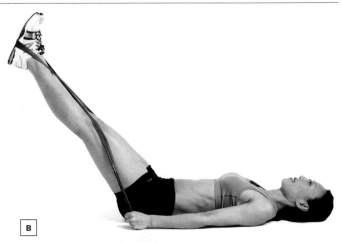

B

- Lie faceup, bend your hips and knees 90 degrees, and loop the band around your feet, crossing the band to create an X. Hold an end in each hand at the side of your hips.

REPS: Do 10 to 12.

- From this position, brace your core and slowly extend your legs into the air straight in front of you.
- Pause, then return to the starting position. That's 1 rep.

Exercise Band Workout 2

Resistance bands allow you to produce specific muscle movements while minimizing the impact on your joints. Highly versatile, they can be used to mimic dozens and dozens of free-weight exercises. Here's a workout of four more moves to alternate with Exercise Band Workout 1.

START HERE:

Move from one exercise to the next without rest. When you complete the last move, rest 30 seconds, then repeat the entire circuit two more times.

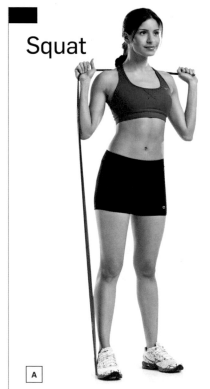

Squat

A

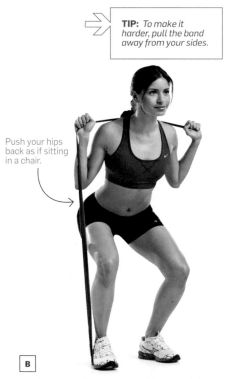

Push your hips back as if sitting in a chair.

TIP: *To make it harder, pull the band away from your sides.*

B

- With your feet shoulder-width apart, step on one end of the band. Stretch the other end up and over your head, place it on your shoulders, and rest it across your upper back.

REPS: Do 10 to 12.

- Now perform a squat by pushing your hips back and lowering your body until your thighs are at least parallel to the floor.
- Push back up to the starting position.

Standing Incline Fly

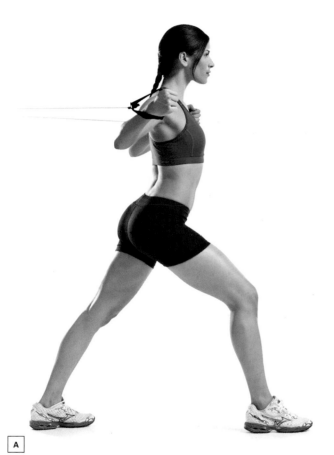

A

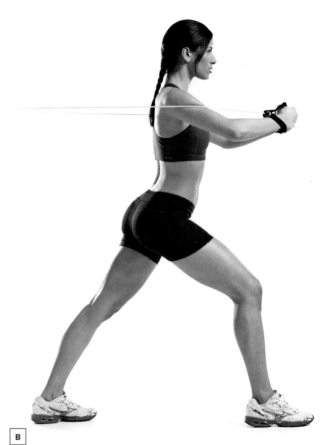

B

- Attach the exercise band securely to a door handle. Turn so your back is to the door and grasp the handles, extending your arms out to the sides to about shoulder level, keeping your elbows soft.

- Step forward until the band is taut. Maintain a staggered stance, with one foot in front of the other, and keep your arms slightly bent.

REPS: Do 10 to 12.

- Without changing the angle of your elbows, pull your hands together in front of your body. Return to the starting position.

Exercise Band Workout 2

Resisted Supine Crunch

- Connect the ends of the band together with a knot or utility strap. Attach the band to the lowest hinge on a door. Lie faceup on the floor with your head closest to the door and your feet farthest from it.
- Grasp the ends of the band. Bend your elbows so your forearms are parallel to the floor and your hands are at eye level above your head.
- Bend your knees with your heels on the floor.

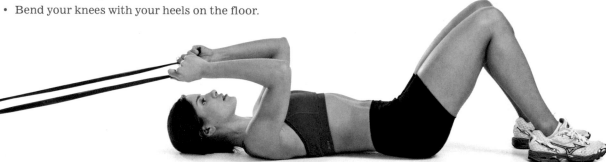

B

- Contract your abs and raise your torso as high as you can off the floor.
- Lower yourself back to the starting position. Perform the exercise as quickly as possible.

Without moving your arms, curl up.

REPS: Do 10 to 12.

Rubber Band Sidesteps

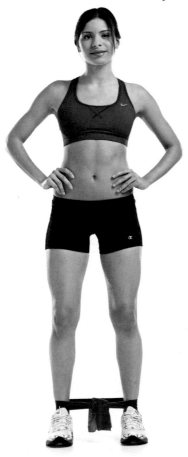

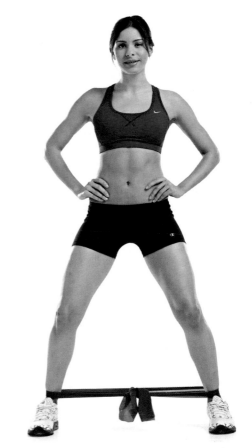

A

- Stand with your legs about hip-width apart. Tie the exercise band into a bow around both legs positioning it just above the ankles. It should be tight enough so it stays in place.

B

- Keeping your knees slightly bent and your back straight, take a giant step with your right foot to the right side.
- Then take a small step to the right with your left foot, returning your feet to about hip-width apart, keeping tension on the band.
- Then take a giant step with your left foot to the left, and a small step to the left with your right. That's 1 rep.

REPS: Do 10 to 12.

Medicine Ball Workout 1

Medicine balls may be the most functional workout gear going. These classic weighted balls (which now come in all shapes, sizes, and materials) allow for a wide range of motion and let you move your arms and legs and core fluidly, as if you were swimming or playing tennis. Medicine ball workouts really stimulate your central nervous system, especially if you're tossing and catching the ball, so you'll actually feel a good buzz when you're done. You'll find two medicine ball workouts below, designed with the help of strength and conditioning coach Jonas Sahratian, who trains the University of North Carolina Tar Heels.

Anatomy of a Medicine Ball

Ancient texts and artwork prove that the medicine ball is one of the oldest pieces of exercise equipment. Three thousand years ago, they were made of sewn animal bladders or skins filled with sand. Your grandfather probably worked out with the hand-stitched leather balls, but today they are usually made of polyeurethane or rubber and are filled with silicone or rubber chips. Today's models come in all sorts of colors, sizes, and weights, typically from 2 to 25 pounds. Med balls are often used for rehabilitation exercise, but they are increasingly employed in core stability and balance training.

START HERE: Complete each exercise back-to-back without resting. After the first circuit, rest for 1 minute, then repeat for a total of three circuits.

■

Big Circles

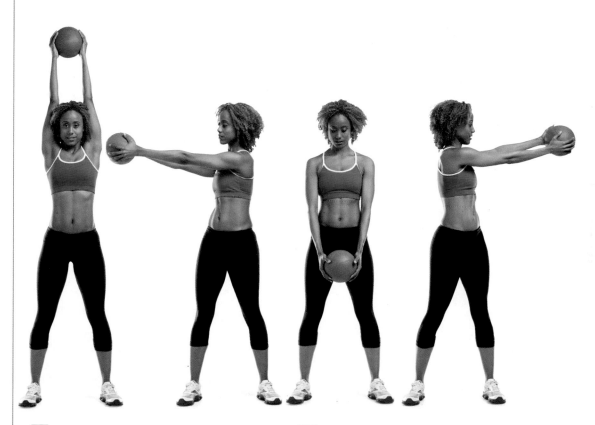

A

- Stand with your feet shoulder-width apart and knees slightly bent, hold the ball with your arms extended above your head.

REPS: Do 10 in each direction.

B

- Without bending your elbows, rotate your arms counterclockwise, using the ball to draw large imaginary circles in front of your body. After completing all reps, repeat circles in a clockwise direction.

231

Medicine Ball Workout 1

Step and Extend

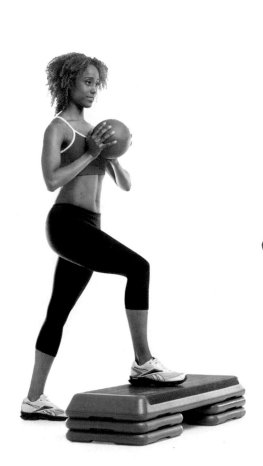

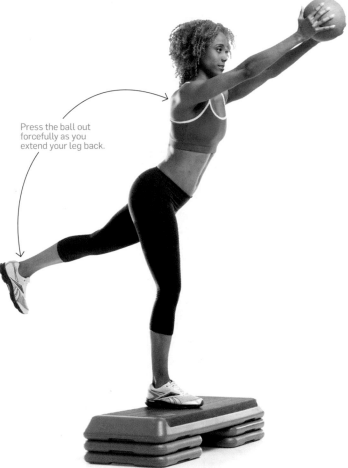

Press the ball out forcefully as you extend your leg back.

A

- Stand about a foot away from a sturdy box or step, feet hip-width apart, holding a medicine ball at chest height in front of you.

REPS: Do 10 to 12, then repeat with the left leg.

B

- Keeping your upper body straight, step up onto the box with your right foot, straightening your right leg and extending the left leg out and back.
- Pause, and reverse motion, stepping back down to the floor.

Wood Chopper

> **TIP:** *The Wood Chopper is an excellent total-body warmup exercise to do before a weight workout.*

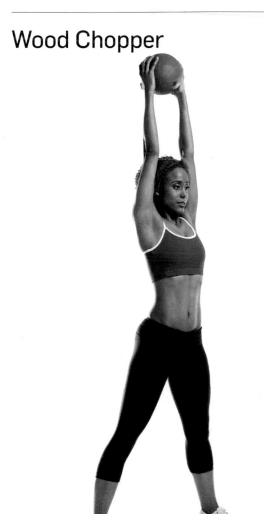

A

- Stand with your feet just beyond shoulder-width apart. With your arms nearly straight, hold the ball above your head.

REPS: Do 15 to 20.

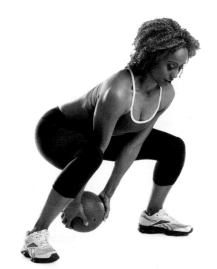

B

- Now, bend forward at your waist and mimic throwing the ball backward between your legs while holding the ball the entire time.

- Quickly reverse the movement with the same intensity and return to the starting position. That's 1 rep.

Medicine Ball Workout 1

Squat To Press

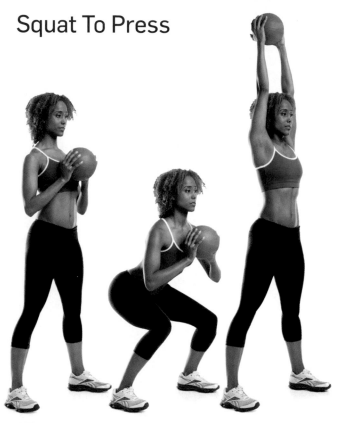

A
- Stand holding the ball close to your chest with both hands, your feet just beyond shoulder-width apart.

B
- Push your hips back, bend your knees and lower your body until the tops of your thighs are parallel to the floor.

C
- Then, drive your heels into the floor to stand as you press the ball over your head.
- Lower the ball back to the starting position. That's 1 rep.

REPS: Do 15 to 20.

Standing Russian Twist

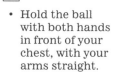

A
- Hold the ball with both hands in front of your chest, with your arms straight.
- Spread your feet greater than shoulder-width apart.

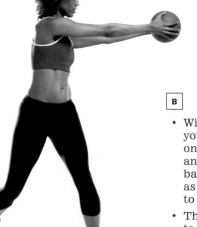

B
- Without dropping your arms, pivot on your right foot and rotate the ball and your torso as far as you can to the left.
- Then do the same to the right. That's 1 rep.

REPS: Do 15 to 20.

Circle Crunches

- Squeeze a ball between your knees and lie on your back with your legs bent so your thighs are perpendicular and your calves are parallel to the floor. Hold your hands behind your head with your elbows out to the sides.
- Contract your abs and raise your upper back, shoulders, and head off the floor about 30 degrees.

- Slowly move your knees in a circular motion counterclockwise 5 times.
- Pause. Then slowly move your knees 5 times in a clockwise motion.

REPS: Do 5 in each direction.

Medicine Ball Situp

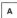

- Grab a medicine ball with both hands and lie on your back. Bend your knees 90 degrees, place your feet flat on the floor, and hold the medicine ball against your chest.

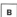

- Now, perform a classic situp by raising your torso into a sitting position.
- Lower back to the starting position. That's 1 rep.

REPS: Do 15 to 20.

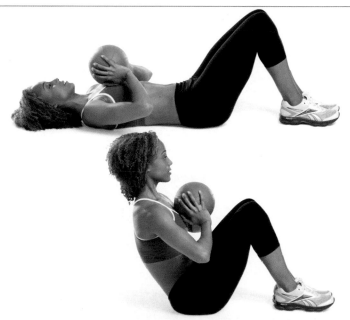

Medicine Ball Workout 2

Here's another "med ball" workout for variety. If you like the range of motion benefits of this piece of gear, supplement your ball with lighter and heavier models.

START HERE: ■

Starting with the first move, complete each exercise back-to-back without resting. After the first circuit, rest for 1 minute, then repeat for a total of three circuits.

Walking Lunge

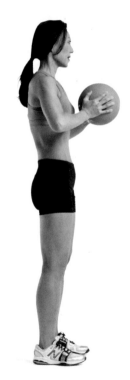

Keep hips facing forward as you twist, your upper body.

A

- Grab a medium-weight medicine ball and stand with your feet shoulder-width apart.

REPS: Do 10 to 12.

B

- Step forward with your left leg and lower into a lunge, so your left thigh is parallel to the ground.
- Twist from your waist as far as you can to the right.
- Step forward and up, bringing the ball back to center. Repeat with your right leg and twist left to complete 1 rep.

Toe Touch

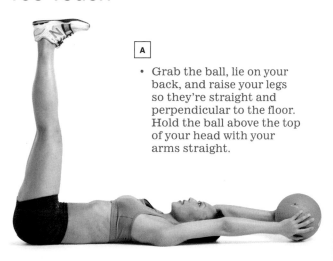

A

- Grab the ball, lie on your back, and raise your legs so they're straight and perpendicular to the floor. Hold the ball above the top of your head with your arms straight.

B

- Without moving your legs or bending your elbows, simultaneously lift your arms and torso until the ball touches your toes.
- Lower yourself back to the starting position. That's 1 rep.

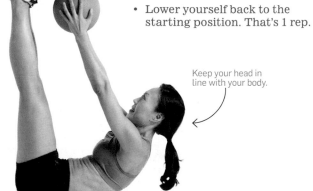

Keep your head in line with your body.

REPS: Do 15 to 20.

Rising and Setting Sun

A

- Stand with feet in a wide straddle stance, toes pointed out about 45 degrees. Hold a medicine ball above your head.

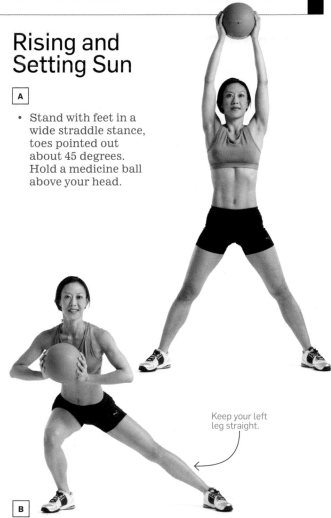

Keep your left leg straight.

B

- In one move, bend your right knee and your elbows, bringing the ball down over your right thigh as you squat back in that direction. Your left leg should stay extended throughout the move.
- Push off your right leg and extend the ball back overhead, returning to the starting position.
- Immediately repeat the motion in the opposite direction without resting. That's 1 rep.

REPS: Do 15 to 20.

Medicine Ball Workout 2

Decline Toss

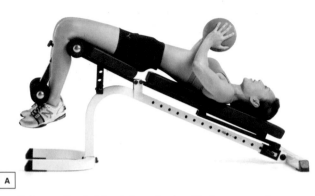

A

- Set an adjustable ab bench at a 45-degree angle. Lie down on it with your head toward the floor and hook your feet under the padded support bar. Hold a medicine ball at your chest as you lower yourself.

REPS: Do 15 to 20.

B

- As you curl up, chest-pass the ball straight up.
- Catch it at the top of the movement, then lower yourself and repeat.

Suitcase Crunch

A

- Lie on your back with your legs straight. Use both hands to hold the ball behind your head, arms straight back and barely off the floor.

B

- Simultaneously raise your torso and bend your right knee toward your chest, as you bring the ball over your knee and toward your foot.
- Repeat but reverse the movement, this time bending your left knee. That's 1 rep.

REPS: Do 15 to 20.

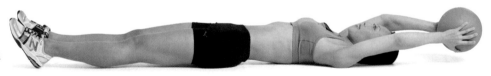

Bring the ball over your knee.

Ditch Digger

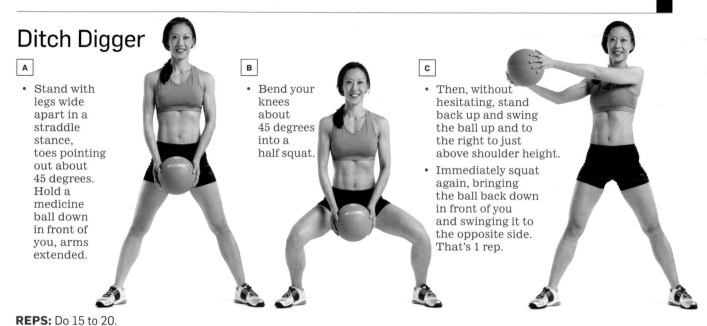

A

- Stand with legs wide apart in a straddle stance, toes pointing out about 45 degrees. Hold a medicine ball down in front of you, arms extended.

B

- Bend your knees about 45 degrees into a half squat.

C

- Then, without hesitating, stand back up and swing the ball up and to the right to just above shoulder height.
- Immediately squat again, bringing the ball back down in front of you and swinging it to the opposite side. That's 1 rep.

REPS: Do 15 to 20.

Medicine Ball Inchworm

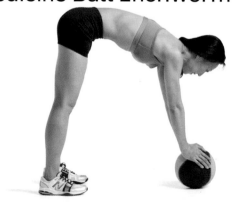

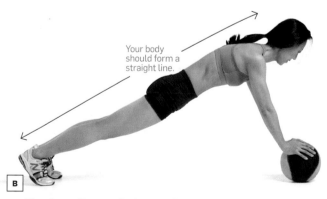

Your body should form a straight line.

A

- Stand with your feet shoulder-width apart and lean forward, knees slightly bent, to place both hands on a medicine ball on the floor.

REPS: Do 10.

B

- Slowly walk your feet away from your hands until your body is in a straight line from head to heels.
- You should move about an inch or two with each step.
- Hold for 1 second, then walk your feet back to the starting position. That's 1 rep.

Stability Ball Workout 1

These versatile, large inflated balls (also known as Swiss balls) make flattening your belly a breeze, as they crank up the effectiveness of crunches and other core moves. In fact, stability ball moves work better than any crunch. In a California State University study of 18 men and women, researchers found that just doing pushups on a ball worked the abs and obliques as well as situps and crunches, while also toning the chest, shoulders, and arms as well.

For these routines, be sure to use a ball that "fits" you properly and isn't too small or too large. As a rule of thumb, when you sit on top of the ball, your hips and legs should be bent 90 degrees. You'll find two stability ball workouts in this chapter, both designed with the help of Ashley Ntansah, personal-training manager at Club H Fitness in New York City, and Micheal A. Clark, DPT, president of the National Academy of Sports Medicine.

START HERE:

Go from one exercise to the next without resting. When you've finished the last move, take a 60-second break, then do the circuit again.

Rollout

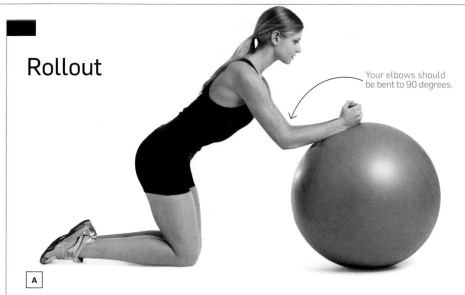

Your elbows should be bent to 90 degrees.

A

- Kneel in front of a stability ball. Place your hands on top of ball, clenched in loose fists, palms facing each other. Keep your feet together. Lean forward slightly.

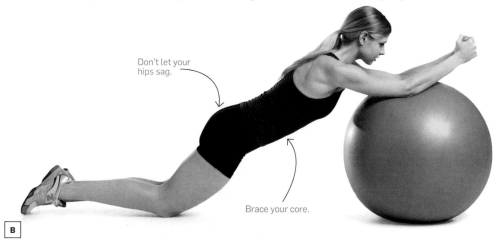

Don't let your hips sag.

Brace your core.

B

- Pivoting from your knees, lean forward and roll your forearms along the ball as you extend your hips and drop your chest toward the ball.
- Stop when your body nearly forms a straight diagonal line from your shoulders to knees.
- Contract your abs, and pull the ball back to the starting position.

REPS: Do 10 to 15.

Stability Ball Workout 1

Pike

A

- Lie facedown on a stability ball with both hands on the floor. Walk your hands out, allowing the ball to roll beneath your body until the ball is under your shins.
- Your hands should be directly below your shoulders, so it looks like you're ready to do a pushup. Your body should form a straight line from your heels to your head.

B

- Keeping your legs straight, tighten your abs, exhale, and lift your hips toward the ceiling while pulling the ball toward your hands, as far as comfortably possible.
- Hold for a second. Then lower back to the starting position.

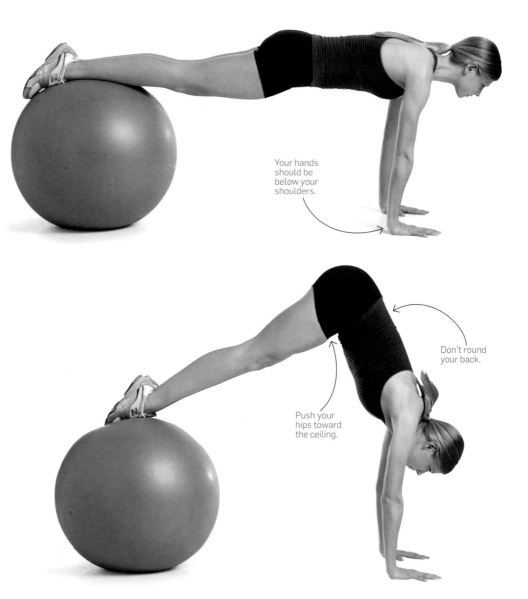

Your hands should be below your shoulders.

Don't round your back.

Push your hips toward the ceiling.

REPS: Do 10 to 15 reps.

Cobra

- Lie facedown on a stability ball and hold a pair of light dumbbells (no more than 5 pounds) with your arms hanging down to the floor, palms facing each other.

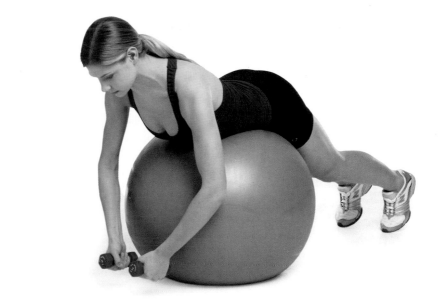

B

- Raise your arms back until they're in line with your body, and pull your shoulder blades down and together.
- Hold for 2 to 3 seconds, then lower the weights.

Lift your chest.

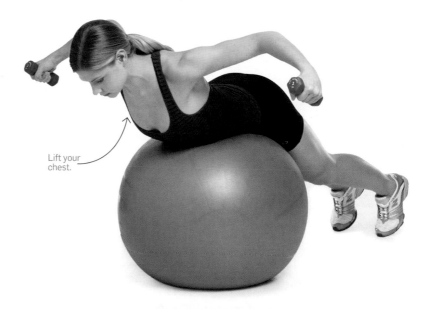

REPS: Do 10 to 15.

Stability Ball Workout 1

Skier

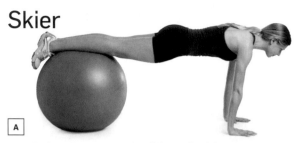

A

- Lie facedown on a stability ball with both hands on the floor. Walk your hands out, allowing the ball to roll beneath your body until the ball is under your shins. Position your hands slightly wider than shoulder-width apart.

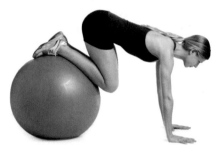

B

- Bend your knees, drawing them forward until your knees are on top of the ball and your hips are pointed toward the ceiling.

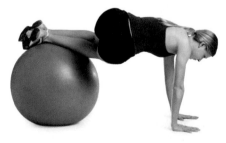

C

- Slowly drop your hips to the right side, allowing the ball to roll to the left; then immediately pull your hips back to the starting position and drop them to the left.
- That's 1 rep. As you become more comfortable with the move, you can perform it at a slightly faster pace.

REPS: Do 10 to 15.

Incline Pushup

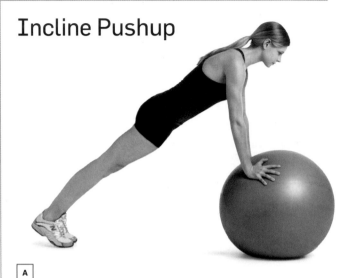

A

- Assume a pushup position by placing your hands on a stability ball, with your arms extended straight.
- Your body should form a straight line from your ankles to your head.

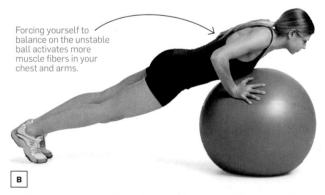

Forcing yourself to balance on the unstable ball activates more muscle fibers in your chest and arms.

B

- Brace your abs, bend your elbows, and lower your chest toward the ball. Stop when your chest touches the ball. Pause, then push yourself up.

REPS: Do 10 to 15.

Leg Curl

> **TIP:** *Make the move harder by doing it one leg at a time.*

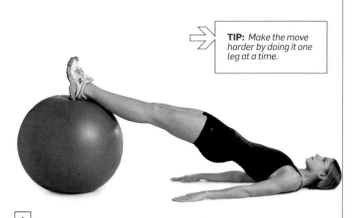

A

- Lie on the floor with your arms at your sides and place your heels on the ball. Press up, so that your hips are in the air and your torso forms a straight line.

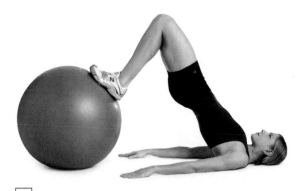

B

- Next, pull the ball toward you, squeezing your hamstrings, and then roll it back out without dropping your hips to the ground.

REPS: Do 10 to 15.

Stretch Lunge

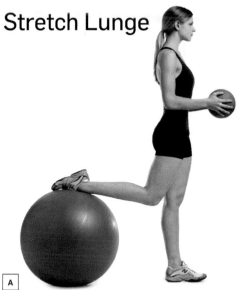

A

- Hold a medicine ball in both hands. Place the top of your right foot on top of a stability ball and your left foot flat on the ground.

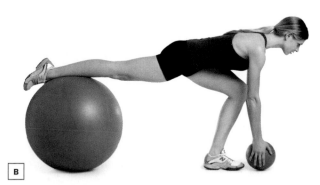

B

- Bend your left knee and lower your hips toward the floor, bending forward and touching the medicine ball on the floor in front of you. Press back to the starting position.

REPS: Do 10 to 15. Then repeat the exercise with the other leg.

Stability Ball Workout 2

You can do dozens of different moves on a stability ball. Here are some more that target your core, hips, and hamstrings. Alternate between workouts 1 and 2 during the week.

START HERE:

Go from one exercise to the next without resting. When you've finished the last move, take a 60-second break, then do the circuit again.

Walk-Up Crunches

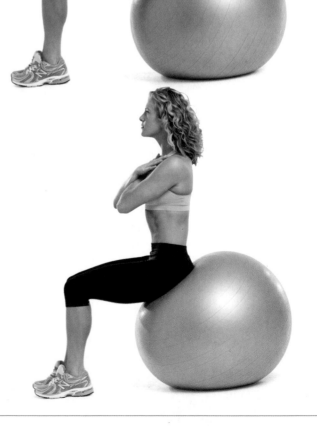

A

- Lie back with your shoulders on a stability ball, hands crossed in front of your chest, with your feet flat on the floor and knees bent 90 degrees.

B

- Contract your abs and move your feet inward as you sit up.
- Reverse the move by slowly walking your feet outward until you're back in the starting position, keeping your abs engaged throughout the exercise. That's 1 rep.

REPS: Do 20.

Hand Walks

TIP: *Try to walk as far out as you can; the farther you go, the harder it is.*

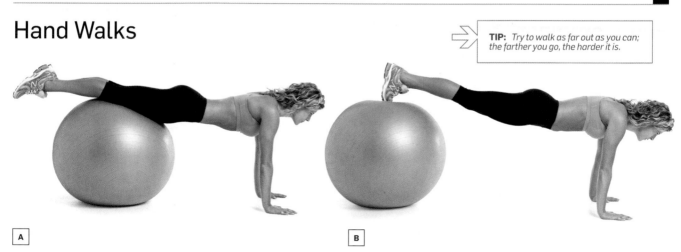

A

- Lie facedown with your torso on the ball, place your hands on the floor, raise your legs, and walk your hands out until just your thighs are on the ball.

REPS: Do 10 to 15.

B

- Squeeze your glutes and walk out until you're in the plank position, with just your feet on the ball.

- Pull your abs in tight to keep your body stable. Hold for 5 seconds, then walk your hands back to the starting position. That's 1 rep.

Leg Raise

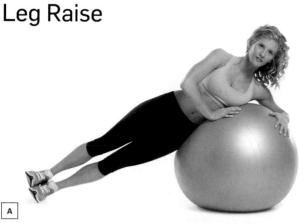

A

- Lie on your left side on the stability ball, legs extended straight out and feet stacked. Position your left hand in a comfortable spot on the ball, and lift your hips so that your body forms a straight line.

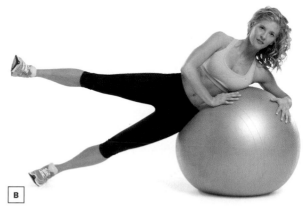

B

- Keeping your body in that position, slowly raise your right leg. Pause, then slowly return to the starting position.

REPS: Do as many reps as you can in 1 minute, then repeat on the other side.

Stability Ball Workout 2

Row Combination

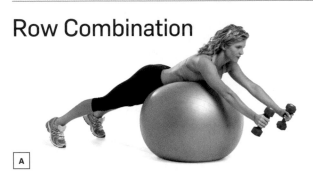

A

- Lie facedown on a stability ball and hold a pair of light dumbbells (no more than 5 pounds) with your arms hanging down and forward, with thumbs up, at 45-degree angles to the floor.

After rowing the dumbbells to the sides of your chest, extend your arms as if doing a chest fly.

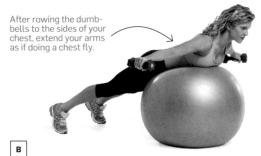

B

- Pull the weights to your chest, then lift them out to your sides.

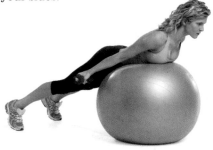

C

- Finally, pull the weights back to the sides of your butt.
- Return the weights to the starting position. That's 1 rep.

REPS: Do 10 to 15.

Jackknife

 TIP: *To make it harder, perform the move with your hands on a step or bench.*

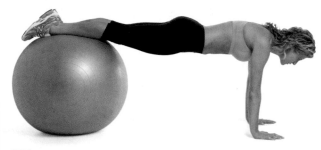

A

- Lie facedown on an exercise ball with both hands on the floor.
- Walk your hands out, allowing the ball to roll beneath your body until the ball is under your shins. Your hands should be directly below your shoulders, so it looks like you're ready to do a pushup.

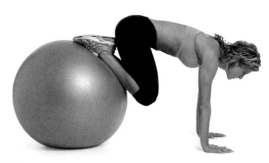

B

- Tighten your abs, and bend your knees, drawing them forward, so you bring your legs and the ball under your torso. Hold for a second.
- Straighten your legs and uncoil as you press back to the starting position.

REPS: Do 10 to 15.

Single-Leg Balance Bridge

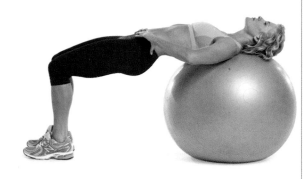

A

- Lie faceup on a stability ball with your legs bent, hips raised, and feet flat on the floor. Extend your arms out to the sides and down toward the floor.
- Walk your feet out until you are balanced with the ball between your shoulder blades. Position your feet close together, thighs parallel.

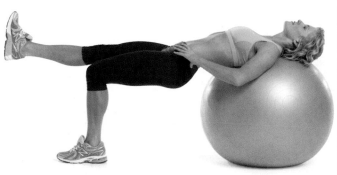

B

- Contract your glutes and slowly raise your right foot and extend your right leg.
- Hold for a count of 10. Repeat to the other side. That's 1 rep.

REPS: Do 5 to 6.

Balancing Bicycle

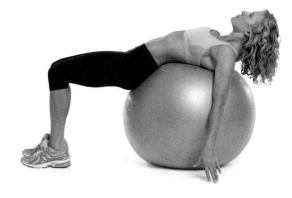

A

- Lie faceup on a stability ball with your legs bent and feet flat on the floor. Place your right hand behind your head and extend your left arm to the side and down, placing your fingertips on the floor for balance.
- Extend your left leg, foot flexed.

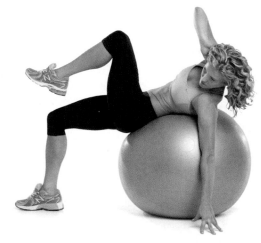

B

- Contract your abs and simultaneously lift your right shoulder up and to the left while drawing your left knee toward your right elbow. Return to the starting position.

REPS: Do 10 to 15, then switch sides.

Slider Workout

A little instability makes all your muscles work harder. Performing exercises on sliding surfaces, such as plastic sliders known as ValSlides, or even paper plates, fires up more fibers, especially in your stabilizing muscles and core, for faster tone and a greater calorie burn. This total-body toner was designed by trainer Valerie Waters, author of *Red Carpet Ready*.

START HERE:

Do the prescribed number of reps of each exercise in the order shown. Move from one exercise to the next without resting. When you've finished the last move, pause 60 seconds, then repeat the circuit.

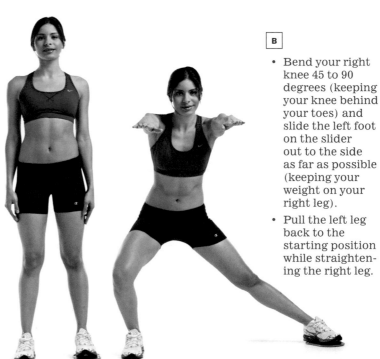

Sliding Side Lunge

A

- Place a slide underneath your left foot and stand with your feet hip distance apart. Shift your weight to your right leg and extend your arms out in front of you, palms down, for balance.

B

- Bend your right knee 45 to 90 degrees (keeping your knee behind your toes) and slide the left foot on the slider out to the side as far as possible (keeping your weight on your right leg).

- Pull the left leg back to the starting position while straightening the right leg.

REPS: Do 10 to 15, then switch sides.

Seated Side Slide

Curtsy

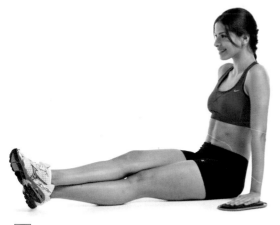

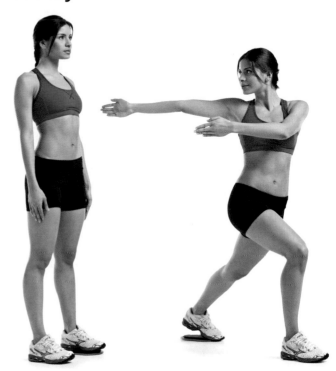

A

- Sit with legs crossed. Rest your right hand on your hip. Extend the left arm down to your side, palm on top of a slider.

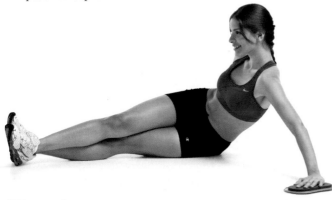

B

- Lean to the left while sliding the left arm straight out in that direction.
- When the right hip lifts off the floor, press into the slide and pull yourself back into an upright position. That's 1 rep.

REPS: Do 10, then switch sides.

A

- Stand with your feet hip-width apart, knees soft, with a slider under your left foot, arms at your sides.

B

- Press into the floor with your right heel and slide the left foot behind you to the right until the right thigh is almost parallel to the floor.
- Simultaneously, raise your arms and reach them across your body toward the right, turning to look in that direction. That's 1 rep.

REPS: Do 12 to 15, then switch sides.

Slider Workout

Pedal Crunch

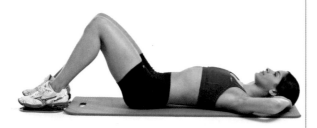

A

- Lie on your back with your knees bent, feet on the floor, and a slider under each foot. Place your hands behind your head so your elbows point out to the sides.

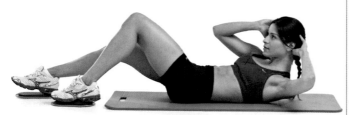

B

- Extend your right leg, sliding the foot along the floor as you contract your abs and lift your head and shoulders off the floor, twisting toward the left knee.
- Slide your right leg back to the starting position and repeat with your left leg. That's 1 rep.

REPS: Do 12 to 15.

Sliding Bridge

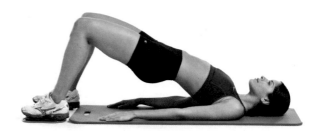

A

- Lie faceup with your knees bent, feet flat, and a slider under each foot. Place your arms at your sides, palms facing down. Squeeze your butt to lift your hips off the floor so your body forms a straight line from your knees to your shoulders.

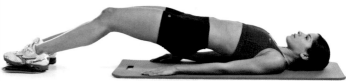

B

- Keeping your abs and butt contracted, slide through your heels and straighten your legs until your butt almost touches the floor.
- Bend your knees and slide back into the bridge position. That's 1 rep.

REPS: Do 8 to 12.

Mountain Climber

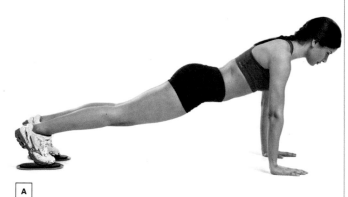

A

- Assume a push up position, arms extended, hands on the floor directly beneath shoulders, legs extended, balancing on toes, with a slider under each foot.

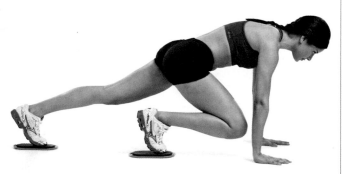

B

- Keeping your body in a straight line, slide the right knee toward your chest.
- Return to start and repeat with the left leg. That's 1 rep.

REPS: Do 12 to 15 at a brisk pace.

Slider Pushup

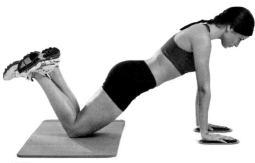

A

- Assume a modified pushup position from your knees, arms extended, hands on the floor on sliders, directly beneath your shoulders.

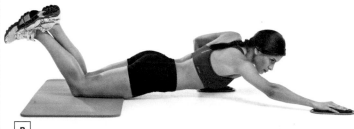

B

- Bend your arms and lower your chest toward the floor as you slide your left hand back toward your ribs and your right hand out at a diagonal.
- Push up and slide both hands to start. Immediately repeat to the opposite side. That's 1 rep.

REPS: Do 12 to 15.

Chapter 11:
15-Minute (Or Less!) Anywhere Workouts

There's No Reason Your Busy Life
Should Keep You From Staying Fit and Trim.
Not When You Have a Plan to Take With You.

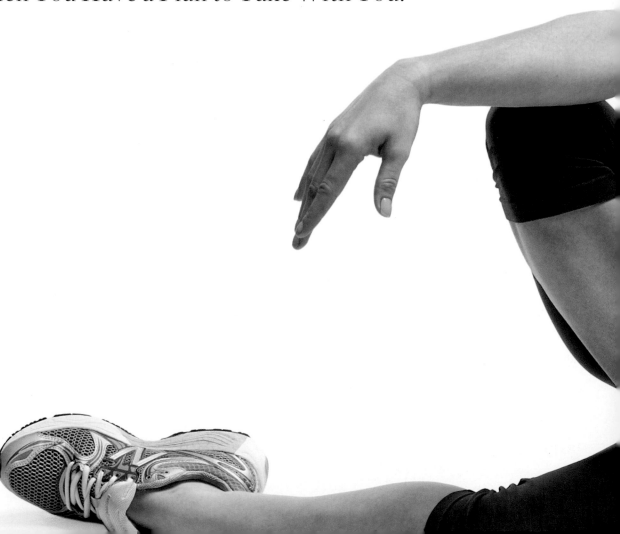

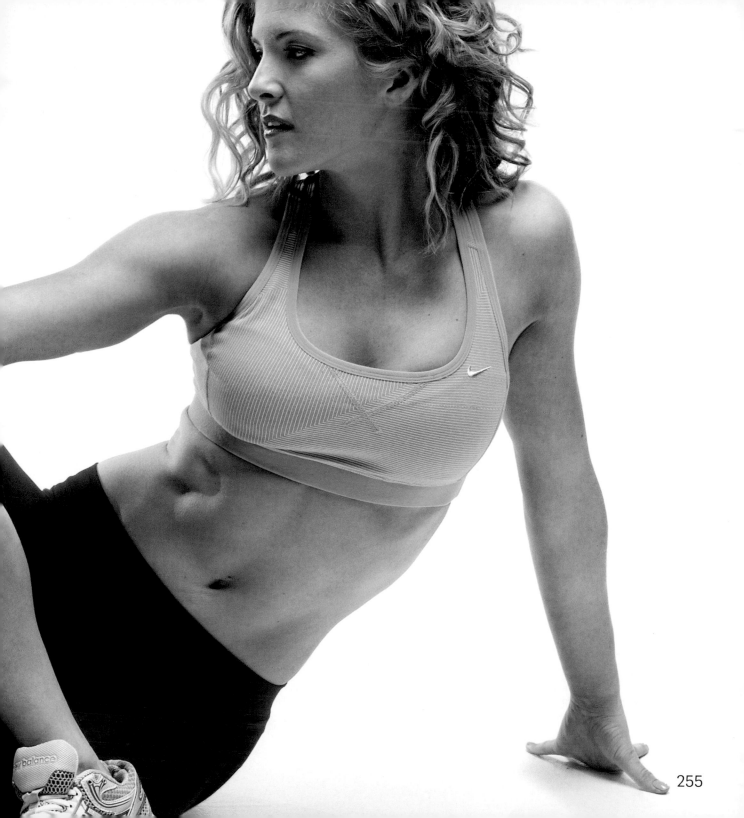

Superfast Workouts To Go!

Let's face it, life often gets in the way of our workouts. There are holidays and travel days and snow days and sick-children-at-home days that leave us stranded with not a gym in sight. Then there are the regular old marathon-day-at-work days that have you chained to your desk for 12 hours at a stretch. But you can make finely toned muscle in 15 minutes' time, wherever you are—all you need are your arms and legs (and maybe a chair and a swing.) These exercise plans can be done at the office, in a hotel room, on the playground with your kids, even 35,000 feet in the air, which is why they're also known as no-more-excuses workouts.

Start with the basics...

Chances are you spend the vast majority of your day working, which probably means you're parked in a chair behind a desk. Even if you do plan to go to the gym at the end of the day, your body needs a break during the work hours. So we've broken from our usual routine to give you five mini office-warrior workouts (lasting 1 to 5 minutes). Try these first and get into the habit of doing them every day whenever you need a lift. Do all five at once and you've done your 15-minute workout for the day.

Find it Quick: Your Do-Them-Anywhere Circuits

YOUR 15-SECOND REFRESHER

Feeling tired and tense? Get out of that chair and stand in a corner—and try this quick stretch: Facing the corner of a room, raise your hands to shoulder height and place forearms, elbows, and hands against each wall. Lean inward to stretch tight chest and back muscles. Hold the stretch for 15 seconds while taking in deep lungfuls of oxygen. You'll feel better in no time. Now, back to work before the boss sees you.

Office Warrior: 1-Minute Super Stretch

Unless you take your muscles though a healthy range of motion regularly, they will get stuck in the hunched over and shortened positions that desk work puts them in. This routine unties knots in the back, chest, and shoulders. Even just 20 seconds away from your computer screen reduces fatigue and increases blood circulation, according to Cornell University researchers.

START HERE: ▮

Repeat the moves one after another without resting.

Rag Doll

- Sit on the edge of your chair and slump your upper body forward over your legs so your chest rests on your knees and your arms hang down.

- Wrap your arms under your knees and press your back up toward the ceiling (your chest will lift off of your legs).

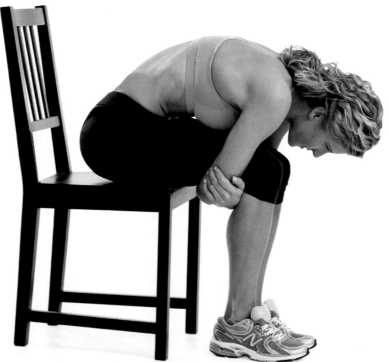

REPS: Hold for 10 to 20 seconds.

Seated Twist

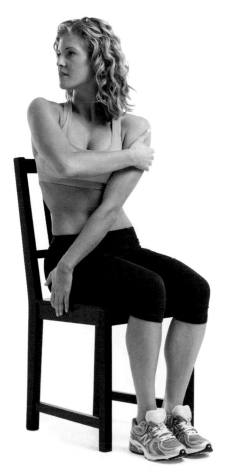

A

- Sit up tall in a chair with your feet flat on the floor.
- Reach across your body with your right arm and place your hand on your left upper arm.
- Reach across your chest with your left arm; then immediately twist to the right and grab the edge or back of the chair with your left fingers. Bring your chin over your right shoulder as you turn.

REPS: Hold for 15 seconds. Repeat on the other side.

Hunch Buster

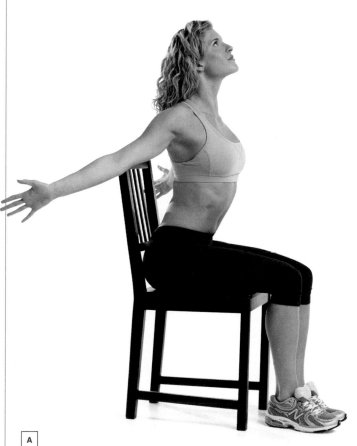

A

- Sit on a chair with your pelvis tilted slightly forward.
- Lift your chest and squeeze your shoulder blades together and down, away from your ears.
- Extend your arms at 45-degree angles and reach slightly behind you, palms facing forward.

REPS: Hold for 10 to 20 seconds.

259

Office Warrior: 1-Minute No-One-Will-Ever-Guess Workout

Give your bored body a break during your next long-winded brainstorming meeting in the conference room. Perform this mini isometric circuit while putting on your best "I'm thinking" expression. You'll stimulate your muscles and boost blood flow, and no one will be the wiser.

START HERE: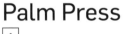

Perform these moves as a circuit, breathing normally throughout. Do it twice.

Palm Press

A

- Place your palms together in front of your chest and press as hard as you can for 10 seconds.

Seat Press

- Sit with your arms at your sides, hands on the chair seat, palms down. Press into your palms as hard as you can for 10 seconds.

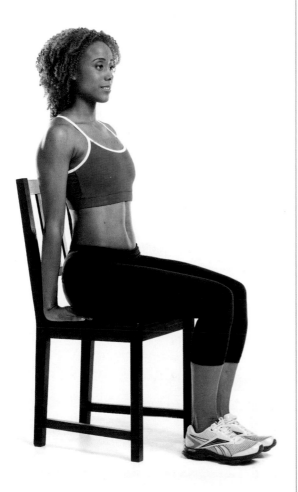

Table Press

A

- Sit straight with your arms at your sides, hands under the table, palms up, about shoulder-width apart. Push up as hard as you can into the underside of the table for 10 seconds.

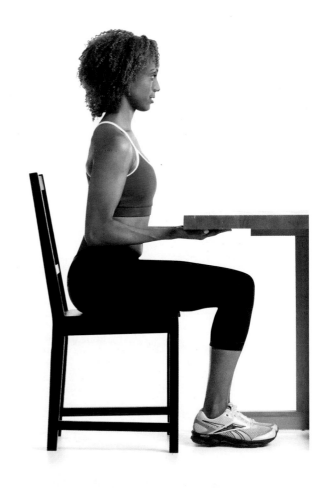

Office Warrior: 4-Minute Total-Body Tune-Up

Got a desk and a chair? That's all you need to tone those trouble spots even when there's no hope for a gym escape in sight.

START HERE:

Do the following moves one after another for 60 seconds each.

Chair Dip

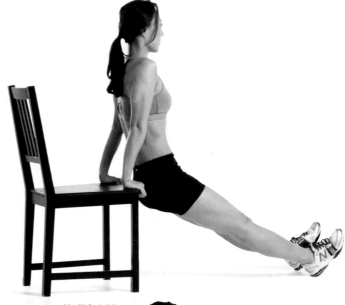

A

- In a stable chair (if yours has wheels, lock them out and back it against the wall to be safe), hold onto the chair seat with both hands on either side of your hips and inch your butt off the seat. Extend your legs straight in front of you.

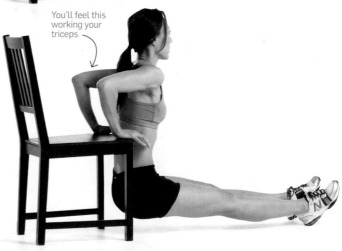

You'll feel this working your triceps

B

- Bend your elbows straight back and lower your hips toward the floor until your shoulders are in line with your elbows. Press back to the starting position and repeat.

Chair Hover and Squat

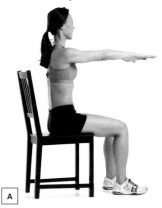

A

- Sit tall on the edge of your seat with your feet flat on the floor, hip-width apart. Extend your arms straight out in front of your chest, palms facing the floor.

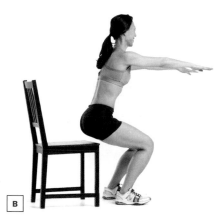

B

- Press into your feet and raise your butt off the chair, so your hips are hovering over the seat.
- Hold for 3 seconds. Stand all the way up.
- Then sit down and repeat.

Desk Pushup

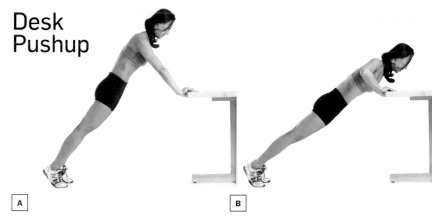

A

B

- Stand facing your desk. Place both hands on the edge of your desk about shoulder-width apart. Walk your feet back until you are in a plank position with your body forming a straight diagonal line from your head to your heels.

- Bend your elbows out to the sides and lower your chest toward the desk until your arms are bent 90 degrees and elbows are in line with your shoulders. Hold for 2 to 3 seconds. Return to the starting position. Repeat.

Leg Extensions

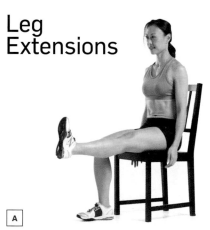

Lift your thigh off the chair a few inches while squeezing your glutes.

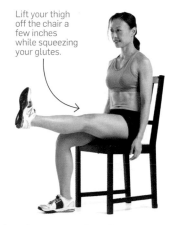

A

B

- Sit up tall in your chair seat, arms down at your sides or behind your back for support. Extend your left leg straight out in front of you until it's parallel to the floor and level with your hip.

- Contract your quad and, using your hip flexor, lift your leg slightly higher.
- Lower and repeat for 30 seconds. Then repeat the exercise with your right leg.

Office Warrior: 5-Minute Water Bottle Workout

Everyday items like books, bottles, and quarterly reports can work just as well as and weights for many moves. Here are some exercises you can do using that water bottle on your desk. Fill it up and fire up some muscle fibers. Do each move for 60 seconds (unless otherwise indicated).

START HERE: ■

Perform these moves as a circuit, breathing normally throughout.

Oblique Bend

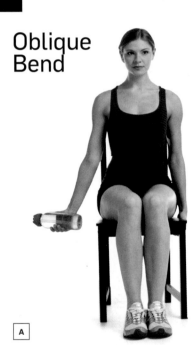

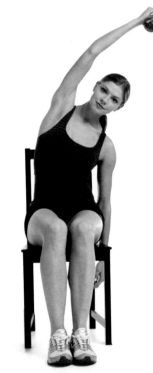

A

- Sit up straight and hold a filled water bottle in your right hand, palm facing out, arm down by your side.

REPS: Do as many as possible in 60 seconds.

B

- In one smooth motion, keeping your arm extended, raise your arm out to the side and overhead to the left, bending to the left as far as comfortably possible. After doing this for 30 seconds, hold the bottle in your left and repeat the exercise.

Inner-Thigh Squeeze

A

- Sit up straight on the edge of your seat. Place the bottle between your knees.
- Contract your inner thighs and slowly squeeze the bottle as hard as you can. Hold the contraction for 5 to 10 seconds.
- Relax slightly (but not completely, or you'll drop the bottle). Squeeze again.

TIP: *Contract your abs with each squeeze of your thighs.*

This exercise targets muscles called the hip adductors, located on the inside of your upper thigh.

Make sure the cap's on tight before you squeeze!

REPS: Do as many as possible in 60 seconds.

Office Warrior: 5-Minute Water Bottle Workout

Overhead Raise, Triceps Press

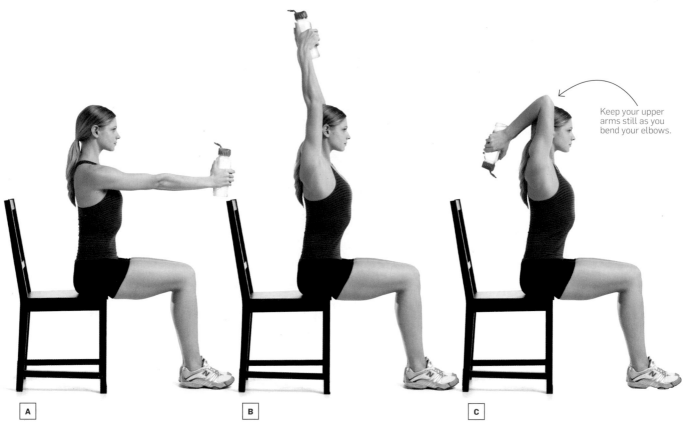

Keep your upper arms still as you bend your elbows.

A

- Sit up straight on the edge of your seat. Hold the bottle with both hands and extend your arms straight out from your chest, so they're at shoulder level.

B

- Keeping your arms straight, raise the bottle straight overhead until your upper arms are by your ears.

C

- Keeping arms tight against your head, bend your elbows to lower the bottle behind your back. Straighten your arms and return to the starting position.

REPS: Do as many as possible in 60 seconds.

Leg Curl

Ab Twist

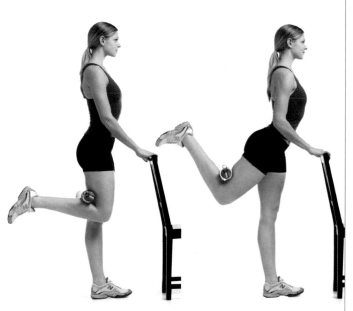

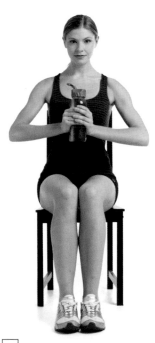

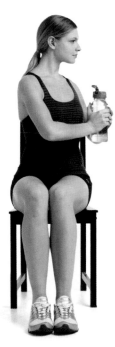

A
- Stand facing your desk or chair. Bend your right leg and place the water bottle behind your right knee. Hold the chair or desk for support.

B
- Squeeze your hamstrings to pull your heel closer to your butt, and contract your glute to press your heel toward the ceiling. Continue for 30 seconds, then repeat with other leg.

REPS: Do as many as possible in 60 seconds.

A
- Sit up straight on the edge of your seat. Hold the bottle with both hands in front of your chest, arms bent, elbows pointing out to the sides.

B
- Contract your abs and slowly twist to the left as far as comfortably possible. Return to center. Repeat to the right.

REPS: Do as many as possible in 60 seconds.

Office Warrior: 5-Minute P.M. Slump Workout

Sometimes, no amount of coffee is going to keep you awake after lunch. This 5-minute workout revs your heart rate, keeping you alert and enhancing your cognitive functioning.

START HERE: ■

Do each move for 60 seconds, unless otherwise indicated.

Desk Mountain Climber

A

- Stand facing your desk. Place both hands on the edge of your desk about shoulder-width apart.
- Walk your feet back until you are in a plank position with your body forming a straight diagonal line from your head to your heels. Bend your arms 45 to 90 degrees.

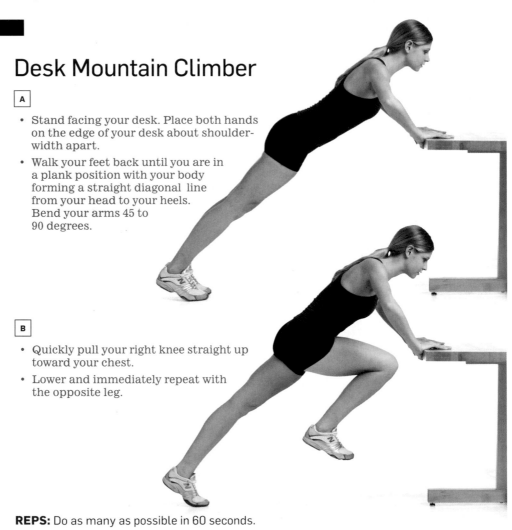

B

- Quickly pull your right knee straight up toward your chest.
- Lower and immediately repeat with the opposite leg.

REPS: Do as many as possible in 60 seconds.

Arm Pumps and Punches

TIP: *If you don't have dumbbells, just do the move with your fists.*

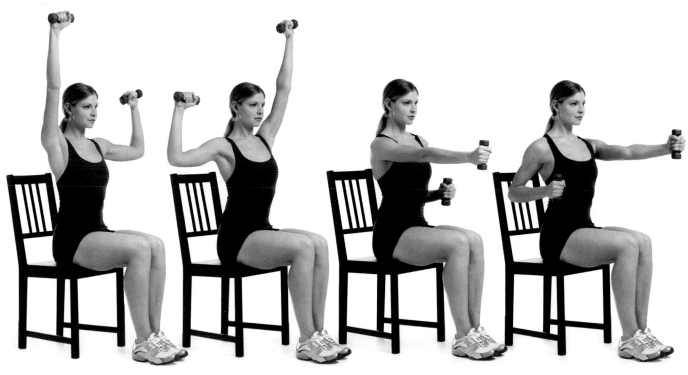

A

- Sit up straight on the edge of your seat. Grasp lightweight dumbbells and place them on the sides of your shoulders, palms facing out. Quickly punch toward the ceiling with your right hand.

B

- Quickly pull the right hand down while simultaneously punching up with your left. Immediately repeat with your right hand. Continue pumping your fists up and down for 30 seconds.

C

- Turn your fists so your palms are facing in and place your hands at either side of your chest.
- Jab forward with your right fist.

D

- Pull back to the starting position, then immediately jab foward with the left. Continue jabbing right and left for 30 seconds.

REPS: Do as many punches up and out as possible in 60 seconds.

Office Warrior: 5-Minute P.M. Slump Workout

T Tip

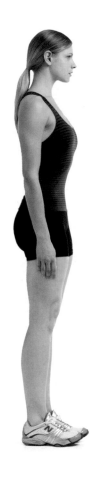

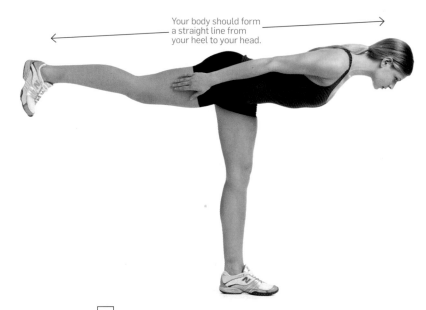

Your body should form a straight line from your heel to your head.

A

- Stand tall with arms at your sides.

B

- Keeping your back straight, hinge forward from the hips and lower your torso toward the floor while lifting and extending your right leg off the floor straight out behind you until your body forms a T with your torso and leg parallel to the floor.
- Pause. Return to the starting position, then repeat while lifting the left leg.

REPS: Do as many as possible with both legs in 60 seconds.

Pendulum Lunges

 A

- Stand tall with feet hip-width apart. Take a giant step back with your right leg, bending the left knee so the left thigh is parallel to the floor and the right knee dips toward the floor.

B

- Press into the left foot and bring your right leg up and immediately swing it in front of you into a forward lunge, bending your right knee, so your right thigh is parallel to the floor, and allowing the left knee to dip toward the floor.

REPS: Continue to alternate lunging forward and back for 30 seconds; then switch legs.

Chair Lift

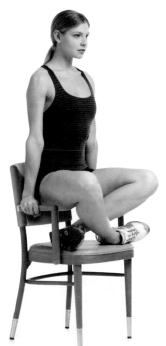
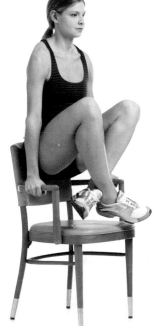

A

- Sit all the way back in your chair and cross your legs so your feet are on the seat. Place your hands on the armrests.

B

- Contract your abs as you lift your knees toward your chest, lifting your feet a few inches above your seat. Pause; then lower.

REPS: Do as many lifts as you can in 60 seconds (you may need to rest a few seconds between reps).

Hotel Room Workout 1

Laid up in a hotel without a gym? (Or worse, one that charges you 30 bucks to use dusty dumbbells and old LifeCycles?) Here's an effective workout that uses only your bodyweight, so you can do it just about anywhere. It's designed to load up every muscle system.

START HERE:

Do these moves one after another with no rest in between. When you finish the last move, pause 60 seconds, then repeat the circuit. This workout comes from **Juan Carlos Santana**, CEO of the Institute of Human Performance, in Boca Raton, Florida.

Side Bridge Abduction

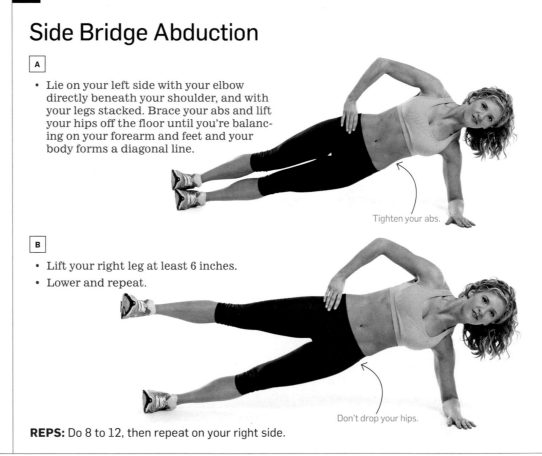

A

- Lie on your left side with your elbow directly beneath your shoulder, and with your legs stacked. Brace your abs and lift your hips off the floor until you're balancing on your forearm and feet and your body forms a diagonal line.

Tighten your abs.

B

- Lift your right leg at least 6 inches.
- Lower and repeat.

Don't drop your hips.

REPS: Do 8 to 12, then repeat on your right side.

Wraparound Ankle Touch

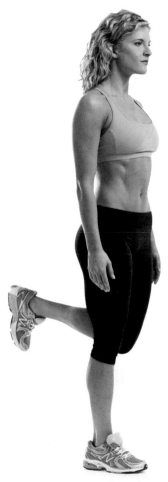

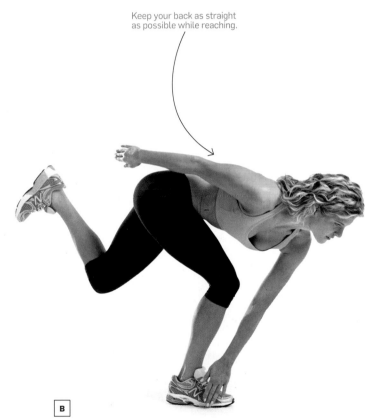

Keep your back as straight as possible while reaching.

A

- Stand with your legs together and bend your left knee 90 degrees so you're balancing on your right leg.

B

- As you squat, reach your left arm across your body and try to touch the outside of your right foot with your fingertips.
- Press back up to the starting position and repeat.

REPS: Do 8 to 12, then repeat while balancing on your left leg.

Hotel Room Workout 1

Double-Stop Pushup

TIP: *Make the move easier by doing it with your knees on the floor.*

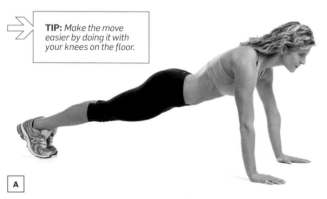

A

- Assume a pushup position with your hands slightly wider than your shoulders and your back straight.

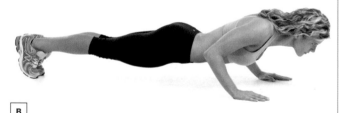

B

- Keeping your neck in line with your spine, lower yourself halfway and hold for 1 second.

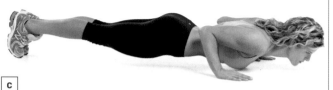

C

- Continue lowering until your chest is only a couple of inches from the floor.
- Pause, then push back up to the halfway point and pause again before finally pressing all the way up.

REPS: Do 8 to 12.

Plank Bird Dog

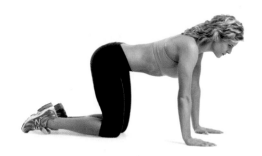

A

- Get on your hands and knees, hands beneath your shoulders with your back straight.

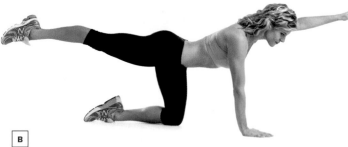

B

- Brace your abs as you simultaneously extend your left arm and right leg.
- Lower them both and repeat, lifting your right arm and left leg.

REPS: Do 8 to 12 on each side.

Windshield Wiper

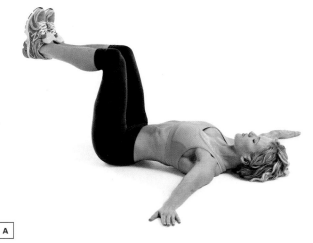

A

- Bend your knees and lift your legs until your thighs are above your hips.

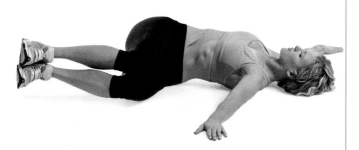

B

- Press your palms into the floor and lower your legs to the left. Go as far as possible while keeping your right shoulder glued to the floor.
- Then bring your legs back to center. Next, lower them to the right.

REPS: Do 8 to 12 on each side.

Supine Row

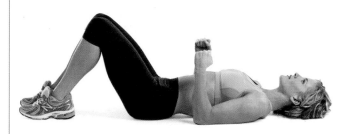

A

- Lie on your back with your knees bent, feet flat on the floor, and arms at your sides with elbows bent 90 degrees.

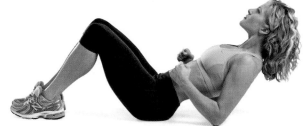

B

- Pinch your shoulder blades together as you dig your elbows into the mat and lift your head and torso a few inches off the floor. Lower and repeat.

REPS: Do 8 to 12.

Hotel Room Workout 2

This killer head-to-toe toning workout was designed with the help of Amy Dixon, an exercise physiologist and group fitness manager at Equinox in Santa Monica, California. It's perfect when you're stuck somewhere with no access to a gym.

START HERE:

Do these moves one after another with no rest between them. When you've finished the last move, pause 30 to 60 seconds, then repeat the circuit twice more.

One-Leg Squat Floor Reach and Press

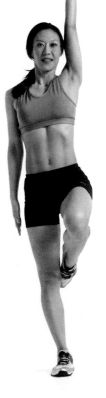

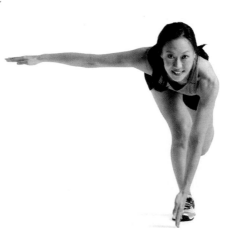

A

- Stand with your feet hip-width apart and your arms at your sides. Bend your left knee, lifting your foot behind you.
- Squat and raise your right arm out to the side to shoulder height, then reach your left hand down across your body, touching the floor outside your right toes.

B

- Stand up as you lift your left hand toward the ceiling, lower your right arm to your side, and raise your left thigh to hip level in front of you.
- Lower your left leg and repeat on the other side. That's 1 rep.

REPS: Do 12 to 15.

Pushup Crawl

- Get in plank position with your hands wider than shoulder-width apart.

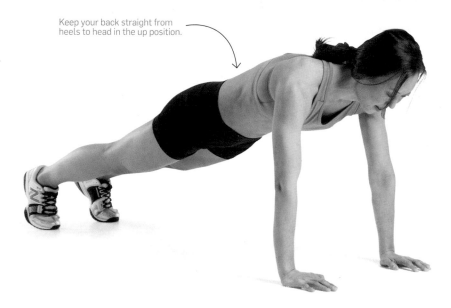

Keep your back straight from heels to head in the up position.

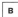

- Lower your chest as close to the floor as you can. Holding that position, lift your right knee to the outside of your right elbow.

- Return to plank position, then push back up to the starting position; repeat on the other side. That's 1 rep.

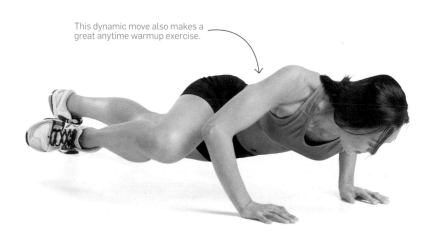

This dynamic move also makes a great anytime warmup exercise.

REPS: Do 12 to 15.

Hotel Room Workout 2

Front Lunge Floor Reach and Reverse Twist

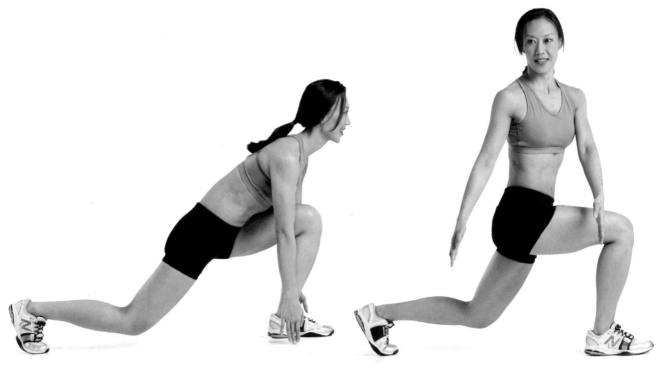

A

- Stand with your feet hip-width apart and your arms at your sides. Lunge forward with your left leg so your right knee is nearly touching the floor and your left thigh is parallel to the floor. Bending forward, try to touch the floor on either side of your left foot.

REPS: Do 12 to 15.

B

- Push off your left foot; using that momentum, step forward with your right foot, shifting your weight to that foot, and swing your left leg behind you. As you sink backward into a lunge, rotate your torso 45 degrees to the right.
- Return to standing. That's 1 rep.

Grand Plié Squat Reach and Jump

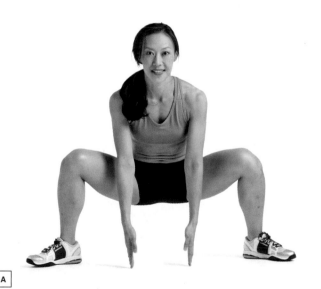

A

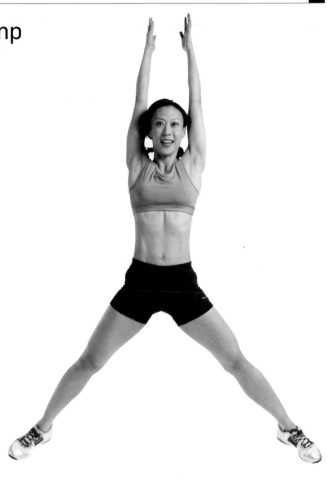

B

- Stand with your legs wide apart, toes turned out, and arms at your sides. Squat until your thighs are parallel to the floor and you're low enough to touch it with your fingertips.

- Immediately jump up as high as you can, keeping your legs wide and extending your arms straight overhead. That's 1 rep.

REPS: Do 12 to 15.

Playground Workout

No reason to just park yourself on a bench while your kids get all the exercise. The playground has great tools, like swings, monkey bars, and yes, that bench you're planted on, to bust out all your favorite moves and a few new ones, too. This workout will keep you in shape all summer.

START HERE:

Perform the moves one after another without rest. When you've completed the last move, pause for 60 seconds. Then repeat the circuit two more times.

Swing Lunge

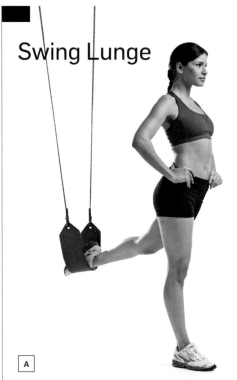

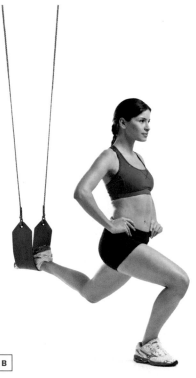

A

- Stand with your back about one giant step from a 1- to 2-foot-high swing seat. Reach back with your left foot and place your toes on the seat .

REPS: Do 10, then repeat with the other leg.

B

- With your arms on your hips, sink into a lunge until your right thigh is parallel to the ground.
- Slowly return to the starting position. That's 1 rep.

280

Monkey Up

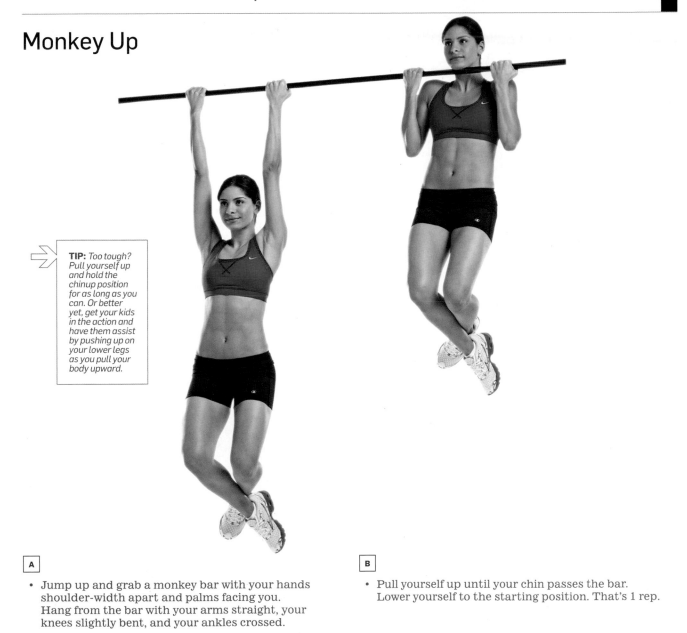

TIP: *Too tough? Pull yourself up and hold the chinup position for as long as you can. Or better yet, get your kids in the action and have them assist by pushing up on your lower legs as you pull your body upward.*

A

- Jump up and grab a monkey bar with your hands shoulder-width apart and palms facing you. Hang from the bar with your arms straight, your knees slightly bent, and your ankles crossed.

REPS: Do as many as you can.

B

- Pull yourself up until your chin passes the bar. Lower yourself to the starting position. That's 1 rep.

Playground Workout

Bench Jump

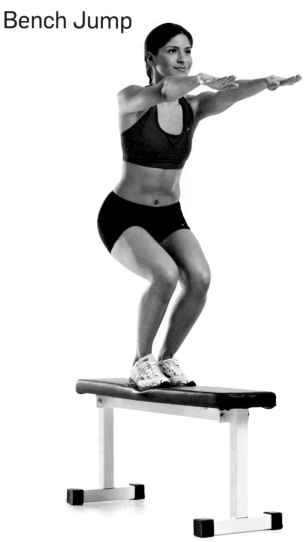

A

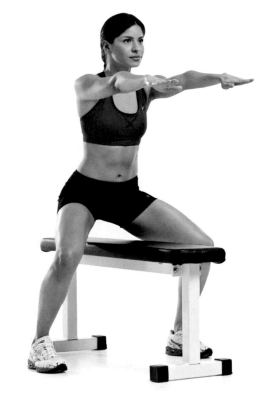

B

- Begin by standing on a 1- to 2-foot-high backless park bench with your knees slightly bent and your arms straight out in front of you at shoulder height.

REPS: Do as many as you can in 20 seconds.

- Jump down so you're straddling the bench. Jump back onto the bench, landing with your feet together.

Swing Pike Pushup

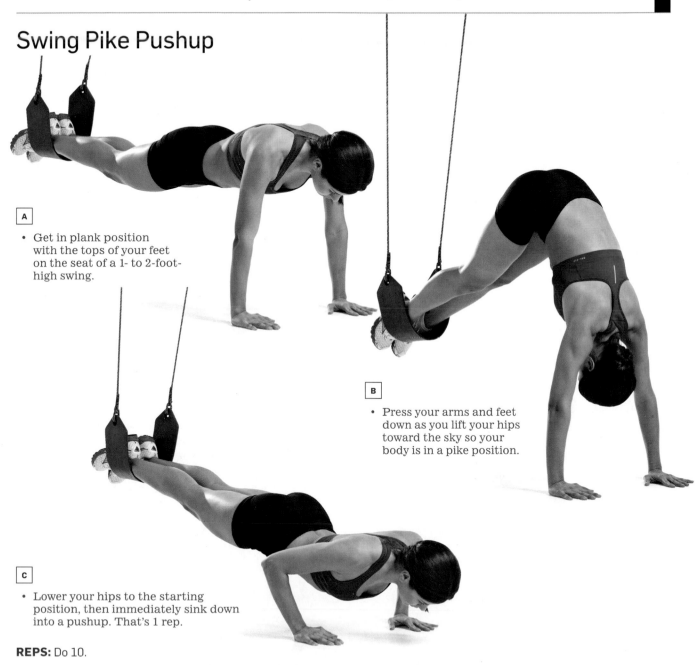

A

- Get in plank position with the tops of your feet on the seat of a 1- to 2-foot-high swing.

B

- Press your arms and feet down as you lift your hips toward the sky so your body is in a pike position.

C

- Lower your hips to the starting position, then immediately sink down into a pushup. That's 1 rep.

REPS: Do 10.

35,000-Feet-in-the-Air Workout

Even when you can't walk the aisle in the plane for exercise (because you're flanked by two huge snoring businessmen), you can still get the blood flowing and tone your body. The following moves will boost circulation throughout your body while you target every key muscle group.

START HERE:

Do the sequence as a circuit, performing each move for about 60 seconds, unless other-wise indi-cated. Rest 30 seconds and repeat the circuit.

Core Lifts

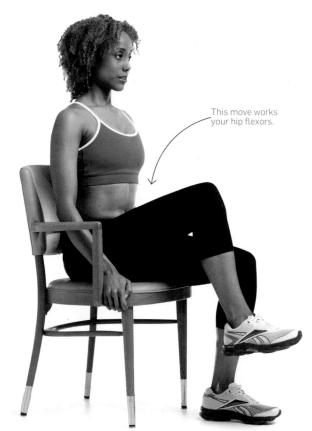

A

- Sit up tall in your seat. Contract your abs and lift one foot off the floor about 6 inches.
- Hold for 10 seconds and slowly lower it while relaxing your abs. Repeat with the opposite leg. Alternate throughout the exercise.

This move works your hip flexors.

REPS: Do as many as you can with each leg for 60 seconds.

Wrist and Ankle Circles

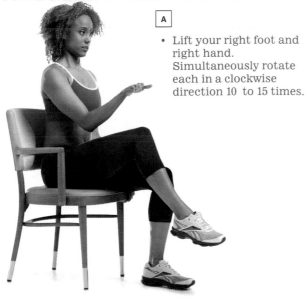

A

- Lift your right foot and right hand. Simultaneously rotate each in a clockwise direction 10 to 15 times.

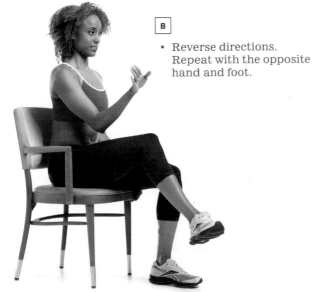

B

- Reverse directions. Repeat with the opposite hand and foot.

REPS: Do as many as you can in 60 seconds.

Armrest Arm Boosters

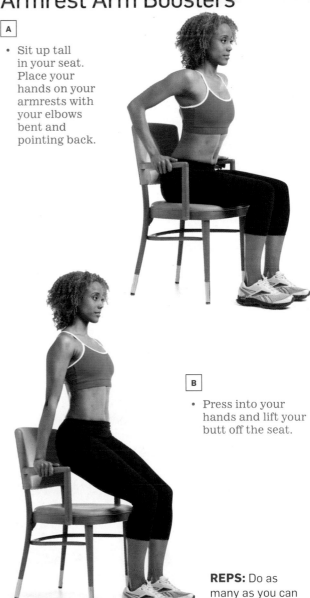

A

- Sit up tall in your seat. Place your hands on your armrests with your elbows bent and pointing back.

B

- Press into your hands and lift your butt off the seat.

REPS: Do as many as you can in 60 seconds.

35,000-Feet-in-the-Air Workout

Heel Raises

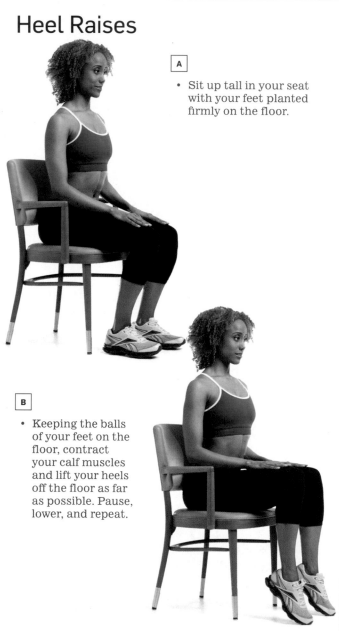

A

- Sit up tall in your seat with your feet planted firmly on the floor.

B

- Keeping the balls of your feet on the floor, contract your calf muscles and lift your heels off the floor as far as possible. Pause, lower, and repeat.

REPS: Do as many as you can in 60 seconds.

Seated Eagle Spine Stretch

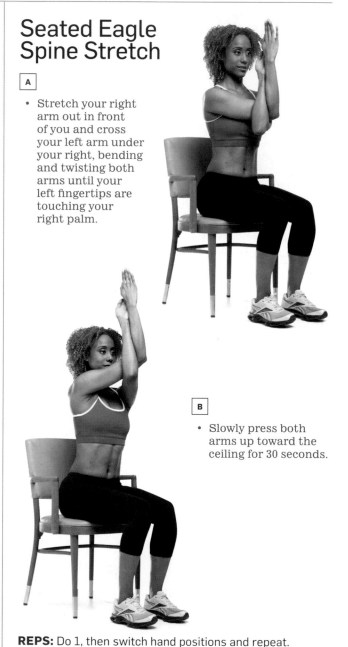

A

- Stretch your right arm out in front of you and cross your left arm under your right, bending and twisting both arms until your left fingertips are touching your right palm.

B

- Slowly press both arms up toward the ceiling for 30 seconds.

REPS: Do 1, then switch hand positions and repeat.

Toe Raises

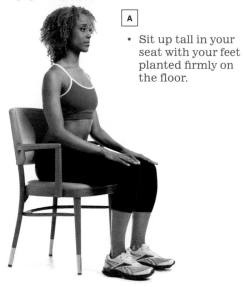

A
- Sit up tall in your seat with your feet planted firmly on the floor.

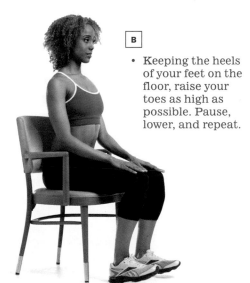

B
- Keeping the heels of your feet on the floor, raise your toes as high as possible. Pause, lower, and repeat.

REPS: Do as many as you can in 60 seconds.

Upright Reverse Crunches

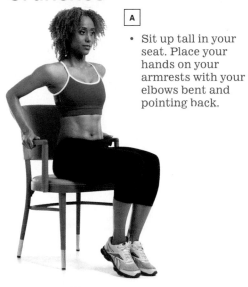

A
- Sit up tall in your seat. Place your hands on your armrests with your elbows bent and pointing back.

B
- Contract your abs and slowly pull your knees toward your chest. Pause, lower, and repeat.

REPS: Do as many as you can in 60 seconds.

Bun Squeeze

(not shown)

- Sit up tall in your seat.
- Contract your glutes and squeeze your buns together as tightly as possible. Hold for 10 seconds. Slowly release.

REPS: Do 6.

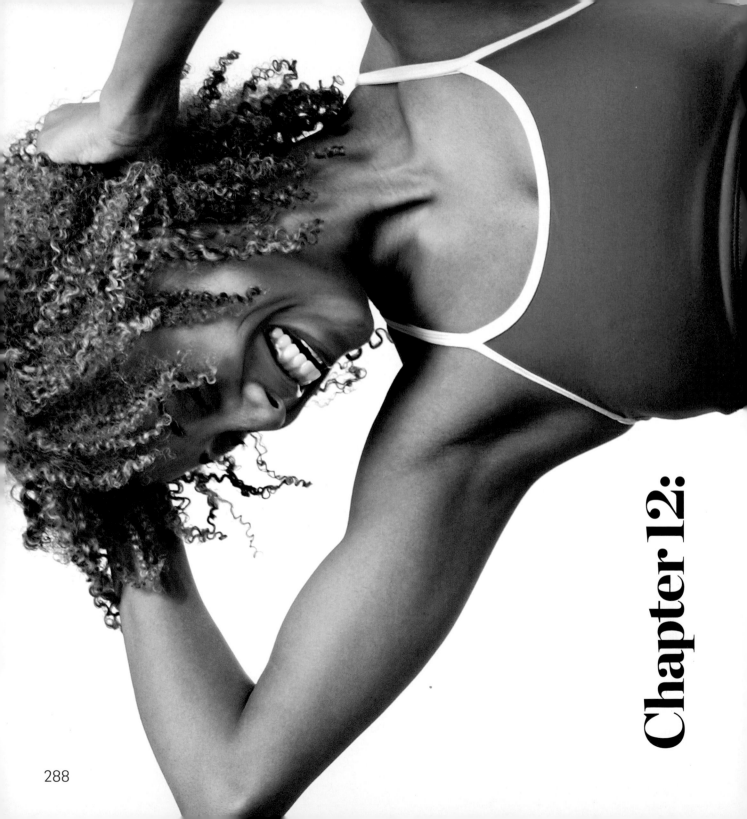

Chapter 12:

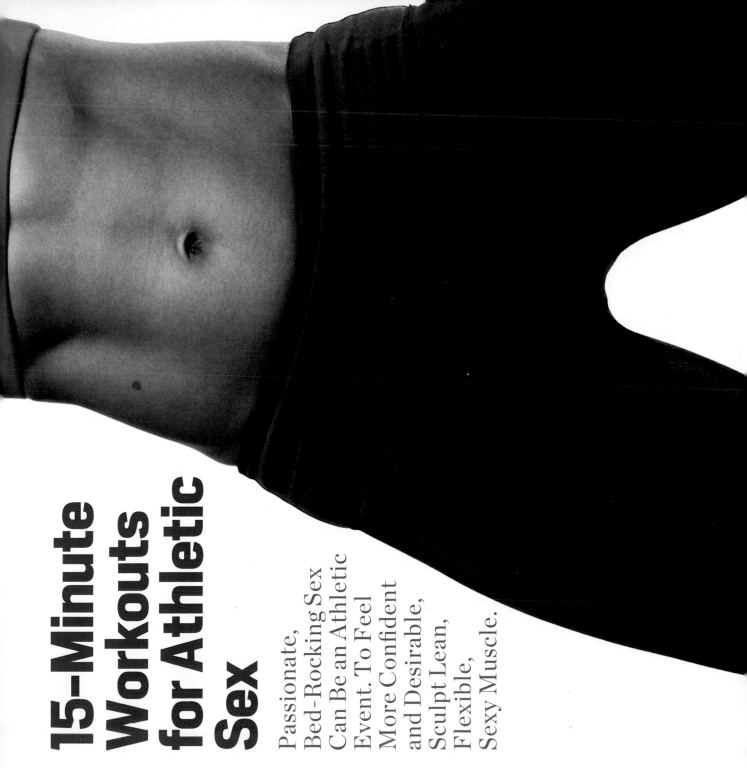

15-Minute Workouts for Athletic Sex

Passionate, Bed-Rocking Sex Can Be an Athletic Event. To Feel More Confident and Desirable, Sculpt Lean, Flexible, Sexy Muscle.

Superfast Better-Sex Workouts

A healthy session in the sack uses every major muscle—including quite a few that you don't see in the mirror. The stronger those muscles, the more likely you are to reach your pleasure peaks. A little sexercising of your inner thighs, glutes, core, upper body, and pelvic floor muscles improves blood flow to key areas, making it more likely that you'll get some satisfaction, again and again. Some women have even reported hitting the big O just by doing some of the moves below (seriously), because of all the pelvic area activation.

These routines are guaranteed to heat things up between the sheets. Just don't try them every day (tempted though you may be). Your love muscles need a break to recover—but feel free to test drive the results anytime!

TOP CONFIDENCE BOOSTERS
The number-one thing that elevates a woman's confidence is a workout, followed by compliments, and third, seeing a flattering photo of herself, according to a poll of *Women's Health* readers.

Begin with the basics...

The original better-sex exercise is one you can do anywhere—at the dinner table, a work meeting, or while driving in a car. You know them: kegels, named after gynecologist Arnold Kegel who prescribed them to his patients. You do them by squeezing the PC, or pubococcygeus, muscle, which you use to stop the flow of urine. Kegels strengthen the pelvic floor muscles and the transverse abdominals, both of which boost blood flow to your nether region, increase the amount of friction you can generate, and intensify contractions during orgasm. While you can do them any time, anywhere, incorporate them into your workouts: Lie on your back with knees bent 90 degrees and feet flat on the floor. Without tighening your glutes, squeeze your PC muscle and hold for 15 seconds. Do 20 or so a day.

FLEX TO FIRE UP LIBIDO

Women who practice yoga regularly report a marked boost in sex drive, according to the *Journal of Sexual Medicine*. You'll find some yogalike moves later in this chapter, as well as yoga-specific workouts in Chapter 15.

▮ Find it Quick: Your 15-Minute Heat-the-Sheets Circuits

p.292
COREgasm Workout

Hanging Straight-Leg Raise

Hanging Side Crunch

Single-Leg Hip Raise

Arm Pullover Straight-Leg Crunch

Medicine Ball Blast

p.296
Pretzel Position Workout

V-Up

Isometric Wall Squat

Fierce Pose

Half Lord of the Fishes

p.298
Cowgirl Workout

Stability Thigh and Fly

Bridge Pose

Frog

Stability Ball Squeeze and Curl

Stability Ball Hip Raise
and Leg Curl

Bear

Reverse Chaturanga

COREgasm Workout

The *what* workout? We know, it sounds strange. But when *Women's Health* asked readers if anyone had ever experienced an orgasm during a workout, women fessed up: yes, many claimed, usually when doing leg-lifting core exercises. And the notion of the COREgasm was born.

How does it work? "When some women exercise, the release of endorphins and dopamine, which are necessary for orgasm, combined with the tension in the abs and lower extremities, can cause the clitoral stimulation that is needed," says sex therapist Victoria Zdrok, PhD, author of *The Anatomy of Pleasure*. Whether you experience an added surprise while doing this workout or not, it's still an amazing routine of waist-whittling moves that will help flatten your belly and give you the pelvic and core strength you need for the main event.

Less Weight, Greater Pleasure

Being overweight can depress your sex life. Researchers studying 1,210 people at Duke University Medical Center say obese people are 25 times more likely to report dissatisfaction with sex as healthy-weight people.

The good news is that good sex can be achieved without a huge change in body composition. Other studies report that people can significantly improve their sexual satisfaction with just a 10 percent reduction in bodyweight.

START HERE:

Do one exercise after another without rest for the recommended number of repetitions. When you've finished the final move, take a 30-second break, then repeat the circuit.

Hanging Straight-Leg Raise

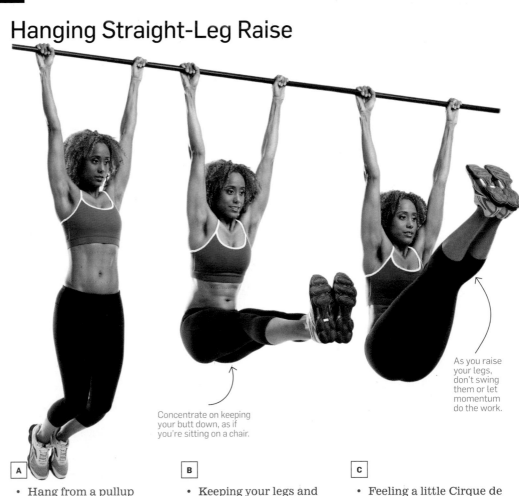

As you raise your legs, don't swing them or let momentum do the work.

Concentrate on keeping your butt down, as if you're sitting on a chair.

A
- Hang from a pullup bar with your hands shoulder-width apart and your hips centered under your body so there's a straight line from your hands to the bottom of your hips.

REPS: Do 4 to 6.

B
- Keeping your legs and back straight and using a slow, controlled motion, raise your legs until they're parallel to the floor. Slowly lower your legs. That's 1 rep.

C
- Feeling a little Cirque de Soleil? Try to raise your feet above 90 degrees.

COREgasm Workout

Hanging Side Crunch

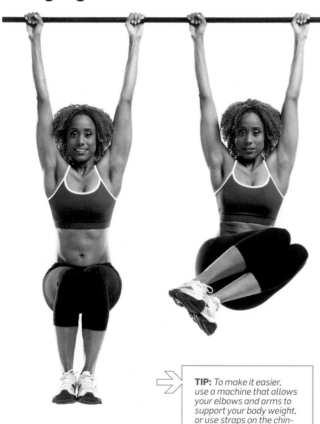

> **TIP:** To make it easier, use a machine that allows your elbows and arms to support your body weight, or use straps on the chin-up bar to add support.

A

- Hang from a chinup bar, holding it with your palms facing forward, and bring your knees up so that your thighs and torso form a 90-degree angle.

REPS: Do 10 to 12.

B

- Next, pinch at your right side, curling your right hip up toward your right shoulder.
- Use your core to keep yourself from swinging, and repeat to the left. That's 1 rep.

Single-Leg Hip Raise

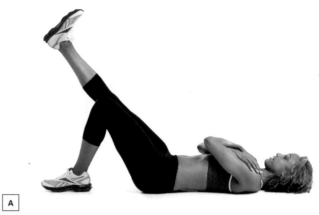

A

- Lie on your back with your knees bent and your feet flat on the floor. Cross your arms over your chest and raise the lower half of your right leg until it's in line with your left thigh.

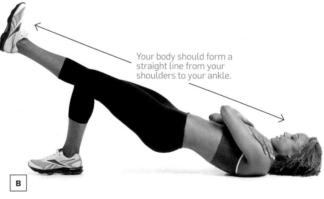

Your body should form a straight line from your shoulders to your ankle.

B

- Press your left foot into the floor and contract your glutes as you lift your torso so it's in line with your thighs.
- Hold for 3 seconds, then repeat, raising the opposite leg. That's 1 rep.

REPS: Do 10 to 12.

Arm Pullover Straight-Leg Crunch

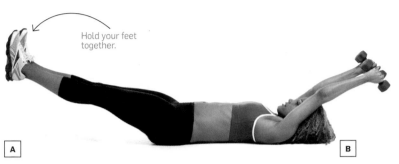

Hold your feet together.

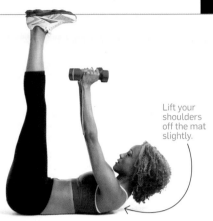

Lift your shoulders off the mat slightly.

A

- Grab a pair of lightweight dumbbells and lie on your back with your arms behind you. Extend your legs at a 45-degree angle.

REPS: Do 10 to 12.

B

- Bring your arms up over your chest and lift your shoulders off the mat while raising your legs until they're perpendicular to the floor.
- Return to the starting position (don't let your legs touch the floor). That's 1 rep.

Medicine Ball Blast

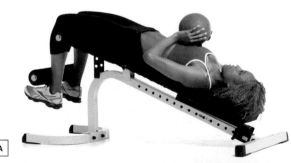

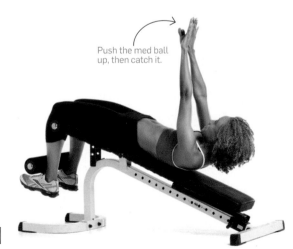

Push the med ball up, then catch it.

A

- Set an adjustable abs bench at a 45-degree angle. Lie down on it with your head toward the floor, and hook your feet under the padded support bar. Hold a medicine ball at your chest as you lower yourself.

REPS: Do 12 to 15.

B

- As you curl up, chest-pass the ball straight up.
- Catch it at the top of the movement, then lower yourself.

Pretzel Position Workout

This routine primes you for all sorts of between-the-sheets configurations—pretzel position (a twisty tangle of legs as the name implies), reverse cowgirl, wheelbarrow...bring it on! It also incorporates some yoga poses to open your hips and stretch your spine to give you flexibility, and it strengthens all those key sex muscles in your pelvic floor, core, and legs.

START HERE:

Do the workout as a circuit. Rest for 1 minute after completing the last exercise in the circuit, then repeat the circuit two more times.

V-Up

- Lie faceup on the floor with legs and arms straight.

- Extend your arms forward, parallel with the floor, palms facing each other. In one movement, lift your torso and legs, your body forming a V shape.

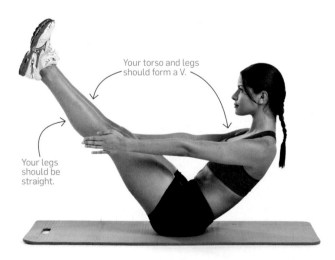

Your torso and legs should form a V.

Your legs should be straight.

REPS: Do 5, holding each pose for 5 to 10 breaths. Relax a few seconds between poses.

Isometric Wall Squat

- Stand and squeeze a stability ball between your lower back and a wall. Lower into a squat (as if you're sitting into a chair), letting the ball roll up your back until your knees are bent 90 degrees.

- Push down into your heels and hold for 60 seconds. Rest for 30 seconds.

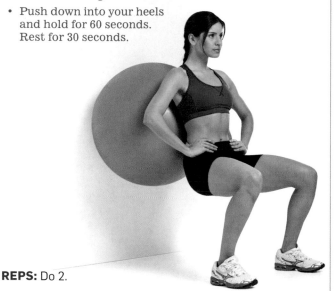

REPS: Do 2.

Fierce Pose

- Stand with your feet hip-width apart. As you raise your arms to the sky, palms facing each another, bend your knees and sit your buttocks back as though you were sitting into a chair.

- Draw your abdomen in to eliminate any curving in the lower back. Put all your weight into your heels and be sure your knees do not extend past your toes.

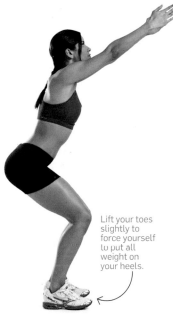

Lift your toes slightly to force yourself to put all weight on your heels.

REPS: Do 2, holding the pose for 5 deep breaths in and out through the nose.

Half Lord of the Fishes

- Sit on the floor with legs outstretched in front of you. Bring the sole of the right foot on the floor outside of the left hip (right knee points to the ceiling). Place your right hand on the floor just behind your right hip. Lift your left arm to the ceiling.

- As you exhale, bend the left arm and place the left elbow to the outside of your right knee. Lengthen your spine with each inhale and twist deeper with each exhale. Press the left elbow into your right leg to help revolve the upper body more. Look to the wall behind you.

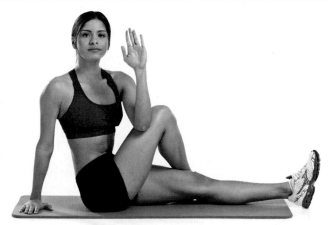

REPS: Do once on each side, holding the pose for 5 to 10 deep breaths.

Cowgirl Workout

It's nice to take the reins and go for a ride. But because our inner thigh muscles can be relatively weak, that giddy-up on top can be woefully short-lived. The following workout targets muscles throughout your groin, inner thigh, hamstrings, and quads, as well as your chest and arms (gotta hold yourself up when you lean in close), so you can saddle up for the long haul.

START HERE:

Perform one exercise after the other without rest for the recommended number of reps. When you've finished the final move, take a 30-second break, then repeat the circuit.

Stability Thigh and Fly

A

- Grab a pair of 8- to 10-pound dumbbells and lie on your back with your arms extended directly above your shoulders, palms facing in, and a stability ball between your legs. Keeping your legs straight, raise them so the bottoms of your feet face the ceiling.

B

- Keeping your elbows slightly bent, slowly lower the dumbbells out to the sides so they're in line with your shoulders. At the same time, slowly lower the ball to within a few inches of the floor.

- Slowly raise the dumbbells and the stability ball back to the starting position. That's 1 rep.

REPS: Do 12 to 15.

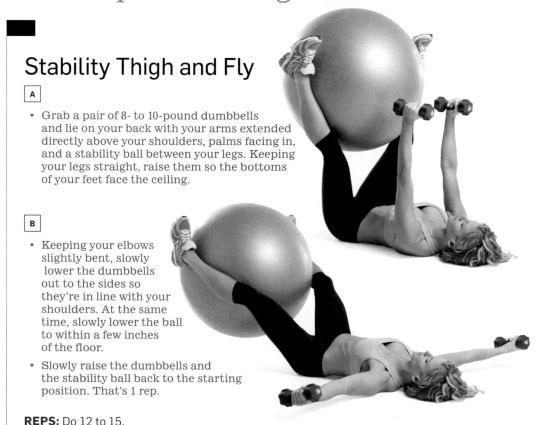

Bridge Pose

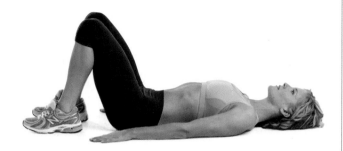

A

- Lying on your back, bend your knees and place the soles of your feet flat on the floor about hip-width apart. Your toes should point straight in front of you. Place your arms straight along your sides.

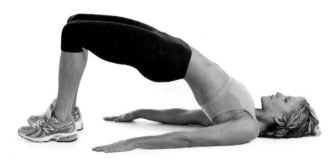

B

- Gently press into your feet as you raise your hips to the sky. Allow the front of your body to slowly expand with each breath. Hold for 5 to 10 breaths. Rest a few seconds.

REPS: Do 3.

Frog

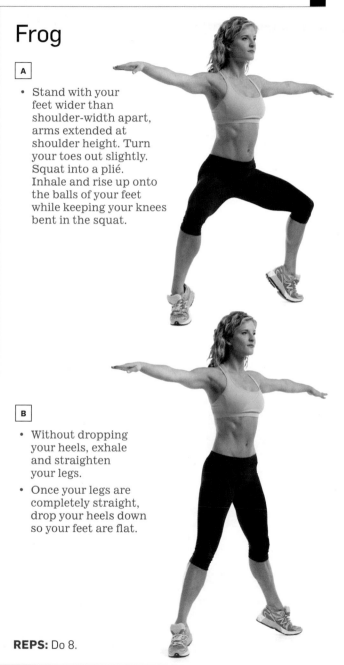

A

- Stand with your feet wider than shoulder-width apart, arms extended at shoulder height. Turn your toes out slightly. Squat into a plié. Inhale and rise up onto the balls of your feet while keeping your knees bent in the squat.

B

- Without dropping your heels, exhale and straighten your legs.
- Once your legs are completely straight, drop your heels down so your feet are flat.

REPS: Do 8.

Cowgirl Workout

Stability Ball Squeeze and Curl

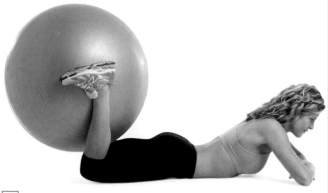

A

- Lie facedown on the floor with your arms crossed in front of you, propping up your upper body. Squeeze a stability ball between your lower legs.

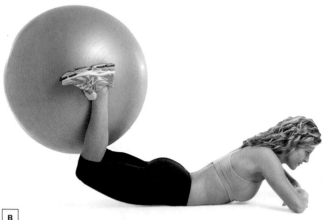

B

- Bend your knees 90 degrees and contract glutes to lift your thighs off the floor.
- Hold for a second. Then return to the starting position.

REPS: Do 12 to 15.

Stability Ball Hip Raise and Leg Curl

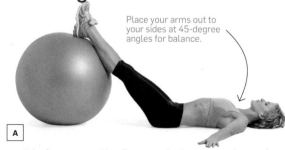

Place your arms out to your sides at 45-degree angles for balance.

A

- Lie faceup on the floor and place your lower legs and calves on a stability ball.

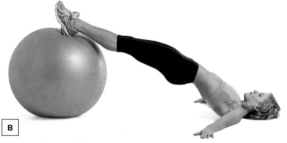

B

- Push your hips up so that your body forms a straight line from your shoulders to your knees.

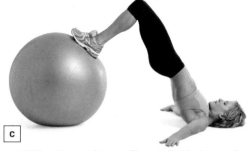

C

- Without pausing, pull your heels toward you and roll the ball toward your butt.
- Pause for 2 seconds, then reverse the motion by rolling the ball back until your body is in a straight line. Lower your hips to the floor.

REPS: Do 12 to 15.

Bear

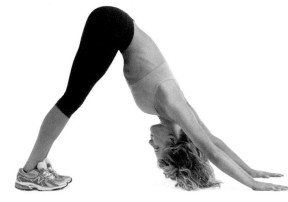

A

- Start in a downward dog, with palms and heels flat on the floor, back straight, body forming an inverted V.
- From downward dog, walk your feet to your hands and separate them about shoulder-width apart.

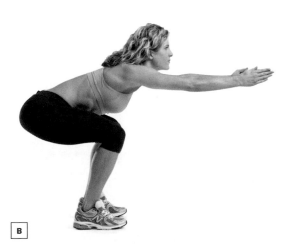

B

- Bend your knees, aligning them with your hips, as you raise your torso to between your thighs, and extend your arms out in front of you.

REPS: Hold for 30 seconds.

Reverse Chaturanga

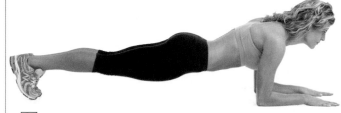

A

- Assume a plank position balancing your body on your toes and forearms with elbows directly beneath your shoulders.

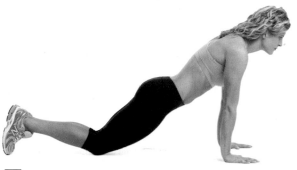

B

- Drop to your knees and straighten your elbows so you are in a modified pushup position.

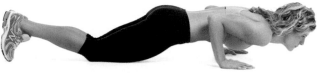

C

- Tighten your biceps and triceps and lower your body, keeping your hips level with your shoulders, and hold yourself just inches above the mat. Return to plank in one slow, fluid motion.

REPS: Do 5.

Chapter 13:
15-Minute Healing Workouts

Who Needs Ibuprofen When You Have Endorphins?
Open This Chapter When Pain Threatens to Derail Your
Workout. It's Exercise for What Ails You.

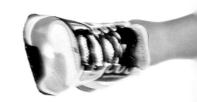

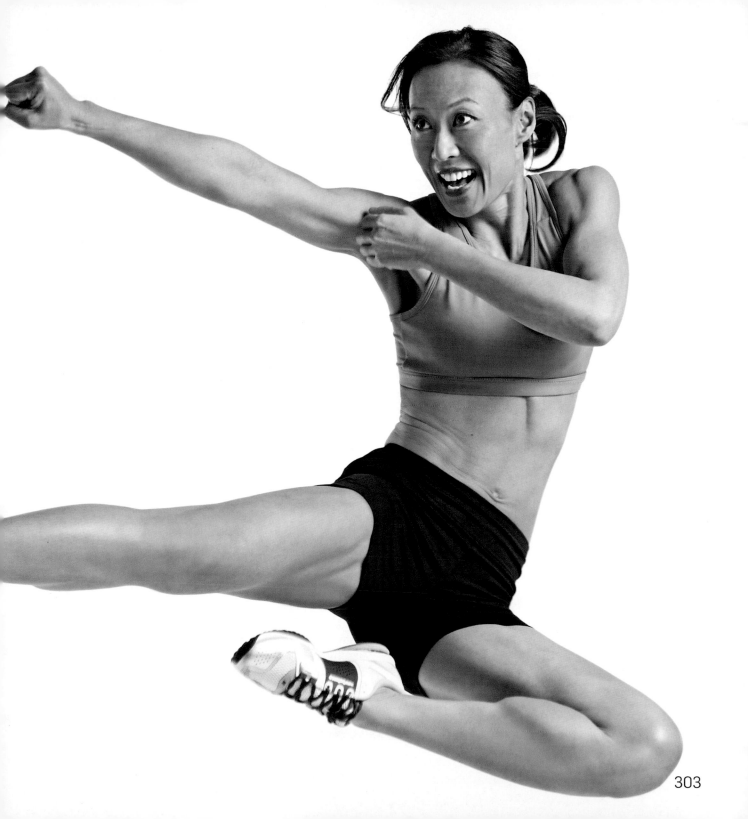

Superfast Workouts That Heal

Exercise has amazing healing properties. Not only does it help fend off heart disease, diabetes, and depression, it can also relieve the everyday woes we battle such as lethargy, headaches, PMS, and back pain. These workouts are to be used in addition to the other 15-minute workouts in this book, or for when you're feeling bloated or achy or otherwise under the weather.

Begin with the basics...

"The best defense is a good offense." Legendary Green Bay Packers coach Vince Lombardi was talking about football, but his famous quote also applies to the human body: being proactive—on the offense—is the best way to defend against pain, illness, and even the passage of time. That's where exercise comes in; studies have shown that people who exercise regularly, eat right, and limit stress have stronger immune systems. So, use the workouts in this chapter not only to treat what ails you, but to prevent health woes from slowing you down.

One 15-minute workout that everyone should try to build into their monthly fitness program is ideal for doing just that: the Age Eraser plyometrics workout starting on page 320. It uses plyometrics—high-energy hops and other jumping exercises—to strengthen your fast-twitch muscles that tend to decline with age. These explosive bounding and leaping movements stress your skeleton, which encourages bone growth, and grow lean muscle mass so you can hang onto that youthful figure as the years go by.

Find It Fast: Your 15-Minute Healing Circuit Plan

CRANK UP YOUR WORKOUT

Use your favorite music to add muscle to these healing workouts. A review of studies in the *American Journal of Public Health* called music "the most accessible and most researched medium of art and healing." The review highlights the physical and psychological benefits of listening to music. Soothing music has been shown to control pain and anxiety in cancer patients as well as improve their immune response. Then there's this research from the University of Maryland: Music that evokes joy can improve blood-vessel dilation by 26 percent. Music also helps us exercise longer by diverting our attention, which lowers our level of perceived effort and makes "hard" seem more like "fun." In one Canadian study, lifters who played music while they pumped iron for 4 weeks completed 56 percent more repetitions than their previous maximum number.

Save-Your-Back Workout

Everyone knows that strong back muscles are good protection against aches and pains. But you also need side (obliques) as well as front (abdominal) muscles and muscular endurance so your back can avoid fatigue during any activity. That means doing isometric contractions such as the ones in the workout below, which help boost endurance in your spine-supporting muscles.

START HERE:

Do two sets of each move, unless otherwise indicated, resting 30 seconds between moves.

Forearm Plank

- Starting at the top of a pushup position, bend your elbows and lower yourself until you can shift your weight from your hands to your forearms.
- Your body should form a straight line. Brace your abs (imagine you're zipping a snug pair of pants) and hold.

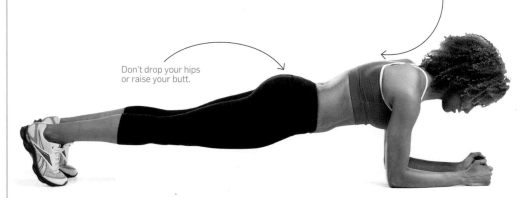

If you were to place a broomstick on your back, it should make contact with your head, upper back, and butt.

Don't drop your hips or raise your butt.

REPS: Do just 1, held for 60 seconds. If you can't make it to 60 seconds, do multiple reps, holding each 5 to 10 seconds, then resting for 5 seconds, and continuing to total 1 minute.

Side Forearm Plank

- Lie on your left side with your legs straight.
- Prop yourself up with your left forearm and stack your feet.

Stack your foot on top of the other.

Your elbow should be directly under your shoulder.

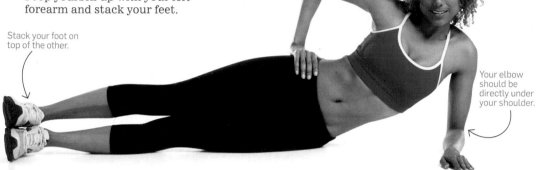

B

- Raise your hips so your body forms a diagonal line. Rest your left hand on your hip. Brace your abs and hold.

Keep your hips and knees off the floor.

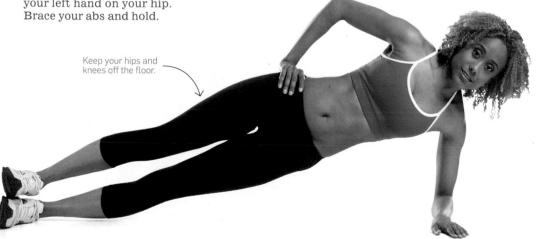

REPS: Hold for 60 seconds. If you can't make it to 60 seconds, hold for 5 to 10 seconds and rest for 5; continue for 1 minute. Repeat the exercise on your left side.

WALK AWAY FROM THE HIP ABDUCTOR

To build true, lasting strength, avoid using machine weights. A study at Georgia State University found that while older adults using exercise machines improved their strength on the machines an average of 34 percent in 2 years, their strength measures for everyday activities actually declined 3.5 percent. Free weights give you more functional strength.

Save-Your-Back Workout

Forearm Plank with Arm Raise

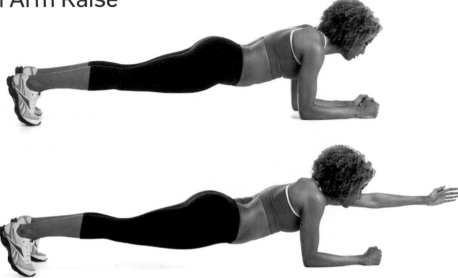

A

- Assume a plank position (toes and forearms on the floor, body lifted). Your body should form a straight line.

B

- Brace your abs and carefully shift your weight to your right forearm. Extend your left arm in front of you for 3 to 10 seconds.

- Slowly bring your arm back in, returning your forearm to the floor. Repeat with the right arm. That's 1 rep.

REPS: Do 6 to 10.

Flat Back Position with Knees Slightly Bent

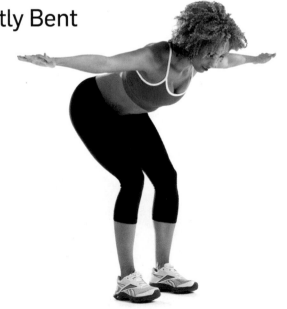

- From standing position, bend your knees slightly and fold at the waist until your back is parallel to the ground. Hold your arms out to the sides to give your back some resistance.

- Imagine that you are holding an orange under your chin and draw your abdomen up toward your spine to create as flat a back as possible. Hold this position for 10 to 20 seconds. Come back to standing with straight legs.

REPS: Do 5.

Superman

- Lying on your stomach, extend your arms in front of you and lift your legs behind you. Keep the insides of your feet touching and turn your palms down.

- Now lift your right arm and your left leg.
- Hold this position for a few seconds.
- Next, lift your left arm and your right leg.

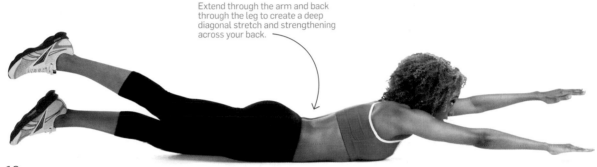

Extend through the arm and back through the leg to create a deep diagonal stretch and strengthening across your back.

REPS: Do 10.

Cobra

- Lying on your stomach with your hands directly underneath your shoulders, inhale and lift your head and torso off the mat into a cobra backbend.

- Keep your elbows in at your waist, your chin into your chest, and your shoulders down. As you exhale, lower back down until your forehead touches your mat.

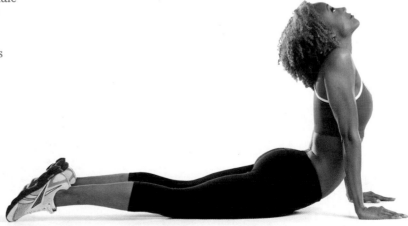

REPS: Hold for 5 breaths.

PMS Workout

A study in the *Journal of the Indian Academy of Applied Psychology* recently found that regular yoga practice can significantly ease symptoms of PMS. To relieve cramps in your pelvis and abdomen, try these moves suggested by Saul David Raye, cofounder of the Center for Sacred Movement in Santa Monica, and Machelle M. Seibel, MD, coauthor of *A Woman's Book of Yoga*.

START HERE:

Go through the moves without rest, holding each for 60 seconds. Repeat the entire sequence three times. For the best results, maintain strong, deep, even breaths that coincide with your movements throughout the workout.

Deep Toe Bend

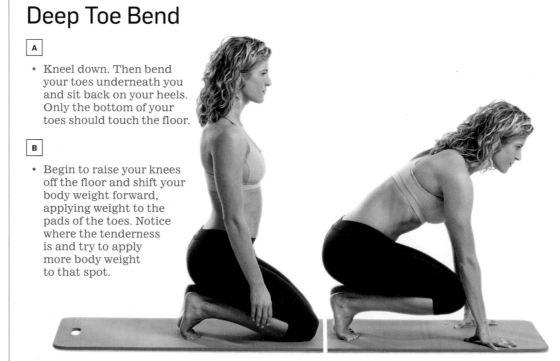

A

- Kneel down. Then bend your toes underneath you and sit back on your heels. Only the bottom of your toes should touch the floor.

B

- Begin to raise your knees off the floor and shift your body weight forward, applying weight to the pads of the toes. Notice where the tenderness is and try to apply more body weight to that spot.

REPS: Hold for 60 seconds.

Garland Pose

Bow Pose

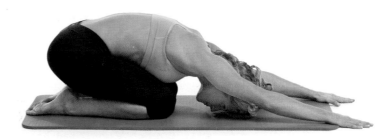

- Begin by lying face down, arms at your sides and chin on the floor. Reach back and grab the inside of your ankles, palms facing in.
- Inhale, pushing your hip bones down into the floor and kicking your legs back and up, which will pull your arms back and lift your chest.
- Keep your head in line with your spine (don't arch your neck) and hug your knees toward each other (try not to let them splay out to the sides).

REPS: Hold for three to six breaths.

Child's Pose

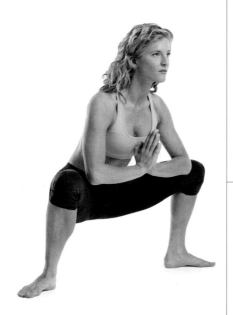

- Kneel on the floor with your big toes touching and knees about hip-width apart. Sit on your heels. Lay your torso between the thighs and bring your forehead to the mat. Extend your arms straight in front of you, palms on the floor. Close your eyes and breathe deeply.

REPS: Hold for 60 seconds.

- Stand with feet slightly wider that hip-width apart. Bring the palms of your hands together in front of your chest as if you're praying. Turn your toes out.
- Deeply bend the knees, squatting down between your legs. Keeping your palms together, gently press your elbows to the insides of your thighs with your spine long and chest open.

REPS: Hold for 60 seconds.

5-Minute Headache Workout

Exercise eases stress and boosts feel-good endorphins, which can help prevent headaches. To really tame the tension that leads to throbbing pain, however, you need focused stretching. This routine, which includes targeted moves recommended by Jyotsna Sahni, MD, a sleep specialist in private practice and former staff physician at the Canyon Ranch Resort and Spa in Tucson, will relax those key tension-holders.

START HERE:

You can do this routine every day, even two or three times a day (it's only 5 minutes long!) or as needed, when times are particularly tense.

Half Roll

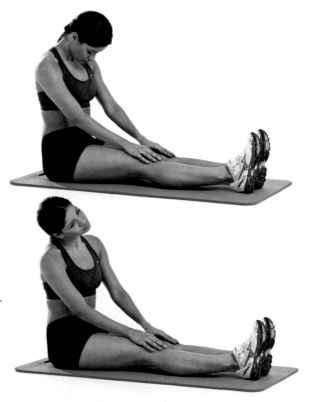

 A

- Sit up tall and straight, eyes forward, chin level to the floor. Keeping your shoulders down and back straight, gently tilt your head forward as far as comfortably possible, trying to bring your chin to your chest.

 B

- Pause here for a few seconds. Then rotate your head toward the right shoulder until your right ear is as near as possible to your shoulder. Hold for 10 seconds.

- Rotate back down. Then rotate your head to the left. That's 1 rep.

REPS: Do 2

Puppy Pose

- Start on your hands and knees with a flat back. Then slide your hands forward and lower your forehead to the floor while keeping your hips elevated.

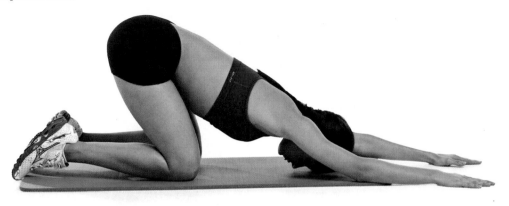

REPS: Hold for 5 to 10 long, deep breaths, feeling tension release from your shoulders and upper back.

Reclining Bound Angle Pose

- Lie on your back with your arms by your side, palms facing up. Bend your knees and place the soles of your feet together, allowing your knees to fall out to either side.

- Inhale as you bring your arms out to the sides and then overhead.

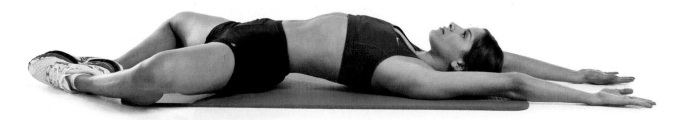

REPS: Hold for 5 to 10 long, deep breaths, relaxing your whole body into the floor with each exhale.

5-Minute Headache Workout

Rabbit Pose

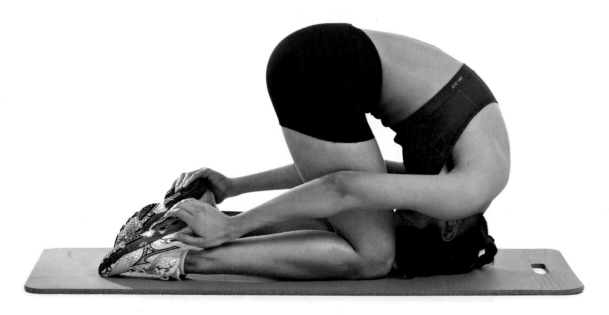

- Kneel on the floor with big toes touching and knees about hip-width apart. Sit on your heels. Lay your torso between your thighs and bring your forehead to the mat. Extend your arms behind you and grab the outside of your ankles.
- Roll from your forehead to the crown of your head. Extend your tailbone up and away from your neck. Shift your body weight forward, feeling the stretch from the back of your neck to your tailbone.

REPS: Hold for 5 to 10 breaths, then slowly sit back on your heels and rest.

Seated Forward Bend

INSTANT UPGRADE

PRESS AWAY PAIN

When you don't have time for the 5-minute headache workout, try triggering a pressure point on your hand between your thumb and index finger for relief. Hold your hand with your palm down, and pinch the webbing with the thumb and forefinger of your opposite hand. Continue to squeeze this point until it is tender, then massage it round and round with your thumb for 15 seconds. Then repeat the process on the opposite hand.

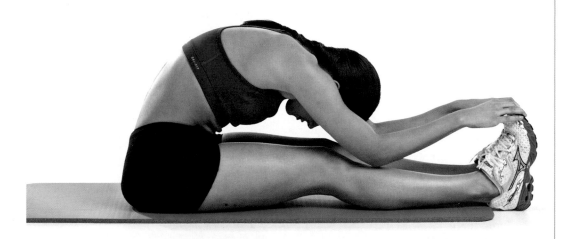

- Sit on the floor with your back straight, arms by your sides, and legs together and extended in front of you. Extend your arms straight overhead, shoulder-width apart.
- Keeping your back straight, reach your chest and arms forward, lowering them about 45 degrees. Grasp your big toes with your thumbs and first two fingers. Extend your spine, bend your elbows and lower your torso closer to your legs. Relax your head toward your knees.

REPS: Hold for 5 to 10 breaths. Slowly lift your torso, reaching your arms overhead, then release them back to your sides.

Post-Partum Workout

It's pretty obvious what body parts get stretched during those nine months of pregnancy: all those deep, abdominal muscles, as well as those in your back and the ever important pelvic floor. The first step in getting your pre-baby body back is targeting, toning, and tightening all those key core muscle groups.

START HERE:

Perform the moves one after another with no rest between them. When you've completed the final move, pause for 30 seconds, then repeat the circuit two more times.

Stability Ball Circles

A

- Place your forearms on a stability ball and extend your legs behind you, hip-width apart. Brace your abs and raise yourself into a plank position.

B

- Using your forearms, roll the ball out to the left, in front of you, and back to the right (like a stirring motion) and then pull it back into the starting position. That's 1 rep.

REPS: Do 8 to 12, then switch directions and repeat.

Long-Arm Crunch

- Lie faceup on a stability ball with your legs bent and feet flat on the floor. Extend your arms overhead with your hands stacked and palms facing up.

B

- Simultaneously lift your arms, head, shoulders, and upper back off the ball. Pause, then return to the starting position.

REPS: Do 12 to 15.

Post-Partum Workout

Stability Ball W

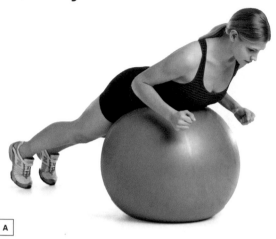

A

- Lie on a stability ball with your back flat and your chest off the ball. Bend your arms and squeeze your elbows in toward your ribs.

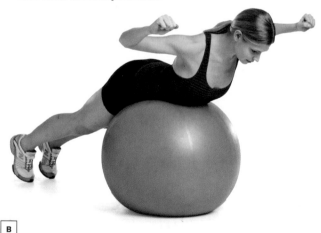

B

- Rotate your arms toward the ceiling, squeezing your shoulder blades together. Return to the starting position.

REPS: Do 12 to 15.

Reverse Curl

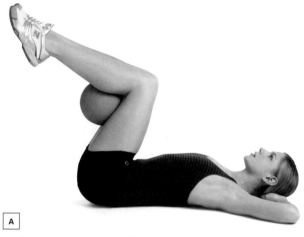

A

- Lie on your back with your legs hooked over a medicine ball, hands behind your head.

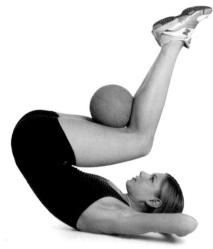

B

- Grasping the ball with your legs, curl your hips up toward your chest as far as possible. Return to the starting position and repeat.

REPS: Do 12 to 15.

Opposite Arm and Leg

A

- Drape yourself over a stability ball so your navel is on the apex. Extend your arms and legs, balancing yourself with your fingertips and toes.

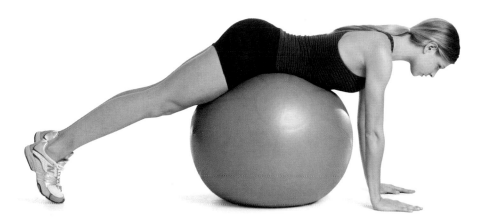

INSIDER TRAINING

Pregnancy and childbirth can weaken your pelvic floor muscles, which can lead to leakage. Get back in shape on the inside with Kegels. Instructions for these pelvic pullups are found on page 291.

B

- Simultaneously lift your left arm and right leg so they form a straight line. Return to the starting position, then repeat using the opposite arm and leg. That's 1 rep.

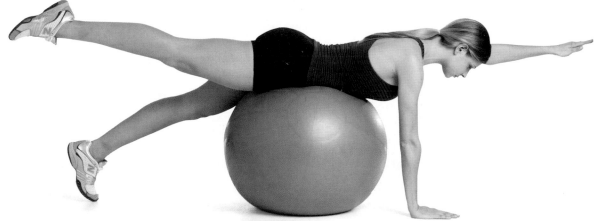

REPS: Do 12 to 15.

Age Eraser Workout

If you want to stop the march of time, strengthen your fast-twitch muscles (the ones that give you speed) and your bones (bone density decreases up to 2 percent a year after age 30). The best workouts to combat aging make use of plyometrics—high energy jumping, hopping, and other explosive exercises such as those shown here.

START HERE: ■

Do all of the moves without resting in between, and then take a 60-second break. Repeat for a total of three circuits.

Skaters

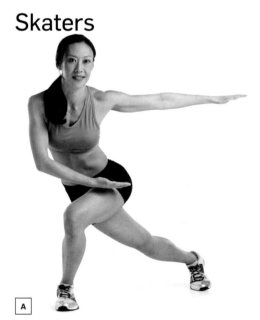

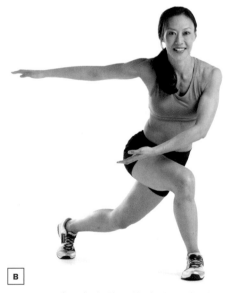

A

- Cross your right leg behind your left leg as you bend your left knee into a half-squat position. Extend your left arm out to the side, and swing your right arm across your hips.

REPS: Do 10.

B

- Hop a few feet directly to the right, switching the position of your legs and arms. That's 1 rep.
- Continue hopping from side to side without pausing or resetting your feet.

Seal Jumping Jacks

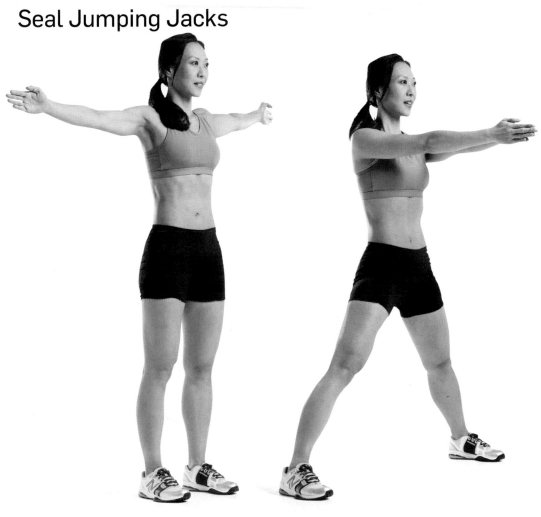

FOOT LOOSE

Flexibility prevents workout injuries, and it often feels really good. Gain greater range of motion with this pre-workout foot massage: Step on a tennis ball or lacrosse ball and roll it around each foot for 45 to 60 seconds. Doing so loosens up the tissue in and around your muscles. And, like a domino effect, it helps trigger the same response up your back side, as well as your calves, hamstrings, and glutes.

A

- Start with your feet about hip-width apart, arms straight out to the sides at shoulder height.

B

- Clap your hands in front of your chest and jump just high enough to spread your feet wide.
- Without pausing, quickly return to the starting position. That's 1 rep.

REPS: Do 20 as quickly as you can with control.

Age Eraser Workout

Clock Walk with Hands

A

- Assume a plank position as if you were ready to do a pushup. Your hands should be direcly under your shoulders.

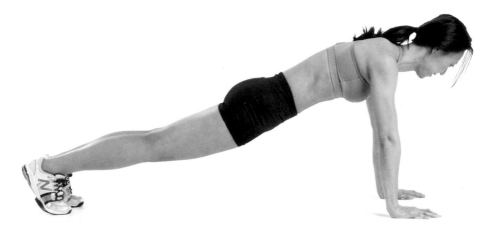

B

- Walk your right hand out wide to the side, then follow with your left hand to return to a shoulder-width stance.
- Continue this pattern to complete one full clockwise rotation leading with your right arm.
- Then do one full counterclockwise rotation leading with your left arm. That's 1 rep.

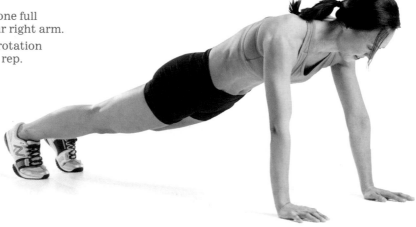

REPS: Do 1.

Low-Step Lateral Shuffle

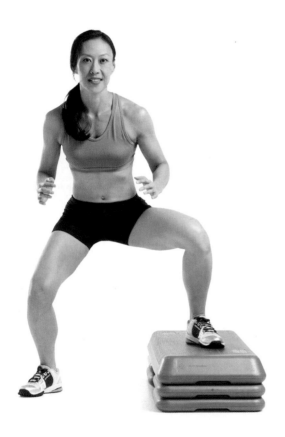

A

- Stand with your left foot on a low box (or step) and your right foot on the floor about 2 feet to the right of the box. Bend your knees slightly, keep your chest up, and bend your arms 90 degrees.

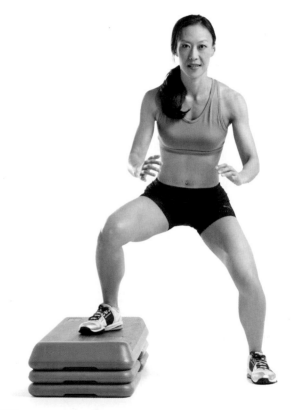

B

- Push off your left foot and jump to your left, landing with your right foot on the box and your left foot on the floor, knees bent.
- Push off your right foot to jump back to the starting position. That's 1 rep.

REPS: Do 10.

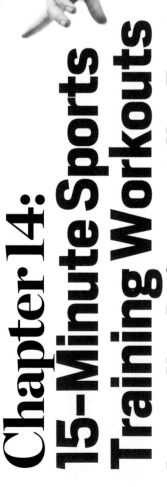

Chapter 14: 15-Minute Sports Training Workouts

Improve Your Performance in Your Favorite Sport (And Avoid Season-Killing Injuries) with Exercises That Mimic How You Move on Your Playing Field.

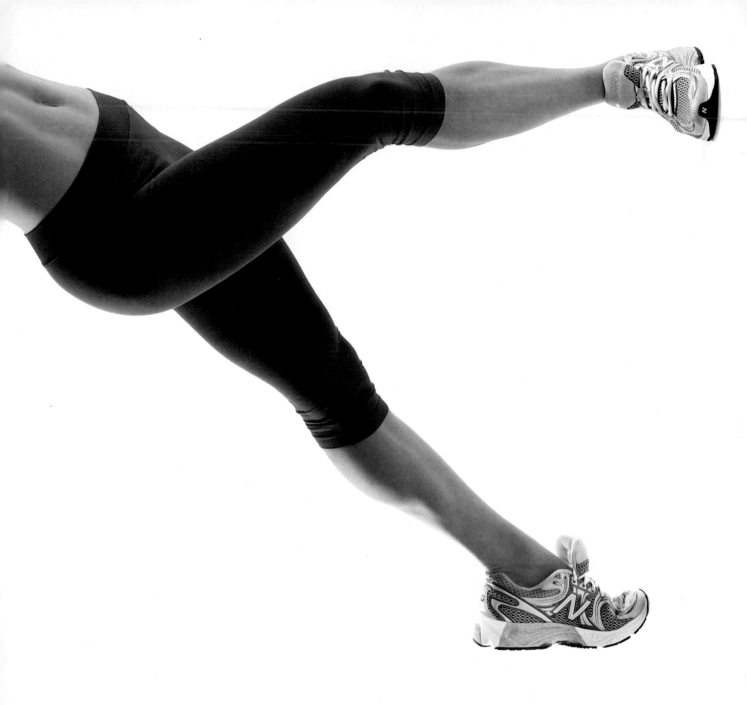

Superfast Sports Training Workouts

Any of the workouts in this book will give you strength, speed, and stamina on the ski slopes, tennis courts, single-track mountain bike trails, or wherever your favorite pastimes take you. But to help you reach the very top of your game, we've designed routines that specifically target the muscles you use for different sports—and re-create the way you need to use them. For the best results, start these workouts at least a month or two before you dive into your sport.

Find It Quick: Your Superfast Sports Training Circuits

CURB CRAMPS

Explosive training exercises for sports can easily trigger charley horses. The remedy? Pickle juice eases muscle spasms, according to a study in *Medicine & Science in Sports & Exercise*. But who carries a jar of gherkins to the playing field? Here are some other ways to keep spasms from cramping your style:

Drink Up: Dehydration messes with your electrolyte balance, causing cramps. Down 20 ounces of water 3 hours before working out .

Stretch: When you feel a charley horse coming on, stop and gently stretch the sore spot for 20 seconds until the pain goes away. Stretching counters the tightening of the muscle.

Add tension: Flexing a cramping muscle may make it release. Massage the muscle vigorously, as if you're kneeding dough. This combines the previous two methods by stretching and compressing the muscle, helping to release the cramp.

Build your athleticism...

Great athletes—especially those who play tennis, basketball, lacrosse, and volleyball—are defined by their ability to change speed and direction quickly. No matter what your sport, you can benefit from adding an old-school agility drill to the end of any workout. Try the T-Drill. **Set it up:** Form a large T with four cones. Place three in a line 8 feet apart (the top of the T) and a fourth 16 feet away from the middle cone (the bottom of the T.

How to do it: Sprint from that bottom T cone to the middle cone. Then immediately shuffle left to the side cone. (Shuffle your feet with short, quick strides, and don't cross them.) Then shuffle right, passing the middle cone to the right cone. Bend down and touch each cone as you pass. Shuffle-step as quickly as possible to the middle cone, and then run backward to the starting cone. Repeat twice more, rest, then repeat the circuit in the other direction.

Golf Workout

Here's one game that looks deceptively easy. But even a leisurely round of golf requires you to twist and turn and generate force with your hips and obliques muscles that go largely unused in daily life. The following moves target those crucial core muscles as well as hips, hamstrings, and shoulders to put power in every drive and stroke.

START HERE:

Do the routine as a circuit, performing the prescribed number of each move and then immediately moving to the next move. Rest a minute, then repeat the circuit twice more.

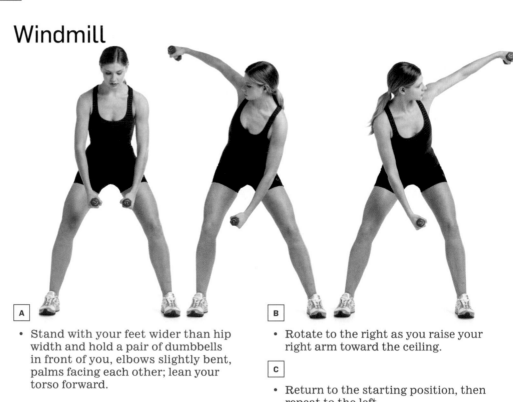

Windmill

A

- Stand with your feet wider than hip width and hold a pair of dumbbells in front of you, elbows slightly bent, palms facing each other; lean your torso forward.

REPS: Do 20, alternating sides.

B

- Rotate to the right as you raise your right arm toward the ceiling.

C

- Return to the starting position, then repeat to the left.

Leaning Hamstring Curl

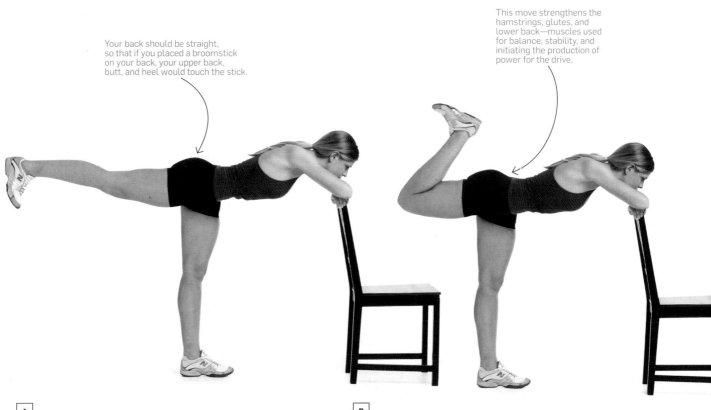

Your back should be straight, so that if you placed a broomstick on your back, your upper back, butt, and heel would touch the stick.

This move strengthens the hamstrings, glutes, and lower back—muscles used for balance, stability, and initiating the production of power for the drive.

A

- Place your forearms on the back of a chair, elbows out, and rest your head on your arms.

REPS: Do 10 to 15, then switch sides and repeat.

B

- Raise your right leg behind you to hip height, left knee slightly bent.

- Slowly bend your right knee, bringing your heel toward your butt. Slowly return to start. That's 1 rep.

Golf Workout

Lawn Mower

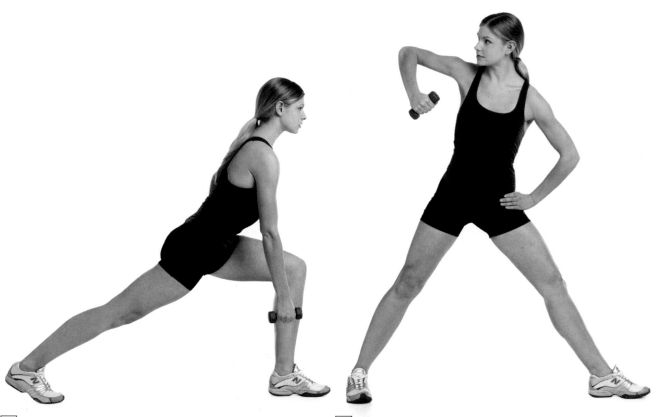

A

- Grab an 8- to 10-pound dumbbell in your right hand and let it hang at your side, palm facing inward. Place your left hand on your left hip.
- Lunge forward with your left leg until your left knee is bent 90 degrees

B

- Straighten your left leg and bend your right elbow, pulling the weight up toward your ribs as you rotate your torso to the right.
- Lower the weight and return to lunge position. That's 1 rep.

REPS: Do 12, then repeat the move with the dumbbell in your left hand.

Low Cross Chop

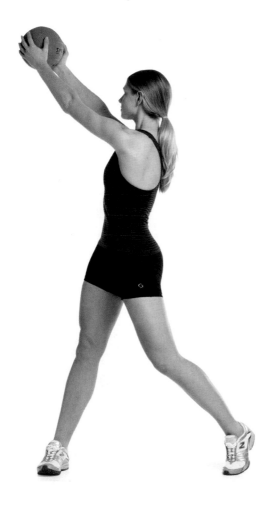

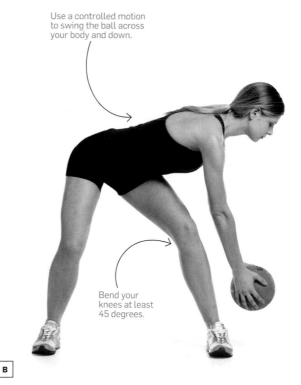

Use a controlled motion to swing the ball across your body and down.

Bend your knees at least 45 degrees.

A

- Grab a 5- to 10-pound medicine ball and stand with your feet shoulder-width apart and your knees slightly bent. Raise the ball above your right shoulder.

B

- Then, bend your knees at least 45 degrees and lower the ball to the outside of your left ankle.
- Repeat from left shoulder to right ankle. That's 1 rep.

REPS: Do 6.

Tennis Workout

Talk about a game that keeps you on your toes. To play sharp, you not only need lightning-fast reflexes, but also the ability to dash from side to side, and slam the ball over the net from each and every direction. That means power, flexibility, and agility through your legs, hips, shoulders, and core. The following moves hit the spot.

START HERE:
Do the routine as a circuit, performing the prescribed number of each move and then immediately moving to the next. Rest a minute, then repeat the circuit again. Go through the entire routine three times.

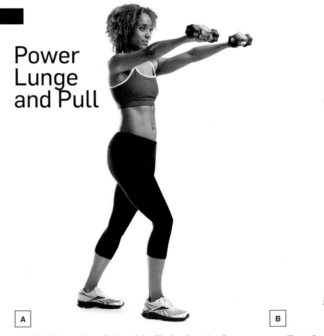

Power Lunge and Pull

A
- Hold a pair of dumbbells in front of you at shoulder height, arms straight, palms facing down. Stand with your right foot in front of your left. This is the starting position.

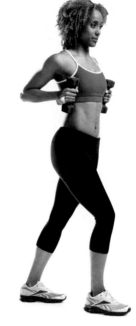

B
- Bend your knees and lean forward slightly. Simultaneously pull the weights to the sides of your torso and rotate your palms toward your body.
- Slowly return to the starting position. That's 1 rep.

REPS: Do 10 to 12. Repeat with your left leg forward.

Calf Raise

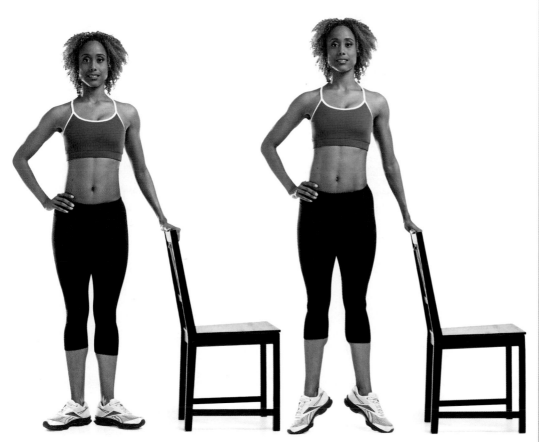

A

- Stand next to a chair with your heels together and toes pointed out to create a wide V shape. Place your left hand on the chair, right hand on your hip.

REPS: Do 10 to 15.

B

- Slowly rise onto the balls of your feet. Hold for 2 seconds, then slowly return to start. That's 1 rep.

Tennis Workout

Rotation Swing

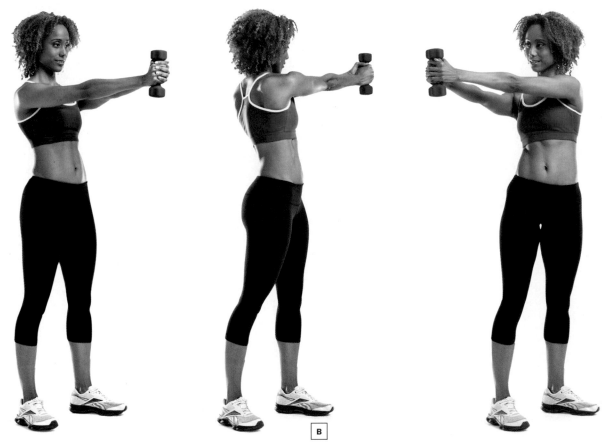

A

B

- Grab a 5- to 10-pound dumbbell with both hands and stand with your feet shoulder-width apart. Extend the dumbbell straight out in front of you at shoulder height.

- Keeping your hips square and your arms straight, rotate your torso and arms to the left as far as you can.

- Then, swing the dumbbell as far to the right as possible.

- Accelerate the weight across the front of your body, then slow it down once it gets to your side. From the right side, slowly return your arms to the center starting position. That's 1 rep. Complete all reps, then repeat, this time swinging first to the left.

REPS: Do 10. Switch sides and repeat.

Lateral Leap with Reach

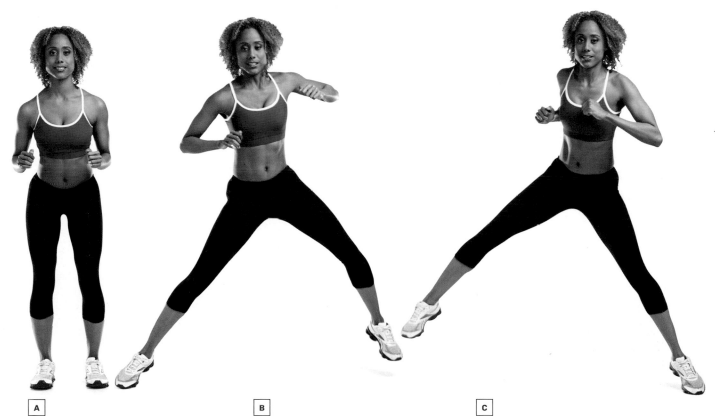

A

- Stand with your feet together, knees slightly bent, with your elbows bent 90 degrees and your hands in front of you.

B

- Jump to the left, landing softly on your left foot. Don't let your right foot touch the floor.
- Immediately push off your left foot to jump to the right, landing on your right foot. That's 1 rep. Do 4 more.

C

- Pause with both feet on the floor. Now jump right. When your right foot touches the ground, squat and touch your right toes with your left hand.
- Immediately push off to jump left, and squat to touch your left foot with your right hand. That's 1 rep. Do 4 more.

REPS: Do 10 total, the last 5 with hand-to-toes touches.

Ski and Snowboard Workout

Anyone who's experienced rubbery legs after a full day on the slopes knows that snow sports demand lower-body power. Those pistonlike legs act as power generators and shock absorbers. The following workout will have you hopping and holding positions to keep your legs steady and strong through the day's very last run.

START HERE: ■

Do the routine as a circuit, performing the prescribed number of each move and then immediately moving to the next. Rest a minute, then repeat the circuit again. Go through the entire routine three times.

Ski Hop

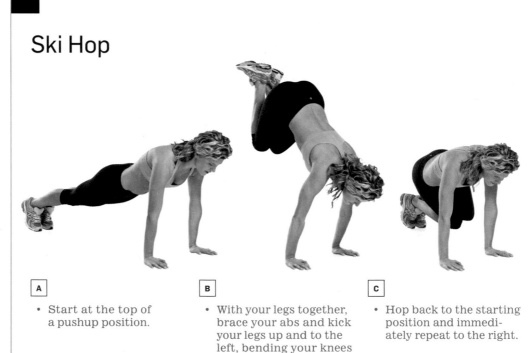

A
- Start at the top of a pushup position.

B
- With your legs together, brace your abs and kick your legs up and to the left, bending your knees toward your butt.
- Your feet should land just outside of your left shoulder.

C
- Hop back to the starting position and immediately repeat to the right.

REPS: Do as many as you can in 1 minute.

Bosu Jumps

TIP: *To make it harder, try jumping 360 degrees.*

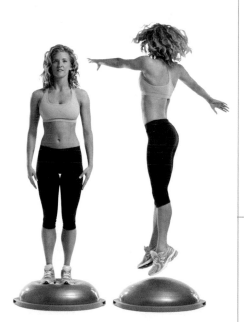

A

- Warm up with some small two-footed bounces on a Bosu for a minute, making sure you keep your hips and knees aligned and using your core to maintain control.

B

- Then jump up higher and turn 180 degrees.

REPS: Do 10 180s, then repeat in the opposite direction.

Lateral Medicine-Ball Hops

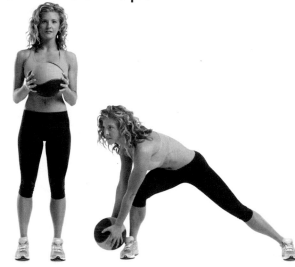

A

- Stand holding a medicine ball in front of your chest.

B

- Bound laterally to your right, bringing the ball down to the outside of your right foot. Next, straighten your body and repeat to the left side. That's 1 rep.

REPS: Do 10 to 12.

Plié Plyometric Jump

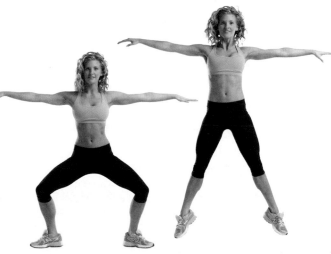

A

- Stand with your feet wider than shoulder-width apart, knees and toes turned out.

B

- Jump in the air, keeping your legs wide. Land with legs wide and knees soft to absorb the shock.

REPS: Do 20.

Race-Running Workout

Running takes way more than your legs. You need strong abs, obliques, and back muscles to keep you from collapsing forward as you start to fatigue. Even your shoulders are star players, because a strong arm swing is key to a powerful stride. This workout bolsters all those muscles and adds explosive power moves for speed.

START HERE: ■

Do the routine as a circuit, performing the prescribed number of each move and then immediately moving to the next. Rest a minute, then repeat the circuit again. Go through the entire routine three times.

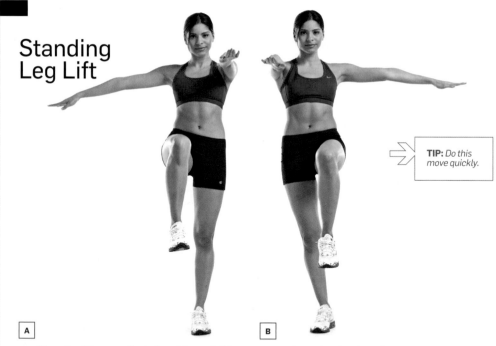

Standing Leg Lift

TIP: *Do this move quickly.*

A
- Stand with your feet shoulder-width apart, arms at your sides. Lift your right knee as high as you can and swing your left arm forward until it's parallel to the floor.

B
- Return to start and repeat with your left knee and right arm.

REPS: Do as many as possible in 1 minute while alternating sides.

Jump Squat

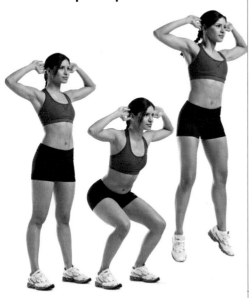

 A

- Stand with your feet shoulder-width apart, arms at your sides or behind your head. Sit back into a regular squat until your thighs are about parallel to the floor.

 B

- Jump up explosively. Land with your knees soft to absorb the impact.

REPS: Do 10 to 15.

Hand Tap

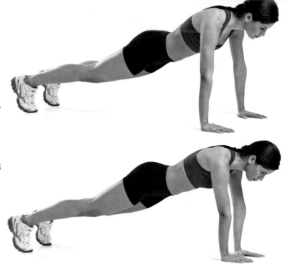

A

- Start at the top of a pushup position, hands wider than shoulder-width apart.

B

- Keeping your abs braced and your arms straight, lift your left hand, put it down next to your right hand, then return to the starting position.
- Repeat with the right hand and return to the starting position.

REPS: Do as many as possible in 60 seconds.

Hip Hike

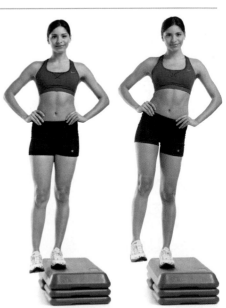

 A

- Stand sideways on a step or box with your left foot planted on the step and your right foot hanging off the edge in the air. Place your hands on your hips.

 B

- Keeping your shoulders level, hips pointed forward, and both legs straight, use your glutes to raise your right hip upward.
- Then lower the leg. Return to the starting position. That's 1 rep.

REPS: Do 12 to 15, then switch sides and repeat.

Triathlon Workout

True to its design, the triathlon—swimming, biking, and running—puts every muscle to the test. This routine does it all with explosive moves to develop power for your run; core stabilizing moves to hold yourself strong on the bike; and full body strength and stretching moves to keep you slicing long and strong through the water.

START HERE:

Do the routine as a circuit, performing the prescribed number of each move and then immediately moving to the next. Rest a minute, then repeat the circuit again. Go through the entire routine three times.

Hindu Pushup

A

- Start in a pushup position, lift your hips, and move into the downward-facing dog pose, keeping your legs straight and pressing your heels into the floor.

B

- From that position, drop your hips toward the floor as you simultaneously sweep your torso forward and up, raising your chest and shifting your weight forward into upward-facing dog.

- Reverse the movement to return to the starting position. That's 1 rep.

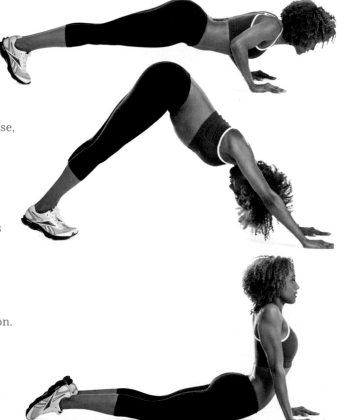

REPS: Do 10.

Switch Lunges

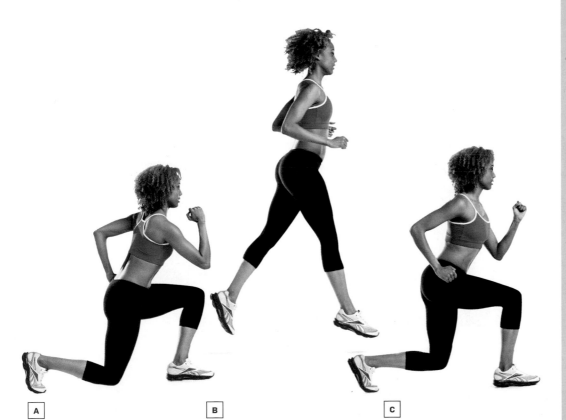

A

- Lunge forward with your left thigh parallel to the floor.

B

- Swinging your arms for balance and momentum, jump up and switch leg positions.

C

- Land in a lunge with your right foot forward.
- Repeat to return to the left-leg forward position. That's 1 rep.

REPS: Do 12 to 15.

THE 15-MINUTE TRIATHLON

Give yourself a mini-triathlon in the gym and get a swimmer's cut shoulders, a cyclist's toned legs, and a runner's lean physique, says Karl Scott, a trainer at The Sports Club/LA in New York City.

HOW TO DO IT: Pedal a bike at a moderate pace—an effort level of 5 or 6 (you're working hard but can still carry on a conversation)—for 5 minutes. Next, run either outside or on a treadmill for 5 minutes, again at an effort level of 5 or 6. Last, head to a rowing machine, which approximates the upper-body demands of swimming, and put in 5 minutes at the same effort level.

Triathlon Workout

INSTANT UPGRADE

SWIM YOURSELF SLIM

If you have time to get to a pool, there's nothing like a swimming workout for slimming down. The body-shaping benefits of swimming come from muscle recruitment and calorie burn. An easy swim burns around 500 calories an hour, while a vigorous effort can torch about 700. Because water is nearly 800 times more dense than air, each kick of the legs and pull of the arms is like a resistance workout for your core, hips, arms, legs, shoulders, and glutes. So in additional to blasting calories as you swim, you build lean muscle, which ignites your metabolism so that you burn more calories once you've showed and dried off.

Deep Chop

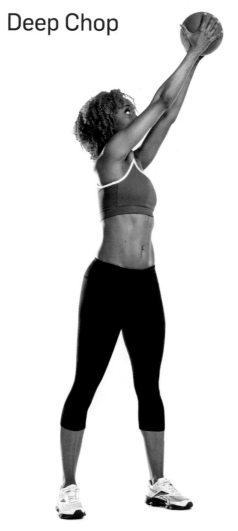

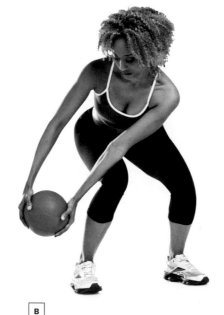

A

- Grab a 5- to 10-pound medicine ball and stand with your feet shoulder-width apart and your knees slightly bent. Raise the ball above your left shoulder.

REPS: Do 10 to 12.

B

- Raise the ball one last time, then bend your knees at least 45 degrees and lower the ball to the outside of your right ankle. Repeat to the other side. That's 1 rep.

Hip Hinge and Rotate

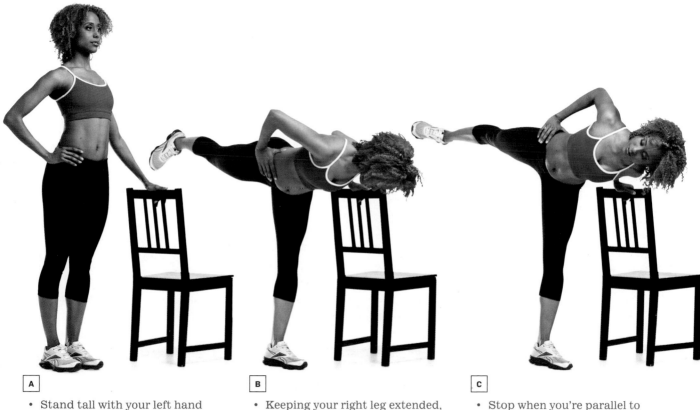

A

- Stand tall with your left hand resting on a chair back or other support, your right hand on your hip.

B

- Keeping your right leg extended, slowly hinge forward from the hips, tipping your torso forward toward the ground while extending your right leg straight behind you, foot flexed, until your body forms a straight line from your head to your heel.

C

- Stop when you're parallel to the floor. Then rotate your body to the right before returning to the starting position.

REPS: Do 10, then switch sides.

Cycling Workout

Your legs might seem like the only thing moving when you ride, but cycling is a full-body event. With each revolution, your upper body acts as a platform for your legs to push off of. Your arms and shoulders help you leverage power going uphill and your hips keep you stable in the saddle. This routine hits the whole cast of characters.

START HERE:

Do the routine as a circuit, performing the prescribed number of each move and then immediately going to the next. Rest a minute, then repeat the circuit twice more for a total of three circuits.

Spider

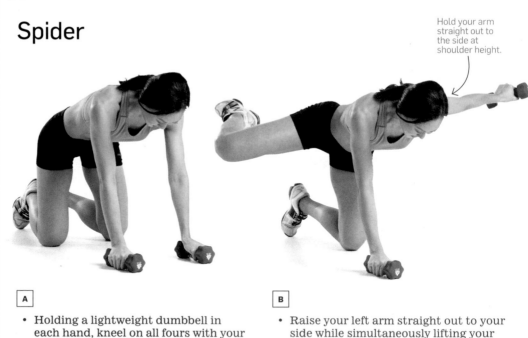

Hold your arm straight out to the side at shoulder height.

A

- Holding a lightweight dumbbell in each hand, kneel on all fours with your back straight, hands directly beneath shoulders (weights should run parallel with body) and knees directly beneath hips.

REPS: Do 10 to 12.

B

- Raise your left arm straight out to your side while simultaneously lifting your bent right leg out to the right. Return to the starting position. Repeat to opposite side. That's 1 rep.

Scoop Squat

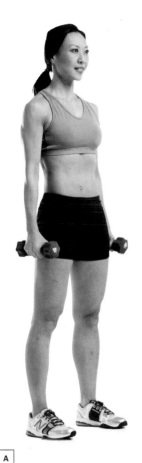

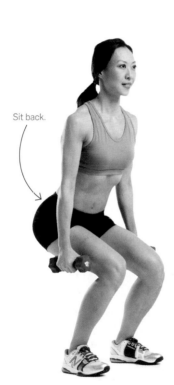

Sit back.

Keep your wrists in a neutral grip throughout the move.

A

- Holding 10- to 20-pound dumbbells at your sides, palms facing your thighs, stand with your feet hip- to shoulder-width apart.

REPS: Do 12 to 15.

B

- In one smooth motion, bend your knees and hips and drop your butt back as if sitting in a chair.
- Immediately push back to start, bending your elbows and curling the weights to your shoulders as you do.

C

- As you reach the standing position, immediately press the weights overhead.
- Lower the weights back to your sides and repeat.

INSTANT UPGRADE

GET YOUR HEAD IN THE GAME

Brain training is an essential part of any sports warmup. "Preparing your central nervous system for activity is just as important as preparing your muscles," says Vern Gambetta, former director of conditioning for the Chicago White Sox. That's because your central nervous system tells your muscles when to contract. Try standing on one leg while you squat down and touch the floor in front of it with your opposite hand. Do 2 sets of 10 to 12 repetitions with each leg.

Cycling Workout

Balance Dip Extend

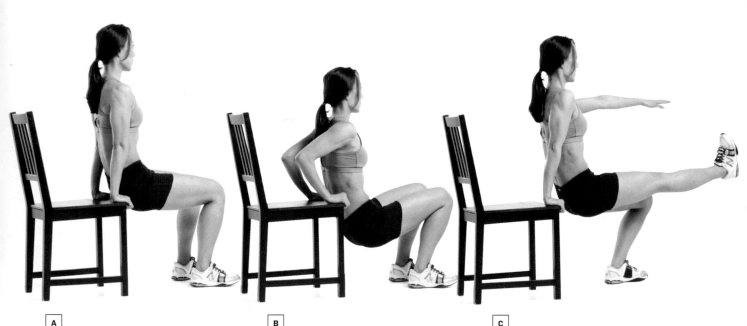

A

- Sit on the edge of a chair, hands grasping the seat on either side of your hips. Keep your knees bent, feet flat on the floor. Scoot your butt off the chair seat.

B

- Bend your elbows and lower your hips toward floor until your upper arms are parallel to the floor.

C

- Straighten your arms, then reach your left arm straight out in front of your body at shoulder height, palm facing down, while simultaneously extending your right leg with the foot flexed.

- Pause. Then bring the arm and leg back to the starting position. Repeat the entire sequence with the other arm and leg. That's 1 rep.

REPS: Do 10 to 12.

Single-Leg Step Down

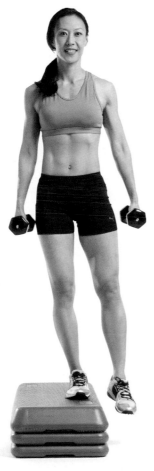

A

9

Number of extra pounds of
fat lost over 10 weeks when
dieters strength trained,
compared with dieters who
did no exercise, according to
the *European Journal of
Applied Physiology.*

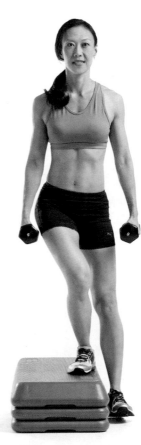

B

- Holding dumbbells, stand on an 18-inch high step
  with only the right foot on top of the step, allowing
  the left leg to hang in the air.

- Pull your navel toward your spine and, keeping
  your chest lifted, slowly step down with the left foot
  and gently tap the left heel on the floor.

- Keeping the right heel firmly planted on the step,
  push up to the starting position. Complete all reps,
  then switch legs.

REPS: Do 10 to 15 with each leg.

Chapter 15: 15-Minute Stretch and Strengthen Workouts

This Series of Flexibilty Exercises Activates Muscle Fibers You Didn't Know You Even Had. It'll Make Your Entire Body Feel Younger, Calmer, and Sexier.

348

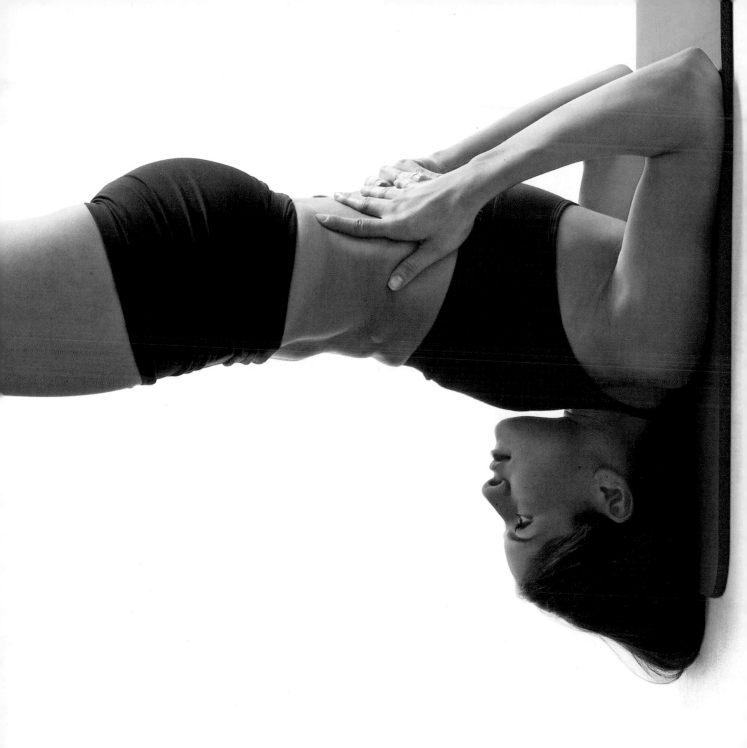

Superfast Stretch and Strengthen Workouts

In the past decade, women have been flocking to yoga and Pilates classes. Smart women. These increasingly popular forms of exercise take a full-body holistic approach to fitness, and they make you feel fabulous afterward. The great news is that yoga and Pilates are strong medicine, and you can reap their benefits even if you don't have the time or the inclination to sign up for a regular class. The workouts here will improve your posture, eliminate muscle aches and soreness, and leave you with a lean, lithe body all in just 15 minutes.

Begin with the basics...

Most of the moves you'll find in this chapter are considered dynamic stretches, meaning they stretch your muscles in various positions while your body is in motion. Dynamic stretches wake up your central nervous system and boost blood flow to your tissues. That makes them ideal warmup exercises for any physical activity. But you can do them anytime to stay strong, limber, and injury-free.

Find It Quick: Your 15-Minute Stretch and Strengthen Circuit Plan

p.352
Yoga Metabolism Workout
Down Dog Split
Half Crow Lift
Knee to Forehead
Warrior III

p.354
Fat-Burning Flow Workout
Plank
Down Dog
Low Lunge
High Lunge with a Twist
Rotated Triangle

p.358
Ballet Workout
Standing Turnout
Scissor Curl
Parallel Extension
Semi Foldover
Curl
High V
Wide Second

p.362
Pilates Workout
Mermaid with Ball
Rollover
Footwork on Ball
Swan on Ball
Back Arm Rolling
Roll Back and Up
Mermaid with Twist
Coordination with Ball

p.366
Perfect-Posture Workout
Foam Roller Snow Angel
Port de Bras
Pilates X
Shrug
Side Angle Pose

p.370
Foam Roller Workout
Calves
Hamstrings
Quads
Back
Outer Hip and Thigh
Shoulder and Side
Butt (Piriformis)

STRETCH INTO A HOT BOD

After a strength-training workout, you should:

A) take a shower
B) stretch
C) down a protein drink

All three are great post-exercise ideas but only one is likely to triple your muscle strength. That would be stretching. In a study reported in the *Journal of Strength and Conditioning Research*, volunteers followed a strength-training regimen three times a week. Half of the group added two stretching sessions to the back end of their workout. After 8 weeks, the group that ended workouts with stretch routines almost tripled their muscle strength. Why? Because stretching, like lifting weights, causes tiny tears in your muscle; as your body repairs them, the tissue becomes stronger, explains study coauthor Jason Winchester, Ph.D., of George Mason University. That's a good reason to tag one of the stretch routines in this chapter onto your strength workouts when you have the time.

Yoga Metabolism Workout

Get ready to rev up your fat-burning muscle fibers and sculpt a sexier shape with this superfast yoga routine.

START HERE:

Complete the moves in order, first on your right side, then on your left. Hold each pose for five to 10 breaths. Then do the series again, holding each pose for one breath. Repeat the one-breath series for a total of six sets. Finally, return to the long holds (five to 10 breaths), alternating sides for three sets.

Down Dog Split

A

- Start in a pushup position, then lift your hips and move into the downward-facing dog pose, keeping your legs straight and pressing your heels into the floor.

B

- Lift your right leg straight back and up, keeping your right foot firmly flexed.

- Imagine you are pressing your foot into the ceiling. This will be the position you return to after each move.

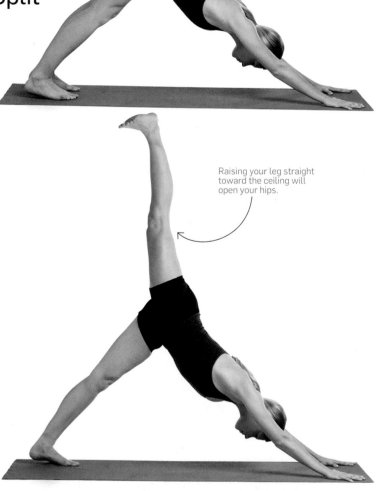

Raising your leg straight toward the ceiling will open your hips.

Half Crow Lift

- From down dog split, lower your right leg and bend your knee in to the outside of your right arm as you raise your chest and shift your weight forward.

- Keep this move slow and controlled.

- Make it harder: Move your shoulders in front of your wrists, bend your elbows, and try to lift your left foot off the ground as much as possible.

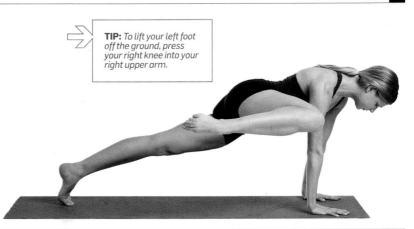

TIP: *To lift your left foot off the ground, press your right knee into your right upper arm.*

Knee to Forehead

- From down dog split, slowly lower your right leg as you raise your stomach and hips, round your back, and bring your knee toward your forehead, keeping your toes pointed and core engaged.

- Tuck your chin toward your chest, and extend your upper back forward through your shoulders.

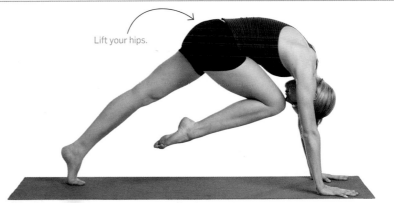

Lift your hips.

Warrior III

- From down dog split with left leg elevated, put your left foot between your hands. Raise your arms off the ground and shift your weight onto your left foot as you raise your right leg.

- At the same time, bring your torso forward until it's parallel to the floor, reaching your arms forward. Flex your right foot, pointing toes down.

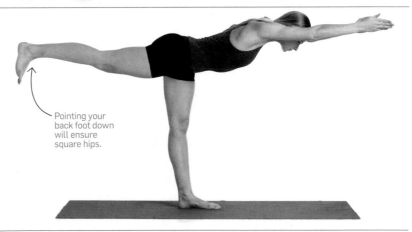

Pointing your back foot down will ensure square hips.

Fat-Burning Flow Workout

Get ready to melt fat as well as boost strength, flexibility, and focus with this challenging sequence of moves that call upon every little sinew in novel ways.

START HERE: ■

Hold each pose for five deep inhales and exhales, unless noted otherwise, then repeat the entire sequence on the other side. Then repeat, so you hit each side twice.

Plank

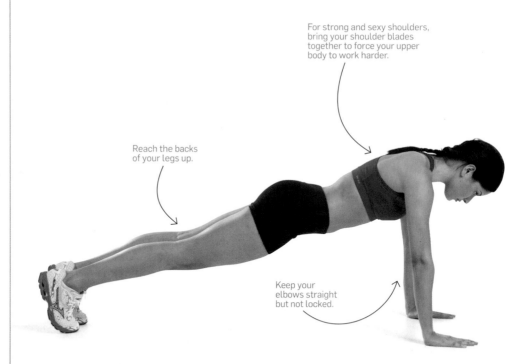

For strong and sexy shoulders, bring your shoulder blades together to force your upper body to work harder.

Reach the backs of your legs up.

Keep your elbows straight but not locked.

- Get on your hands and knees. Tuck your toes under and straighten your legs so you're in a horizontal line.
- Bring your shoulder blades together, extend forward through the top of your head, and reach back through your heels.

Down Dog

70

The percent reduction in low-back pain that study participants reported after attending a weekly yoga class and practicing at home for 3 months.

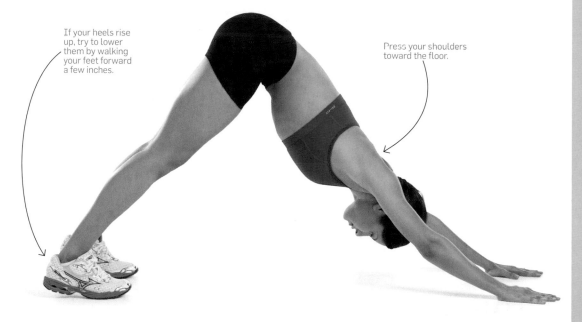

If your heels rise up, try to lower them by walking your feet forward a few inches.

Press your shoulders toward the floor.

- From plank, spread your fingers wide on your mat, lift your hips up and back, and extend your legs. Press your shoulders toward the floor and relax your neck. Press your palms against the floor.
- Walk your feet back, pull up through your hips, and press your heels down.

Fat-Burning Flow Workout

Low Lunge

- From down dog, step forward with your right foot.
- Bend forward from the waist and press your fingertips to the floor on each side of your right foot.
- Bend your knees slightly and step back with your left leg into a low lunge. Push through your left heel and sink your hips low.

Your left leg should be straight and your right leg deeply bent.

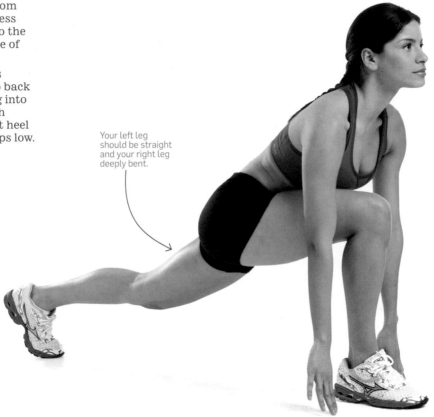

GO WITH THE FLOW

Vinyasa, which is Sanskrit for "flow," is a more challenging style of yoga because you move quickly from one pose to the next. Studies have shown that moving through a series of poses can catapult your heart rate into the coveted aerobic zone and burn up to 9 calories a minute.

High Lunge with Twist

- Reach your left arm forward and your right arm back, and turn your torso to the right.
- Relax your shoulders and look back over your right hand.

Rotated Triangle

- Lower the fingertips of your left hand to the floor outside your right foot. Open your shoulders to the right and extend your right arm up.
- Bring your left foot forward about 12 inches and press your heel down so your toes point a little out to your left side. Straighten your legs.

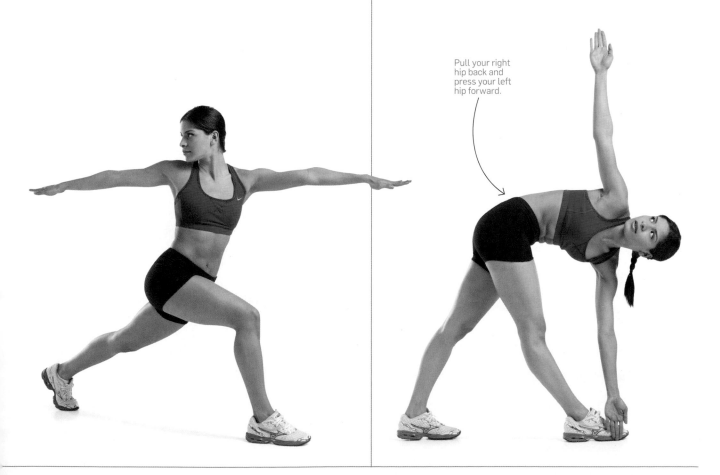

Pull your right hip back and press your left hip forward.

Ballet Workout

Ever wonder how dancers get those incredibly toned bodies? Rather than banging out big moves like squats in the weight room, dancers practice small concentrated movements that place each tiny muscle under tension for a long time. The result is strong, lean, long, and flexible muscles, especially through the core, hips, butt, and arms, with zero bulk.

START HERE:

These moves are intended for a dance barre, but you can do them with a chair or counter. Do each move for the prescribed amount of time with each side of your body before moving on. If you have time, repeat the circuit once or twice.

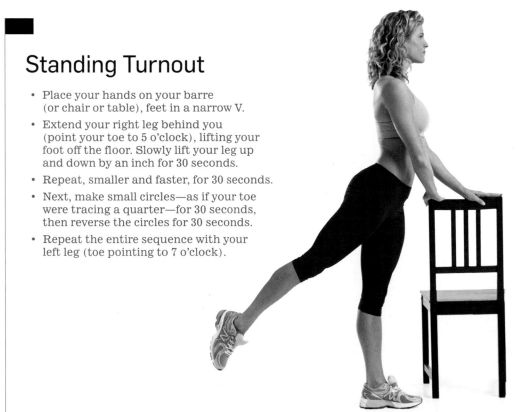

Standing Turnout

- Place your hands on your barre (or chair or table), feet in a narrow V.
- Extend your right leg behind you (point your toe to 5 o'clock), lifting your foot off the floor. Slowly lift your leg up and down by an inch for 30 seconds.
- Repeat, smaller and faster, for 30 seconds.
- Next, make small circles—as if your toe were tracing a quarter—for 30 seconds, then reverse the circles for 30 seconds.
- Repeat the entire sequence with your left leg (toe pointing to 7 o'clock).

Scissor Curl

Parallel Extension

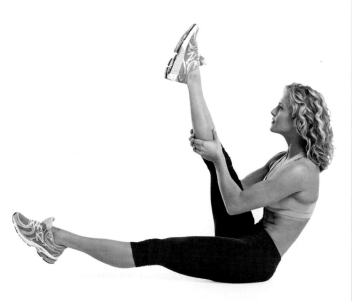

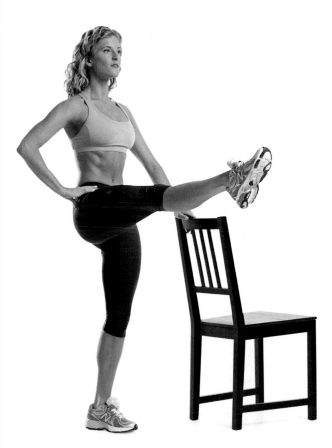

- Lie on your back with shoulders and feet raised, right leg extended up, and hands behind knee.

- Slowly curl up and down by an inch for 30 seconds.

- Continue, smaller and faster, for 30 seconds. Next, bring your left arm to your ear and curl for 30 seconds.

- Then reach your left arm toward your right ankle, curling for 30 seconds. Switch sides and repeat the sequence.

- Stand next to your support, and extend your right leg in front of you, keeping your left knee slightly bent.

- Slowly lift and lower your raised leg by an inch for 30 seconds.

- Repeat, using a smaller, faster motion, for 30 seconds.

- Next, make small circles with your leg (as if your toe were tracing a quarter) for 30 seconds, then reverse the circles for 30 seconds. Switch legs and repeat the entire sequence.

Ballet Workout

Semi Foldover

- Place your forearms on your support and rest your head on your arms.
- Lift your right leg, foot flexed, and bring your heel toward your butt. Press your heel up and down by an inch for 30 seconds.
- Continue, only smaller and faster, for 30 seconds. Extend your leg and slowly lift up and down by an inch for 30 seconds.
- Continue, smaller and faster, for 30 seconds. Repeat the sequence on the other leg.

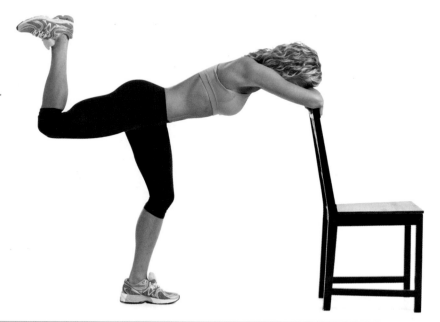

Curl

- Sit with your knees bent, holding the backs of your thighs.
- Round your back and lower it toward the floor, contracting your core.
- Slowly curl down and up inch by inch for 30 seconds. Then bend one arm to bring it up so you can lightly touch your ear with your fingertips. Continue curling for 30 seconds.
- Switch arms and repeat. Finally, bend both arms and lightly touch your ear with your fingertips as you curl up and down for 30 seconds.

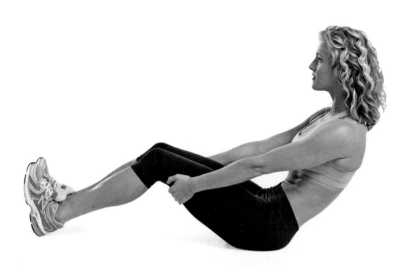

High V

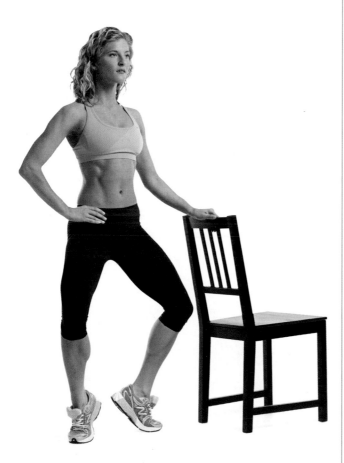

- Stand next to your support, feet in a narrow V.
- Rise onto the balls of your feet. Bend your knees, bringing your butt down.
- Slowly move down and up by an inch for 30 seconds. Repeat, using smaller, faster up-down movements, for another 30 seconds.

Wide Second

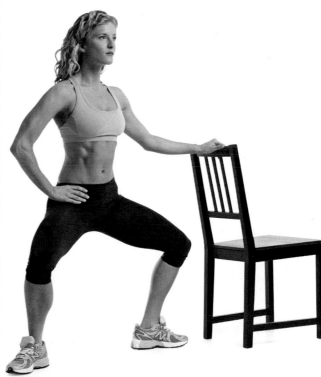

- Stand next to the support, feet more than shoulder-width apart, toes turned out.
- Lower your body about 6 inches.
- Slowly move down and up by an inch for 30 seconds. Continue, smaller and faster, for 30 seconds.
- With knees bent, rise onto the balls of your feet, then lower your feet; continue for 30 seconds. Repeat, faster, for 30 seconds.

Pilates Workout

Pilates is fabulous exercise but classes can be expensive. This program will help you achieve a tight tush, abs, and lean legs for much less money. Created by Lauren Piskin, owner of Physicalmind Studio in New York City, it is to be done with a Pilates ball, which mimics the resistance of the reformer machine used in studios.

START HERE:

Starting with the first move, do eight to 10 reps of each exercise with little to no rest between exercises.

Mermaid with Ball

- Sit with the Pilates or medicine ball at your left side, and bend your left leg in front of you, your right leg behind you. Place your left hand on the ball, elbow slightly bent, and extend your right arm out to your side at shoulder level.

- Brace your core and roll the ball out to the left as far as you can while reaching your right arm over your head.

- Hold for 2 or 3 seconds, then roll the ball back toward your body and return to the starting position. That's 1 rep. Finish all reps, then switch sides and repeat.

REPS: Do 8 to 10 on each side.

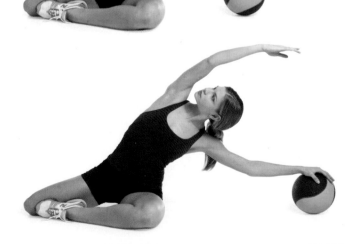

Rollover

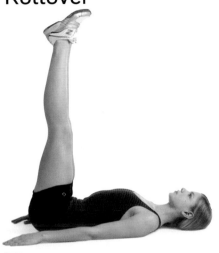

A

- Lie faceup on the floor or an exercise mat with your arms at your sides, palms down, legs straight.
- Lift your legs until they're perpendicular to the floor, feet flexed.

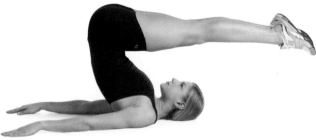

B

- Keeping your shoulders relaxed and legs straight, brace your core and raise your hips, slowly reaching your legs behind your head as far as you possibly can and pointing your toes behind you.
- Slowly reverse the movement to return to the starting position. That's 1 rep.

REPS: Do 8 to 10.

Footwork on Ball

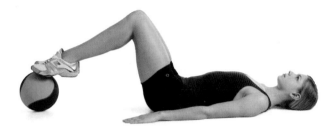

A

- Lie faceup, arms by your sides, palms facing down. Bend your knees and place the balls of your feet on top of the ball, heels together and toes pointing slightly outward in a small V shape.

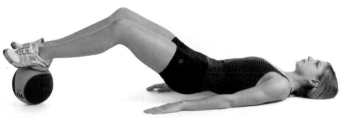

B

- Engage your core and contract your glutes to lift your hips an inch off the floor, then roll the ball away from you until your heels are on the ball.
- Pause, then bend your knees to roll the ball back to the starting position. That's 1 rep.

REPS: Do 8 to 10.

Pilates Workout

Swan on Ball

Keep your core engaged throughout the movement to prevent putting pressure on your lower back.

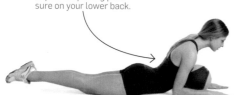

A

- Lie facedown with your legs extended shoulder-width apart behind you, feet slightly off the floor. Position the ball under your chest and rest your forearms on the floor, palms down, elbows close to your body.

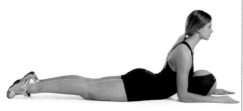

B

- Bring your shoulder blades back and down, press your palms lightly on the floor, and slowly lift your head and chest as you lengthen your spine.
- Hold for 2 or 3 seconds (imagine trying to create as much space between your ears and toes as possible), then return to the starting position. That's 1 rep.

REPS: Do 8 to 10.

Back Arm Rowing

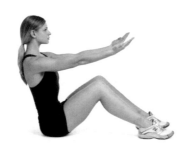

A

- Sit with your knees bent and feet flat on the floor about hip-width apart. Extend your arms straight in front of you, palms up. Your back should be straight, your chest up.

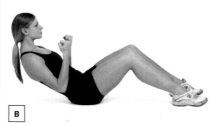

B

- Brace your core, curl your tailbone under, and slowly lower your upper body to a 45-degree angle.
- At the same time, bend your arms to bring your elbows close to your body, closing your hands into fists and pulling them toward your shoulders at chin level.
- Pause, then reverse the motion to return to the starting position. That's 1 rep.

REPS: Do 8 to 10.

Roll Back and Up

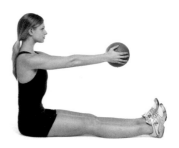

A

- Sit with your legs extended straight out in front of you, feet flexed. Hold the ball in front of you at shoulder level, arms straight. Keep your chest up and your back straight.

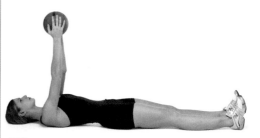

B

- Contract your core and glutes, then slowly roll back until your back is flat on the floor and the ball is directly overhead.
- From that position, bring your chin to your chest and slowly roll back up to the starting position. That's 1 rep.

REPS: Do 8 to 10.

Mermaid with Twist

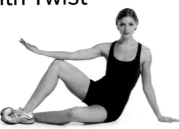

A

- Sit on your left hip with your left leg flat on the floor, knee bent 90 degrees, and your left palm on the floor.
- Bend your right knee toward the ceiling and place your right foot flat on the floor in front of your left foot; rest your right arm on your right knee.

B

- Shift your weight onto your left arm and straighten both legs to raise your hips toward the ceiling while extending your right arm directly over your head.

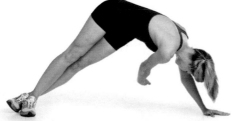

C

- From this position, twist your torso down and to the left, reaching your right arm underneath your body.
- Reverse the movement to return to the starting position. That's 1 rep. Finish all reps on that side, then switch sides and repeat.

REPS: Do 8 to 10.

Coordination with Ball

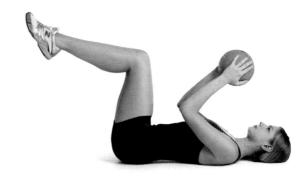

A

- Lie faceup with your hips and knees bent 90 degrees; hold the ball with both hands, arms straight.
- Bend your elbows and lower the ball toward your chest, pressing your hands firmly against the ball.

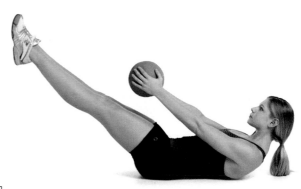

B

- Brace your abs, extend your arms in front of you, curl your shoulders off the floor, and straighten your legs.
- Hold for 1 or 2 seconds, then reverse to return to start. That's 1 rep.

REPS: Do 8 to 10.

Perfect-Posture Workout

Having poor posture can wreck your waistline (your belly pops out when your shoulders are droopy and your hips are slumped) and can even sabotage your workout results. (Structural imbalances compromise your muscles and cause pain.) This workout strengthens your upper back and shoulders and opens up your chest and hips.

START HERE: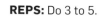

Do the following routine—which borrows from dance, Pilates, and yoga as well as traditional strength and stretching moves—as a circuit, moving from one exercise to the next without rest. Repeat the circuit three times total.

Foam Roller Snow Angel

 A

- Lie back along a 3-foot foam roller so that it runs the length of your spine. Bend your knees and rest your feet flat on the floor. Place your hands next to your hips, palms up, with your arms straight.

B

- Without raising your shoulders, slowly—take 15 seconds—drag your hands along the floor (as if you're making a snow angel) until they're above your head or they lose contact with the floor.

- Hold for 10 to 15 seconds. Take another 15 seconds to drag them back to the starting position. If you feel tightness in a particular spot, pause there for 10 to 15 seconds, then keep moving.

REPS: Do 3 to 5.

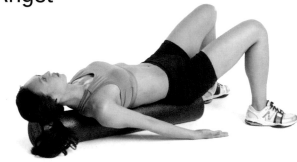

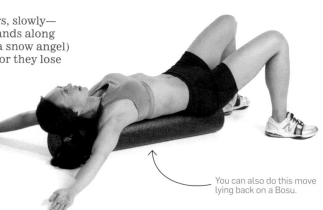

You can also do this move lying back on a Bosu.

Port de Bras

A
- Stand with your feet hip-width apart. Brace your abs. Keeping your shoulders down, raise both arms overhead.

B
- Bend forward, reaching your hands in front of you while keeping your back flat. Go only as far as you can without losing your form.

C
- Brace your abs again, stand up, and, with arms still raised, arch backward slightly.

REPS: Do 8.

Perfect-Posture Workout

Pilates X

A

- Lie on your stomach with your arms and legs extended, forming an X.

B

- Brace your abs and relax your shoulders. Inhale and lift your arms and legs off the floor, making sure your legs go no higher than your arms. Exhale, bending your elbows toward your waist and pulling your legs together.

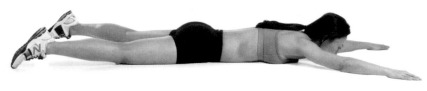

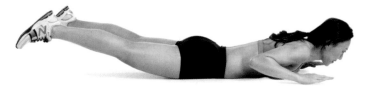

REPS: Do 6 to 8.

Shrug

A

- Grab a 5- to 15-pound dumbbell in each hand and stand with your feet about hip-width apart.

B

- With your arms at your sides, lift your shoulders toward your ears. Hold for 5 seconds, then lower.

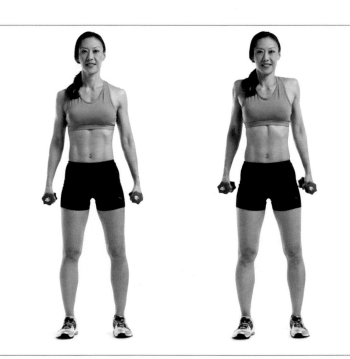

REPS: Repeat for 1 minute.

Side Angle Pose

TIP: *Do this move with your back against a wall to make it even more effective.*

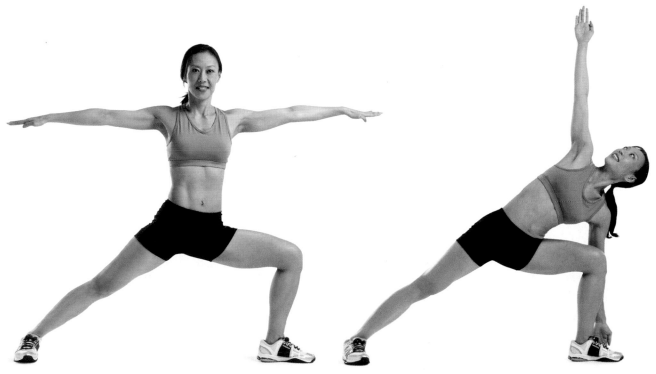

A

- Stand with your feet about 4 feet apart and turn your left foot out about 90 degrees.
- Keeping your back throughout, extend your arms, palms down, at shoulder height.

B

- Bend your left knee until it's over your ankle. Flex from the waist to the left and place your left hand outside your left foot (or your hand on the inside of your foot or ankle if you can't reach the floor).
- Reach your right arm over your ear and turn your chin toward your right armpit.
- Look up and take five slow breaths. Return to standing and switch sides. That's 1 rep.

REPS: Do 5.

Foam Roller Workout

If you work out long enough, eventually you're going to get stuck, literally. Your muscles will develop adhesions—knots that make you stiff and sore. Foam rollers can untie those knots; they're like a massage you give to yourself. They break the adhesions and stretch muscles for instant relief (and they're a lot cheaper than a masseuse).

START HERE:

Follow these directions, rolling each body part over the foam roller five to 10 times. If a spot feels extra tender, try this: Start below the area, work up to it and hold for a few seconds, then roll through it.

Calves

A

- Sit on the floor with your legs straight out, hands on the floor behind you supporting your weight. Place the roller between your knees and upper calves.

B

- Slowly roll along the back of your legs up and down from the backs of your knees to your ankles.

REPS: Do 5 to 10.

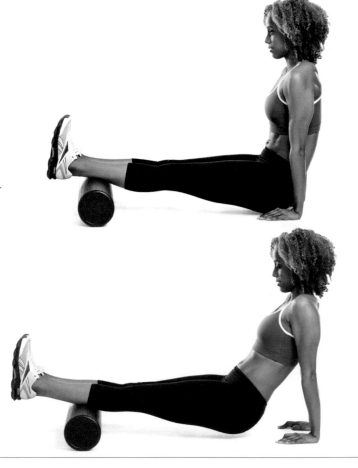

Hamstrings

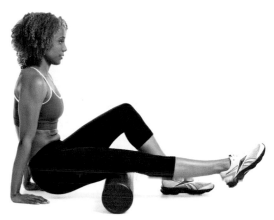

A

- Sit with your right leg on the roller; bend your left knee and put your hands on the floor behind you.

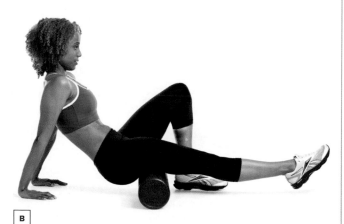

B

- Roll up and down from your knee to just under your left butt cheek.

REPS: Do 5 to 10 on each leg.

Quads

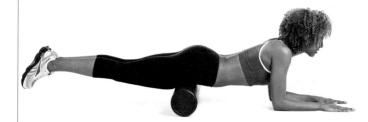

A

- Lie facedown on the floor and place the roller under your hips.

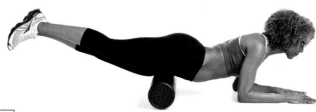

B

- Lean on your left leg.

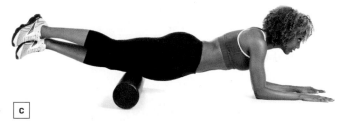

C

- Roll up and down from your hip to your knee.

REPS: Do 5 to 10 on each leg.

Foam Roller Workout

Upper Back

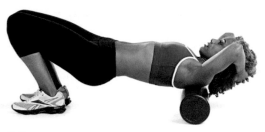

A

- Sit on the floor with the foam roller behind you. Lace your fingers behind your head and lean your upper back onto the roller.

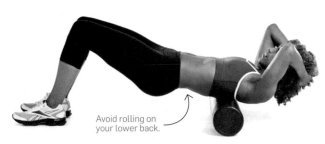

Avoid rolling on your lower back.

B

- Tighten your abs and glutes and slowly move up and down the roller from shoulders to midback.

REPS: Do 5 to 10.

Outer Hip and Thigh

Cross your right leg over your left for support.

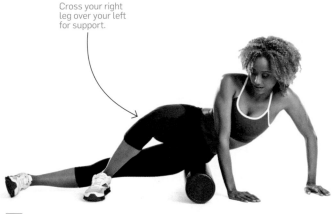

A

- Lie on your side with the roller under your left hip.

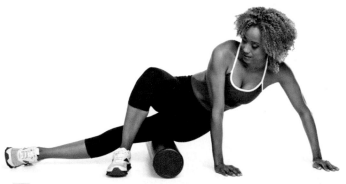

B

- Bracing your abs and glutes for balance, slowly roll down from your hip to your knee. Switch to the other leg and repeat.

REPS: Do 5 to 10 on each leg.

Shoulder and Side

Butt (Piriformis)

TIP: *The piriformis muscle lies deep behind the gluteals and is responsible for the external rotation of the hip joint. When muscle becomes too tight, it can impinge the sciatic nerve, causing pain and numbness in the low back or legs. This stretch can help.*

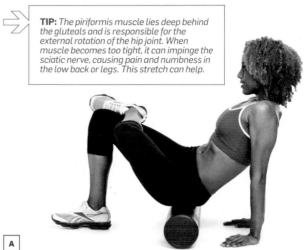

A

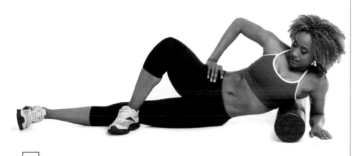

A

- Lie on your left side with the roller under your armpit.

- Sitting on the foam roller, cross your left leg over your right knee and lean toward the left hip, putting your weight on your hands for support.

Cross your right leg over your left for support.

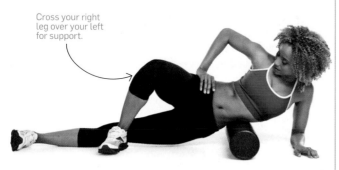

B

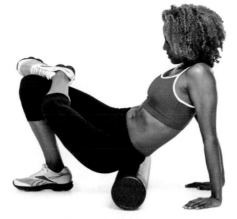

B

- Brace your abs and glutes for stability, and slowly roll down from your underarm to the bottom of your rib cage. Switch sides and repeat.

- Slowly roll one butt cheek over the roller. Switch sides and repeat.

REPS: Do 5 to 10 on each leg.

REPS: Do 5 to 10 on each leg.

Chapter 16:
Your 15-Minute Plan to Fight Fat with Food

Eating Healthy Starts with Being Prepared with
the Right Ingredients, the Best Tools, and Delicious Recipes.
You'll Find It All in this Chapter.

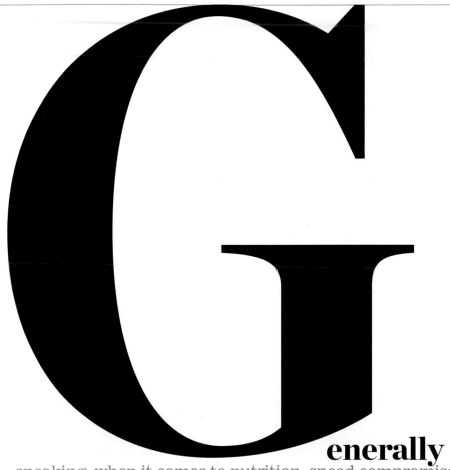

Generally

speaking, when it comes to nutrition, speed compromises health. But there are ways to feed yourself fast other than by heading for the nearest drive-thru. In Chapter 3, you learned the ins and outs of the Superfast Weight-Loss System. But knowing what to eat and applying it to the meals you actually put on your plate can be two different things. That's why we've added this chapter on how to fight fat with food — the chapter will actually tell you how and what to eat. Having the right tools, counter layout, and, of course, meal plans in place will go a long way toward speeding up your success.

The Superfast Kitchen Overhaul

For most women who are scheduled to the gills, time is a precious commodity. To whip up the lightning-quick meals in this chapter, you need a kitchen set up for NASCAR-level speed. That means all the right tools in all the right places. Here's a two-step, 15-minute kitchen makeover that will have you prepared for healthy cooking in less time than it takes to call for take out.

Clean House

The first step in your 15-Minute Kitchen Overhaul is a clean sweep of your fridge, cabinets, and pantry. We're asking you to be ruthless, to toss out perfectly good food (that's bad for you), whether you've opened it or not. The key is to get rid of all of your temptations. Because if the Cheetos aren't there, you can't eat them in a moment of salt-craving weakness. So grab a large trash bag and let's get started: Take all the sweets and treats like candy and cookies and toss them. If you just can't bear to trash those $30 Godiva chocolates, then at least hide them from plain view where they can't be easily reached. Even better, place them in opaque containers before you hide them. Researchers have found that men and women eat far fewer sweets when they're stored in containers that obscure what's inside than when they're in clear jars. In fact, in one study from the University of Illinois, office workers ate 25 percent fewer Hershey's Kisses when they were placed inside a slightly inconvenient spot out of sight, like inside a desk drawer, than when they were within arm's reach in plain view.

Did you get rid of the snack cakes and baked goods? Good. Next, sniff out the white bread, white rice and pasta, boxed and canned pasta meals, and other highly processed foods. The nonperishable stuff can be donated to a local food bank, including juices and sodas. Banish all sugary beverages from your home. Remember, if it's not there, you can't drink it or eat it. Out of sight, out of mind, out of mouth.

Get Ready for Action

Okay, your trash bag is full and your cupboard is bare, but you still have 5 minutes left in your 15-Minute Kitchen Overhaul. Now focus on your tools. You can't make quick meals if you have to spend 10 minutes fumbling through your junk drawer for a measuring spoon. Take the time right now to dig out the following items and place them prominently on your countertops or in easy-to-grab spaces in your cupboards, so you have quick access to your food-prep tools any time of day.

Cutting boards: For chopping fruits and veggies, slicing meats, and general food prep.
Knives: At least one good chef's knife is a must. And make sure it's sharp! All good chefs know that dull knives are dangerous knives. Round out your knife arsenal with a serrated version and a paring knife.
Measuring cups and spoons: They help keep portions (and pounds) in check.
Colander: For rinsing vegetables.
Blender/food processor: To crush ice for smoothies, purée raw ingredients into

silky-smooth soups or sauces, and grind meat or chop nuts.
Shredder: For cheese, of course, but also for shredding ginger and other flavorings. (We also recommend a grater or zester—think tinier teeth—for grating spices and making citrus zest.)
Oven mitts: For handling HOT pots and pans.
Flexible nylon food turner: Because they won't scratch your nonstick pans.
Tongs: A stainless steel model, as well as one with nylon-covered tips for those nonstick pans.
A wooden spoon: For stirring sauces and sneaking tastes.
A pepper mill: Because there's nothing like having fresh ground peppercorns to spice up a meal.

JUST ADD WATER

Replace your can of diet soda with ice cold water. Researchers at the University of Utah found that volunteers who drank 8 to 12 8-ounce glasses of water per day had higher metabolic rates than those who sipped only 4 glasses. Your body may burn a few calories heating the cold water to your core temperature, says Madelyn Fernstrom, PhD, founder and director of the University of Pittsburgh Medical Center Weight Management Center. Though the extra calories you burn drinking a single glass is pretty small, making it a habit can add up to pounds lost with essentially zero additional effort.

YOUR STAPLES: Restock your fridge and pantry with these mainstays of healthy eating

HIGH-QUALITY PROTEINS	LOW-STARCH VEGETABLES*		NATURAL FATS
Beef	Artichokes	Mushrooms	Avocados
Cheese	Asparagus	Onions	Butter
Eggs	Bok choy	Peppers	Coconut
Fish	Broccoli	Radishes	Cream
Pork	Brussels sprouts	Salad greens	Nuts and seeds
Poultry	Carrots	Spinach	Olives, olive oil, and canola oil
Soy	Cauliflower	Tomatoes	
Whey and casein proteins	Celery	Turnips	Full-fat salad dressings
	Cucumbers	Zucchini	

Any vegetables besides potatoes, peas, and corn are fair game.

377

15 Delicious Muscle-Building, Fat-Fighting Meals You Can Make in 15 Minutes or Less

Let's get something straight: The following recipes won't turn you into the next Food Network star. But they will help you to eat better for good health and weight loss. And they won't keep you kitchen-bound for hours up to your elbows in wheat grass. Oh yeah, most important: These meals taste great. That's a promise.

In the spirit of this book—simplicity and quarter-hour speed—we've compiled recipes for 15 nutrient-dense meals that you can make in 15 minutes or less. When you tire of these meals or for days when you have more time to spend in the kitchen, grab a copy of *The New Abs Diet Cookbook*, also from *Women's Health*. It's packed with more than 200 recipes utilizing the same healthy ingredients recommended in this book. Meanwhile, grab a plate and try these.

BREAKFAST

GREEN EGGS OMELET

2   large eggs
2   egg whites
1   tablespoon milk
1   teaspoon butter
¾   cup baby spinach, washed
¼   cup reduced fat shredded
      Cheddar cheese
      ground black pepper

- Beat the eggs and milk
  together in a bowl.
- Melt the butter in a skillet
  over medium heat. Add
  the eggs and cook until it
  begins to set.
- Add the spinach and
  shredded cheese on top and
  cook for another minute;
  then, using a spatula or
  nylon food turner, fold into
  an omelet.
- Cook until the eggs are
  thoroughly set.
- Season with salt and pepper
  and serve.

Makes 1 serving.

*Per serving: 260 calories,
23 g protein, 4 g carbohydrates,
15 g fat (7 saturated), 1 g fiber*

SUPERFAST HUNGER BUSTER

¼   cup cottage cheese
½   cup fresh blueberries
1   tablespoon crushed walnuts

- Mix all together in a bowl.

Makes 1 serving.

*Per serving: 198 calories,
10 g protein, 14 g carbohydrates,
12.5 g fat (2.5 g saturated), 3 g fiber*

NUKED OATMEAL

1   cup rolled oats
1   cup low-fat milk
½   cup frozen strawberries
      dash of salt
      teaspoon of sugar (optional)
      dash ground cinnamon
1   scoop vanilla whey protein
      powder

- Combine the oats and milk
  in a microwavable bowl.
- Microwave for 1 minute,
  stir, and then microwave for
  1 more minute.
- Allow to cool for a minute
  before mixing in the protein
  powder, salt, cinnamon,
  and sugar.

Makes 1 serving.

*Per serving: 585 calories,
43 g protein, 80 g carbohydrates,
11 g fat (3.6 g saturated), 10 g fiber*

10 WAYS TO SNEAK FIBER INTO YOUR DIET

The golden number for daily grams of dietary fiber is between 20 and 35, according to the USDA. But few of us consume that much. To get more of the belly-filling, cholesterol-lowering, metabolism-boosting good stuff, try these tricks:

1. Sprinkle garbanzo beans into your salad. A half-cup delivers up to 6 grams of extra fiber.

2. Drop a handful of berries to add flavor to plain or vanilla yogurt. Half a cup provides 4 grams of fiber.

3. Eat the skin of your next baked potato for 2 extra grams of fiber.

4. Add fiber to chips and salsa by dumping some black or kidney beans into jarred salsa.

5. Crunch on 1 ounce (about a handful) of almonds, peanuts or sunflower seeds for 2 to 4 grams of fiber.

Continued on page 380

Your 15-Minute Plan to Fight Fat With Food

6. Bite an apple, spread on some almond butter, bite again, and repeat.

7. Add lentils to soups. One-quarter cup of these tiny legumes is crammed with 11 grams of fiber.

8. Munch on 2 cups of low-fat popcorn for 2 grams of fiber.

9. Drop a whole orange into the blender to flavor your morning smoothie. (Uh, peel it first.) One orange has nearly 3 grams more fiber than even the pulpiest orange juice.

10. Doctor your favorite jarred pasta sauce with ½ cup of frozen chopped spinach. The spinach will adopt the flavor of the sauce and pad the fiber count by more than 2 grams.

LUNCHES, SNACKS

A LITTLE ITALY

2   Wasa Crispbreads
4   thin slices prosciutto
6   basil or baby spinach leaves
2   slices ripe red tomato
2   slices part-skim mozzarella cheese (about 2 ounces)
1   teaspoon extra virgin olive oil
     Cracked black pepper to taste

- Top each crisp with 2 slices of prosciutto, 3 basil leaves, 1 tomato slice, and 1 mozzarella slice.
- Drizzle with olive oil and grind some black pepper on top.

Makes 1 serving.

Per serving: 409 calories, 23 g protein, 15.5 g carbohydrates, 26.5 g fat (5.3 g saturated), 3 g fiber

SPICY TUNA SANDWICH

⅛   cup mayonnaise
¼   teaspoon wasabi paste
4   ounces canned tuna
4   slices whole-wheat bread
2   thin slices red onion
2   thin rings red bell pepper, seeded
½   cup avocado, sliced
¼   cup pickled ginger, sliced
4   romaine lettuce leaves

- In a small bowl, mix the mayonnaise and wasabi paste. Fork the tuna into the bowl and mix well.
- Spread an equal amount of the spicy tuna on 2 slices of bread.
- Top the tuna with an onion slice, pepper ring, avocado, some ginger, and 2 lettuce leaves. Then add the second slice of bread.

Makes 2 servings.

Per serving: 315 calories, 22 g protein, 35 g carbohydrates, 10 g fat (2.3 g saturated), 7 g fiber

ZIPPY PITA PIZZA

¼   cup chunky salsa
1   whole-wheat pita pocket
¼   cup cooked ham, diced
¼   cup mozzarella cheese, shredded

- Using a spoon, spread the salsa over one side of the pita.
- Top with the diced ham and shredded mozzarella.
- Place on a microwave-safe plate and microwave for a few seconds until the cheese melts.

Makes 1 serving.

Per serving: 360 calories, 23 g protein, 39 g carbohydrate, 13 g fat (5.5 g saturated), 5 g fiber

ZIPPY NO-DOUGH PIZZA

1 large Portobello mushroom cap
1 tablespoon thick spaghetti sauce
½ cup mozzarella cheese
5 thin slices pepperoni

• Preheat an oven to 400 degrees.
• If the stem is still attached to the mushroom, remove it. Also cut some of the gills out of the inside of the cap to make more room for the sauce and cheese.
• Place the mushroom cap side down on an oiled baking sheet and bake in the preheated oven for 4 minutes to remove some of the moisture.
• Take the baking sheet out of the oven and top the mushroom with spaghetti sauce, shredded mozzarella, and pepperoni slices.
• Bake for another 10 minutes or until the cheese has melted.

Makes 1 serving.

Per serving: 235 calories, 10.6 grams carbohydrates, 19 grams protein, 13.6 g fat (6.6 g saturated), 2.3 g fiber

SMOOTHIES

ANTIOXIDANT POWER PUNCH

1 green tea bag
1 teaspoon honey
1½ cups frozen blueberries
½ ripe banana
¾ cup vanilla soymilk

• Brew a cup of tea using boiling water and the tea bag. Remove the bag and stir in honey.
• Allow to cool. Add 5 tablespoons of the tea, blueberries, banana, and soy milk to a blender on a "chop" or "crush" setting.
• Blend until smooth.

Makes 2 servings.

Per serving: 151 calories, 5 g protein, 30 g carbohydrates, 1 g fat (0 g saturated), 3 g fiber

VIRGIN CABO DAIQUIRI

½ cup 1 percent milk
2 tablespoons low-fat plain yogurt
¼ cup frozen orange juice concentrate
½ ripe banana
¼ cup strawberries
½ cup cubed mango
2 teaspoons vanilla whey protein powder
3 ice cubes

• In a blender, puree the milk, yogurt, juice concentrate, banana, strawberries, mango, protein powder, and ice cubes.

Makes 2 servings.

Per serving: 154 calories, 7 g protein, 31 g carbohydrates, 1 g fat (0.5 g saturated), 2 g fiber

(From The New Abs Diet Cookbook.)

PROTEIN MAKES A MEAL

Building every meal around protein helps build and maintain lean muscle mass. Muscle burns more calories than fat does, even at rest, says Donald Layman, PhD, professor of nutrition at the University of Illinois. Aim for about 30 grams of protein—the equivalent of about 1 cup of low-fat cottage cheese or a 4-ounce boneless chicken breast—at each meal.

Your 15-Minute Plan to Fight Fat With Food

DINNERS

CORNED BEEF AND CABBAGE

It cooks in a slow cooker while you're at work. Prep takes less than 15 minutes.

8   small red potatoes (keep skin on)
4   medium carrots cut in half
3   cloves garlic
1   tablespoon brown sugar
1   bay leaf
3   pounds corned beef brisket
3   cups water
1   bottle Guinness beer
1   medium green cabbage cut into quarters

- Combine potatoes, carrots (not the cabbage), garlic, sugar, and bay leaf in a slow cooker.
- Add the brisket on top of the vegetables and pour the water and beer over the beef.
- Cover and cook on low for up to 10 hours.
- An hour before serving, add the cabbage.
- Remove the beef and vegetables from the cooker and place on a large platter.
- Discard the bay leaf. Serve with mustard and horseradish.

Makes 8 servings.

Per serving: 350 calories, 19 g protein, 23 g carbohydrates, 17 g fat (6 g saturated), 4 g fiber

STUFFED CHEESE LAMB BURGER

1   pound ground lamb
¼   pound smoked mozzarella cheese
4   large romaine lettuce leaves
    Salt and pepper to taste

- Cut the mozzarella into quarters.
- Form four burger patties by dividing the ground lamb evenly and molding each around a hunk of the cheese.
- Grill for about 4 minutes per side over high heat.
- Wrap each burger in a romaine leaf to serve.

Makes 4 servings.

Per serving: 397 calories, 26 g protein, 2 g carbohydrates, 31 g fat (14.5 g saturated), 1 g fiber

GRILLED TUNA KEBABS WITH ASIAN SAUCE

For the Asian sauce (make beforehand)

¼   cup low-sodium soy sauce
½   cup hoisin sauce
½   teaspoon sesame oil
½   teaspoon sugar
2   garlic cloves, minced
1   teaspoon fresh ginger, minced

- Combine all ingredients in a saucepan. Cook over medium heat until bubbly.
- Cool and store in a covered glass jar in refrigerator for up to 2 weeks.

For the kebabs

1   pound tuna steak
12 white button mushrooms
12 cherry tomatoes
6   scallions cut into 2-inch pieces
4   bamboo or wooden skewers

- Soak the skewers for 30.
- Cut the tuna into cubes a little larger than bite-sized.
- Divide the tuna cubes and vegetables into four even groups and thread the pieces alternately onto each skewer.
- Brush with the Asian sauce to cover. Grill or broil for 6 minutes, turning once, and brushing with the remaining dressing after 2 minutes of cooking.

Makes 4 servings.

Per serving: 220 calories, 30 g protein, 14 g carbohydrate, 5 g fat (0.5 g saturated), 2 g fiber

ROAST RATATOUILLE

1 medium eggplant, peeled and cut into ½-inch pieces

1 large zucchini, cut into ½ -inch pieces

1 medium red onion, chopped

1 red bell pepper, seeded and cut into large 2-inch pieces

1 yellow bell pepper, seeded and cut into large 2-inch pieces

½ medium fennel bulb, cored and thinly sliced

1 can (15 ounces) diced tomatoes

1 tablespoon olive oil

1½ teaspoons oregano

½ teaspoon coarse kosher or sea salt

¼ teaspoon freshly ground black pepper

• Preheat an oven to 500 degrees.

• Coat a large roasting pan with cooking spray.

• Place eggplant, zucchini, onion, peppers, fennel, and tomatoes in the roasting pan.

• Toss with olive oil, oregano, salt, and pepper to coat.

• Roast, stirring occasionally, for about 15 minutes or until vegetables are tender.

Makes 4 servings.

Per serving: 127 calories, 3.5 g protein, 19 g carbohydrates, 4 grams fat (1 g saturated), 7 g fiber

SALAD FOR DINNER

This salad is loaded with muscle-building protein and quality carbs, plus fats that will satisfy your hunger, roughly 30 grams of each. Made with leftover grilled skirt steak, it can be built in just minutes.

4 ounces grilled skirt or hanger steak, sliced thinly against the grain

2 cups chopped romaine lettuce

1 hard-boiled egg, halved

6 cherry tomatoes, halved

¼ avocado, sliced

1 tablespoon blue cheese, crumbled

1 cup sugar snap peas, steamed and halved

1 tablespoon extra-virgin olive oil

1 strip pre-cooked bacon, heated

• Toss all ingredients together and serve.

Makes 1 serving.

Per serving: 650 calories, 49 grams protein, 32 g carbohydrates, 35 g fat (13.5 g saturated), 8 fiber

HEALTHY OPTION: *Trim extra calories by eating half of this salad with a bowl of soup and saving the rest for tomorrow's lunch.*

A SIDE OF LEMONY SPROUTS

1 16-ounce package frozen petite Brussels sprouts

1 tablespoon butter

1 teaspoon extra-virgin olive oil

½ teaspoon lemon zest

1 teaspoon lemon juice
   Salt and ground pepper to taste

• Toss the Brussels sprouts into a large pan with ¼ cup of water. Bring to a boil, cover, reduce heat, and simmer for 10 minutes or until tender.

• While the sprouts are cooking, heat 1 tablespoon of butter in a small saucepan until almost melted.

• Stir in the olive oil, finely grated lemon zest and lemon juice.

• Drain the sprouts and toss with the lemon-butter. Season with salt and fresh ground pepper.

Makes 4 servings.

Per serving: 187 calories, 3 grams protein, 8 g carbohydrates, 16 g fat (8 g saturated), 3 g fiber

INSTANT UPGRADE

RECHARGE WITH MILK

Milk is the new post-workout drink. And it helps torch fat. In a study in the journal *Medicine & Science in Sports & Exercise,* women who drank skim milk after exercising lost 3.5 pounds of fat in 12 weeks. Those who sipped sports drinks after working out actually gained weight. Milk's protein improves the body's ability to burn calories and build muscle.

Index

INDEX

INDEX